Cardiomyopathies: Current Treatment and Future Options

Cardiomyopathies: Current Treatment and Future Options

Editor

Stefan Peters

MDPI

Basel • Beijing • Wuhan • Barcelona • Belgrade • Novi Sad • Cluj • Manchester

Editor
Stefan Peters
Chair Internal
Medicine—Cardiology
Norden
Germany

Editorial Office
MDPI
St. Alban-Anlage 66
4052 Basel, Switzerland

This is a reprint of articles from the Special Issue published online in the open access journal *Journal of Clinical Medicine* (ISSN 2077-0383) (available at: https://www.mdpi.com/journal/jcm/special_issues/Cardiomyopathies_Treatment_Future_Options).

For citation purposes, cite each article independently as indicated on the article page online and as indicated below:

Lastname, A.A.; Lastname, B.B. Article Title. *Journal Name* **Year**, *Volume Number*, Page Range.

ISBN 978-3-7258-0373-6 (Hbk)
ISBN 978-3-7258-0374-3 (PDF)
doi.org/10.3390/books978-3-7258-0374-3

Contents

Stefan Peters
Editorial: Cardiomyopathies: Current Treatment and Future Options
Reprinted from: *J. Clin. Med.* **2020**, *9*, 3531, doi:10.3390/jcm9113531 . . . . **1**

Matthias Eden and Norbert Frey
Cardiac Filaminopathies: Illuminating the Divergent Role of Filamin C Mutations in Human Cardiomyopathy
Reprinted from: *J. Clin. Med.* **2021**, *10*, 577, doi:10.3390/jcm10040577 . . . . **3**

Michał Marchel, Agnieszka Madej-Pilarczyk, Agata Tymińska, Roman Steckiewicz, Ewa Ostrowska, Julia Wysińska, et al.
Cardiac Arrhythmias in Muscular Dystrophies Associated with Emerinopathy and Laminopathy: A Cohort Study
Reprinted from: *J. Clin. Med.* **2021**, *10*, 732, doi:10.3390/jcm10040732 . . . . **11**

Nicolò Martini, Martina Testolina, Gian Luca Toffanin, Rocco Arancio, Luca De Mattia, Sergio Cannas, et al.
Role of Provocable Brugada ECG Pattern in The Correct Risk Stratification for Major Arrhythmic Events
Reprinted from: *J. Clin. Med.* **2021**, *10*, 1025, doi:10.3390/jcm10051025 . . . . **22**

Heinz-Peter Schultheiss, Thomas Bock, Heiko Pietsch, Ganna Aleshcheva, Christian Baumeier, Friedrich Fruhwald and Felicitas Escher
Nucleoside Analogue Reverse Transcriptase Inhibitors Improve Clinical Outcome in Transcriptional Active Human Parvovirus B19-Positive Patients
Reprinted from: *J. Clin. Med.* **2021**, *10*, 1928, doi:10.3390/jcm10091928 . . . . **32**

Birgit J. Gerecke and Rolf Engberding
Noncompaction Cardiomyopathy—History and Current Knowledge for Clinical Practice
Reprinted from: *J. Clin. Med.* **2021**, *10*, 2457, doi:10.3390/jcm10112457 . . . . **43**

Federico Migliore, Giulia Mattesi, Alessandro Zorzi, Barbara Bauce, Ilaria Rigato, Domenico Corrado and Alberto Cipriani
Arrhythmogenic Cardiomyopathy—Current Treatment and Future Options
Reprinted from: *J. Clin. Med.* **2021**, *10*, 2750, doi:10.3390/jcm10132750 . . . . **71**

Irfan Vardarli, Manuel Weber, Christoph Rischpler, Dagmar Führer, Ken Herrmann and Frank Weidemann
Fabry Cardiomyopathy: Current Treatment and Future Options
Reprinted from: *J. Clin. Med.* **2021**, *10*, 3026, doi:10.3390/jcm10143026 . . . . **88**

John E. Madias
Takotsubo Cardiomyopathy: Current Treatment
Reprinted from: *J. Clin. Med.* **2021**, *10*, 3440, doi:10.3390/jcm10153440 . . . . **98**

Jan Koelemen, Michael Gotthardt, Lars M. Steinmetz and Benjamin Meder
RBM20-Related Cardiomyopathy: Current Understanding and Future Options
Reprinted from: *J. Clin. Med.* **2021**, *10*, 4101, doi:10.3390/jcm10184101 . . . . **125**

Andreas Brodehl and Brenda Gerull
Genetic Insights into Primary Restrictive Cardiomyopathy
Reprinted from: *J. Clin. Med.* **2022**, *11*, 2094, doi:10.3390/jcm11082094 . . . . **140**

Carsten Tschöpe and Ahmed Elsanhoury
Treatment of Transthyretin Amyloid Cardiomyopathy: The Current Options, the Future, and the Challenges
Reprinted from: *J. Clin. Med.* **2022**, *11*, 2148, doi:10.3390/jcm11082148 . . . . **165**

Riccardo Bariani, Maria Bueno Marinas, Ilaria Rigato, Paola Veronese, Rudy Celeghin, Alberto Cipriani, et al.
Pregnancy in Women with Arrhythmogenic Left Ventricular Cardiomyopathy
Reprinted from: *J. Clin. Med.* **2022**, *11*, 6735, doi:10.3390/jcm11226735 . . . . **179**

Gassan Moady, Otman Ali, Rania Sweid and Shaul Atar
The Role of Stress in Stable Patients with Takotsubo Syndrome—Does the Trigger Matter?
Reprinted from: *J. Clin. Med.* **2022**, *11*, 7304, doi:10.3390/jcm11247304 . . . . **190**

Juan David López-Ponce de Leon, Mayra Estacio, Natalia Giraldo, Manuela Escalante, Yorlany Rodas, Jessica Largo, et al.
Hypertrophic Cardiomyopathy in a Latin American Center: A Single Center Observational Study
Reprinted from: *J. Clin. Med.* **2023**, *12*, 5682, doi:10.3390/jcm12175682 . . . . **199**

Journal of
Clinical Medicine

MDPI

Editorial

Editorial: Cardiomyopathies: Current Treatment and Future Options

Stefan Peters

Internal Medicine-Cardiology, Ubbo Emmius Hospital Norden, Cardiology, Osterstr. 110, 26506 Norden, Germany; stefan.peters@u-e-k.de; Tel.: +49-4931-181-435

Received: 28 October 2020; Accepted: 29 October 2020; Published: 31 October 2020

Abstract: Cardiomyopathies are an essential component in clinical cardiology. The number of different cardiomyopathies have increased a lot due to genetics and newer insights in pathomechanism. The current treatment and future options are demonstrated in advance.

Keywords: cardiomyopathy; hypertrophic; dilated; arrhythmogenic

---

Cardiomyopathies are an essential factor in cardiology with important progress in genetics, medical treatment and treatment with devices. Ablation in order to treat various forms of arrhythmias plays a more and more increased role.

In 1995, the most important cardiomyopathies were dilated cardiomyopathy, hypertrophic cardiomyopathy, restrictive cardiomyopathy and arrhythmogenic right ventricular cardiomyopathy [1].

A lot of other cardiomyopathies have been described in recent years, such as non-compaction cardiomyopathy, takotsubo cardiomyopathy, and many other subtypes of already known cardiomyopathies [2].

In hypertrophic cardiomyopathy, we must differentiate between various forms of hypertrophy. We can offer articles to various types of hypertrophy due to different causes like Amyloid cardiomyopathy and Fabry cardiomyopathy. The same genes for hypertrophic cardiomyopathy can cause non-compaction left ventricle, which is included in our reviews.

The definition of arrhythmogenic cardiomyopathies has changed in recent years; meanwhile, arrhythmogenic dilated cardiomyopathy, arrhythmogenic right ventricular cardiomyopathy, and arrhythmogenic left ventricular cardiomyopathy are included. What is more important is the fact that different genes play a crucial role, like Filamin C, Lamin A/C, phospholamban and RBM20. We could invite international experts in this field to write important papers.

The importance of ajmaline testing in arrhythmogenic right ventricular cardiomyopathy and hypertrophic cardiomyopathy is worth a particular paper in order to predict the risk of life-threatening ventricular arrhythmias.

Idiopathic dilated cardiomyopathy has gained intensive interest due to different stages of the disease. Arrhythmogenic dilated cardiomyopathy, non-dilated hypokinetic left ventricle, and dilatation without contraction impairment were described in 2016 [3]. The progress in definition are described by experts in the field.

Several cases of rare cardiomyopathies hide under the term of non-ischemic heart failure with preserved left ventricular ejection fraction and benefit from newer treatment options like tafamidis, and in the near future, mavacamten.

A lot has changed in the definition of cardiomyopathies since 1995, summarized in present papers with increased knowledge in genetics, pathophysiology, medical treatment, the use of devices, and ablation techniques, and future options in treatment are developing in the coming years.

Funding: This research received no external funding.

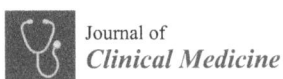

Conflicts of Interest: The authors declare no conflict of interest.

References

1. Richardson, P.; McKenna, W.; Bristow, M.; Maisch, B.; Mautner, B.; O'Connell, J.; Olsen, E.; Thiene, G.; Goodwin, J.; Gyarfas, I.; et al. Report of the 1995 World Health Organization/International Society and Federation of Cardiology Task Force on the definition and classification of cardiomyopathies. *Circulation* **1996**, *9*, 841–842.
2. Maron, B.J.; Towbin, J.A.; Zhiene, G.; Antzelewitch, C.; Corrado, D.; Arnett, D.; Moss, A.J.; Seidman, C.E.; Young, J.B. Contemporary definitions and classification of cardiomyopathies. *Circulation* **2006**, *113*, 1807–1816. [CrossRef] [PubMed]
3. Pinto, Y.M.; Elliott, P.M.; Arbustini, E.; Adler, Y.; Anastasakis, A.; Böhm, M.; Duboc, D.; Gimeno, J.; de Groote, P.; Imazio, M.; et al. Proposal for a revised definition of dilated cardiomyopathy, hypokinetic non-dilated cardiomyopathy, and its implications for clinical practise: A position statement of the ESC working group on myocardial and pericardial diseases. *Eur. Heart J.* **2016**, *37*, 1850–1858. [CrossRef] [PubMed]

Journal of
Clinical Medicine

MDPI

Review

Cardiac Filaminopathies: Illuminating the Divergent Role of Filamin C Mutations in Human Cardiomyopathy

Matthias Eden [1,2] and Norbert Frey [1,2,*]

[1] Department of Internal Medicine III, University of Heidelberg, 69120 Heidelberg, Germany; matthiaseden@web.de
[2] German Centre for Cardiovascular Research, Partner Site Heidelberg, 69120 Heidelberg, Germany
* Correspondence: norbert.frey@med.uni-heidelberg.de

Abstract: Over the past decades, there has been tremendous progress in understanding genetic alterations that can result in different phenotypes of human cardiomyopathies. More than a thousand mutations in various genes have been identified, indicating that distinct genetic alterations, or combinations of genetic alterations, can cause either hypertrophic (HCM), dilated (DCM), restrictive (RCM), or arrhythmogenic cardiomyopathies (ARVC). Translation of these results from "bench to bedside" can potentially group affected patients according to their molecular etiology and identify subclinical individuals at high risk for developing cardiomyopathy or patients with overt phenotypes at high risk for cardiac deterioration or sudden cardiac death. These advances provide not only mechanistic insights into the earliest manifestations of cardiomyopathy, but such efforts also hold the promise that mutation-specific pathophysiology might result in novel "personalized" therapeutic possibilities. Recently, the FLNC gene encoding the sarcomeric protein filamin C has gained special interest since FLNC mutations were found in several distinct and possibly overlapping cardiomyopathy phenotypes. Specifically, mutations in FLNC were initially only linked to myofibrillar myopathy (MFM), but are now increasingly found in various forms of human cardiomyopathy. FLNC thereby represents another example for the complex genetic and phenotypic continuum of these diseases.

Keywords: filamin C; cardiomyopathy; gene mutations

Citation: Eden, M.; Frey, N. Cardiac Filaminopathies: Illuminating the Divergent Role of Filamin C Mutations in Human Cardiomyopathy. *J. Clin. Med.* **2021**, *10*, 577. https://doi.org/10.3390/jcm10040577

Academic Editor: Stefan Peters
Received: 5 January 2021
Accepted: 2 February 2021
Published: 4 February 2021

1. Introduction

Human cardiomyopathies in general can be classified into primary and secondary cardiomyopathies. Within this classification, primary cardiomyopathies can be subdivided into pure genetic forms like hypertrophic cardiomyopathy (HCM), arrhythmogenic right ventricular cardiomyopathy (ARVC), and left ventricular non-compaction cardiomyopathy (LVNCM) as well as Ion channel, conduction, and storage disorders. Dilated cardiomyopathies (DCM) as well as restrictive cardiomyopathy (RCM) are categorized in to mixed primary cardiomyopathies, since a potential genetic etiology explains only a part of these clinical entities [1–5].

As it has been previously described for filamin A (FLNA) and B (FLNB), filamin C (FLNC) is also recognized as an important structural crosslinker of actin rods at the sarcomeric z-disc of both cardiac and skeletal muscle [6]. Moreover, all three filamin variants reveal high sequence similarities indicating similar cellular functions. While FLNA and FLNB are ubiquitously expressed, FLNC is predominantly enriched in cardiac and skeletal muscle. Of note, dimerization of two identical filamins through their Ig-like domains 24 is crucial for correct filamin function (Figure 1) [4,7]. For all three filamins, a subcellular localization at the sarcomeric z-disc, intercalated discs, cell-membranes, and myotendinous junctions has been described. It is speculated that, due to their structural characteristics, in particular filamin A and filamin C also can serve as a nodal point for sarcomeric mechanotransduction in different muscle cells [7,8].

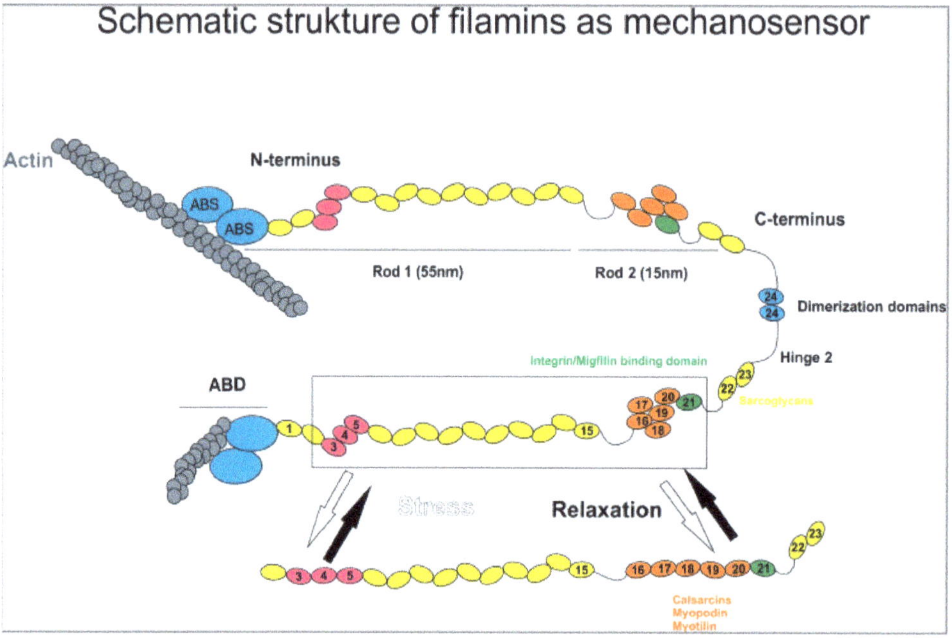

Figure 1. Schematic structure of filamins as mechanosensor.

Schematic structure of Filamins binding and cross-linking F-actin via N-terminal Actin Binding Domains (ABD; blue) containing Actin Binding Sites (ABS). Distinct regions within rod 1 (R3–5; violet) and rod 2 (R16–21) are prone to spring-like conformational changes. Domains highlighted in orange are possible interaction sites for z-disc proteins, domain 21 (green) represents the possible interaction site with integrins. Domains R22–23 interact with sarcoglycans (yellow). The proposed model shows that contractile force and deformation of actin networks induce conformational changes of both filamin dimers. Subsequently, some binding partners are able to interact with exposed binding sites under mechanical stress, whereas some will rather dissociate under conformational change [7,8].

Filamin C was first reported to be associated with various forms of skeletal myopathy (i.e., MFM) [7]. The encoding *FLNC* gene consists of 48 coding exons and is located on chromosome 7q32–35. Two isoforms (one shorter isoform, lacking exon 31 and predicted to be less flexible) have been partially characterized so far. The shorter Isoform is thought to be expressed 3.5 times higher in skeletal than cardiac muscle, whereas the longer filamin C isoform seems less abundant in cardiomyocytes under basal conditions but is rapidly induced upon cardiac stress. More than 90 potential binding partners for filamin C have been denoted in the current literature [6,7]. At sarcomeric z-discs, filamin C interacts with various proteins partially linked to inherited cardiomyopathies like calsarcins (Involved in HCM [9–11]), myopalladin (linked to RCM [12]), cypher (linked to ARVC and DCM [13]), actin (linked to DCM [14]), myotilin, myopodin, and others. Moreover, filamin C binds to the sarcolemma via integrin-1β and sarcoglycan-delta (known as part of the muscular dystrophin complex) [15,16]. Filamin C can be cleaved by the protease calpain in order to differentially regulate the sarcoglycan-filamin interaction.

In mice, loss of *FLNC* function leads to diverse results. Whereas partial FLNC −/− mice, expressing a truncated filamin C by deletion of exons 41–48, show a severe muscular phenotype, leading to lethality due to respiratory failure, before birth, they displayed no obvious cardiac defects [17]. In contrast, a recent publication stressed the crucial role for cardiac filamin C in mice, analyzing multiple, complete FLNC knockout mouse models [18]. In contrast to the partial *FLNC* knockout, they generated conventional and heart restricted knockouts in which Cre-mediated deletion of the *FLNC* region between exons 9 and 13 resulted in subsequent frameshift of *FLNC* and, thereby, complete loss of the protein. Since these global and heart restricted FLNC $-/-$ mice were embryonic lethal, additional inducible heart restricted FLNC knockout mice were generated by crossing *FLNC*-floxed mice with αMHC-MerCreMer mice [18]. Strikingly, these mice developed rapid progressive dilated cardiomyopathy that already occurred after 1 week knockout induced by tamoxifen treatment [18]. In humans, more than 325 unique sequence variants in *FLNC* are known (mainly affecting the longer isoform NM_001458.5), and not always resulting in distinct cardiac phenotypes in human cardiomyopathy [4]. It remains obscure why, in mutant carriers, cardiomyopathies are not accompanied by clinically overt skeletal muscle myopathies.

2. Filamin C Mutations Reveal a Distinct Phenotype of Human Dilated Cardiomyopathy (Dcm) with Increased Risk of Sudden Cardiac Death

DCM is one major cause for terminal heart failure ultimately leading to requirement of cardiac transplantation, left ventricular assist devices, and/or sudden cardiac death. Genetic variants cover more than 40 known genes with encoded proteins spanning a large variety of different cellular compartments [3]. Truncating *FLNC* mutations (stop or frameshift etc.) seem to be enriched in DCM patient cohorts compared to healthy individuals, while the overall prevalence of *FLNC* variants only ranges from 1% to 4.5% in different publications [4]. Interestingly, and consistent with other genetic variants found in cardiomyopathy, *FLNC* variants found in human DCM do not come along with concomitant myofibrillar myopathy. The group of Ortiz-Genga published an analysis in 2016, where 23 new truncating variants of *FLNC* were found in a DCM cohort and they reported that these gene variants were all absent in more than 1000 individuals with HCM, indicating a unique genotype phenotype correlation [19]. Surprisingly, all these patients showed no filamin aggregates in cardiac immunohistological stainings, which normally denotes a typical phenotypic feature of filamin associated MFM.

In their data set, FLNC-DCM phenotypes show marked LV-dilation and systolic dysfunction, a high degree of myocardial fibrosis (assessed by CMR and biopsies) and associated conduction abnormalities (i.e., T-Wave changes and low voltage QRS criteria in ECG recordings). One might speculate that a high degree of myocardial fibrosis and the observed conduction abnormalities in surface ECG could explain a significantly higher risk for ventricular arrhythmias (>80%) and sudden cardiac death in *FLNC* mutation carriers. Judging these typical findings, filaminopathies share some analogy to cardiac laminopathies [20,21] and in particular to desmin-related cardiomyopathies [22]. Mutations in the intermediate filament protein desmin can typically result in formation of large protein aggregates and thereby are linked to dilated cardiomyopathy [23], restrictive cardiomyopathy [24], arrhythmogenic right ventricular cardiomyopathy [25], and rarely HCM [26].

In support of these concepts, Begay et al. reported similar findings in *FLNC* truncated mutation carriers and their DCM cohort. They also speculated about a phenotypic RV involvement (seen in around 38%) and excessive fibrosis deposition assessed by electron microscopy pictures of RV-tissue. Moreover, they saw a biventricular myocardial fibro-fatty infiltration and redistribution of cell-cell junction proteins, a feature that is also typically seen in arrhythmogenic right ventricular cardiomyopathy (ARVC). These results also indicate a potential phenotypic "overlap" of DCM and ARVC in some *FLNC* mutation carriers. Since, unlike desminopathies, no protein aggregates were found in several studies, one potential mechanism of truncated *FLNC* variants affecting cardiac phenotypes is believed to be haploinsufficiency rather than storage myopathy, with reduced protein contents seen in Western blot analysis of affected individuals [27]. Whereas this proposed haploinsufficiency seems to result in late onset DCM beyond the age of 40, biallelic *FLNC* mutations (one missense (318 C > G), one stop gaining (2971 C > T)) were reported to potentially cause severe congenital dilated cardiomyopathy requiring early heart transplantation [28].

3. Filamin C Mutations in Arrhythmogenic Cardiomyopathy

Arrhythmogenic right ventricular cardiomyopathy (ARVC) is a genetic disorder that is diagnosed by clinical criteria affecting mainly the right ventricle and the conduction system [29,30]. In 50% of cases, the underlying genetic variant is known and mainly affecting desmosomal genes (*PKP2, DSP, JUP, DSG2 and DSC2*), genes at the area composite (*CTNNA3, CDH2*) and rarely non-desmosomal genes (*DES, LMNA, PLN, RYR, TGFB3, TTN, SCN5A, TMEM43*) [31,32]. Mutation carriers show a fibro-fatty infiltration of right ventricular myocardium and are affected by a high incidence of life-threatening arrhythmias and sudden cardiac death as well as by progressive dilation and dysfunction of the right ventricle itself [19,33,34]. Very recently, truncating *FLNC* variants were also linked to patients fulfilling ARVC criteria and with excluded genetic variants in all common ARVC genes [34]. Of note, truncating *FLNC* mutations seem to be a rather rare observation in ARVC cohorts (1%). One described genetic variant was a loss of function mutation in exon 40, the other resulted in a *FLNC* frameshift in exon 48. Interestingly, immunohistological analysis revealed altered desmosomal protein localizations but no protein aggregate accumulation in mutation carriers. Although index patients showed no signs of left-ventricular involvements, it remains unclear if these *FLNC* variants clearly are linked to an isolated ARVC phenotype.

4. Missense Filamin C Mutations Can Result in Human Hypertrophic Cardiomyopathy

Hypertrophic cardiomyopathy (HCM) is also a genetic disorder mainly affecting genes encoding for of sarcomeric proteins [3]. The disease is characterized by excessive and sometimes asymmetric thickening of the myocardium in the absence of afterload increasing conditions like arterial hypertension or valvular heart disease (i.e., aortic stenosis). Hypertrophic cardiomyopathy has an autosomal dominant inheritance with several hundred mutations in more than 30 genes reported so far. *MYH7, MYBPC, MYL3, TPM1,* and *TNNT2* are the most frequently mutated genes, accounting for more than 70% of all cases. *FLNC* missense mutations (mainly localized in the ROD2 domain important for cell signaling and interaction to calsarcin, synaptopodin, and nexilin at the sarcomeric z-disc; [4,35]) are believed to explain up to 10% of HCM phenotypes from patients in which common mutations in main sarcomeric genes were excluded [36]. Unlike histological findings in other cardiomyopathies, Valdes-Mas et al. also reported the formation of large mutated filamin C protein aggregates (in patients in vivo and in cell culture expressing mutated *FLNC* variants in vitro) as well as myofibril disarray and fibrosis, but again in the absence of overt skeletal myopathy [36]. Comparable to clinical courses observed in *FLNC* associated DCM and ARVC patients, HCM individuals and families expressing *FLNC* missense mutations seemed to be more prone to ventricular arrhythmias and sudden cardiac death. Mechanistically, it is speculated that, unlike truncating mutations in DCM and ARVC, missense mutations lead to loss of function phenotypes in HCM, although the precise consequences of *FLNC* missense mutations remain unexplained [36]. In a recent screen in HCM cohorts, Gomez et al. revealed that most of the found *FLNC* variants were associated with mild forms of HCM and showed reduced penetrance [37]. Beyond in contrast, one has to take into account that various other publications did not observe an excess of missense variants in HCM cohorts compared to controls, questioning the real relevance of *FLNC* sequence variants in this particular cardiac disease [38,39].

5. Filamin C Mutations in Restrictive Cardiomyopathy (RCM)

Restrictive cardiomyopathy is a very rare primary cardiomyopathy, according to current American Heart Association (AHA) classification, with a rather poor clinical prognosis [40]. RCM is mainly characterized by impaired diastolic function and enlarged cardiac atria, leading to diastolic heart failure, atrial fibrillation (AF), and valvular regurgitation due to severe anular dilation. Few clearly inherited RCM forms are published, and the underlying genetic mutations have only been rudimentarily characterized. Affected genes include MYH7, alpha-actin, as well as troponin T (TNT) and troponin I (TNI) subunits [41]. In 2017, Tucker et al. found a novel *FLNC* mutation in Exon 5 in a family of RCM (pV2297M) resulting in diminished sarcomeric localization, but again without protein aggregate formation [41]. In this publication, the authors speculate that like in HCM, rather "loss of function" and not haploinsufficiency explains the phenotype of the assessed *FLNC* genotype variants.

Overall, *FLNC* mutations can be also regarded as a potential target for newborn genetic testing for myopathy and cardiomyopathy (known sequence variants related to their phenotypes summarized in Figure 2) [42].

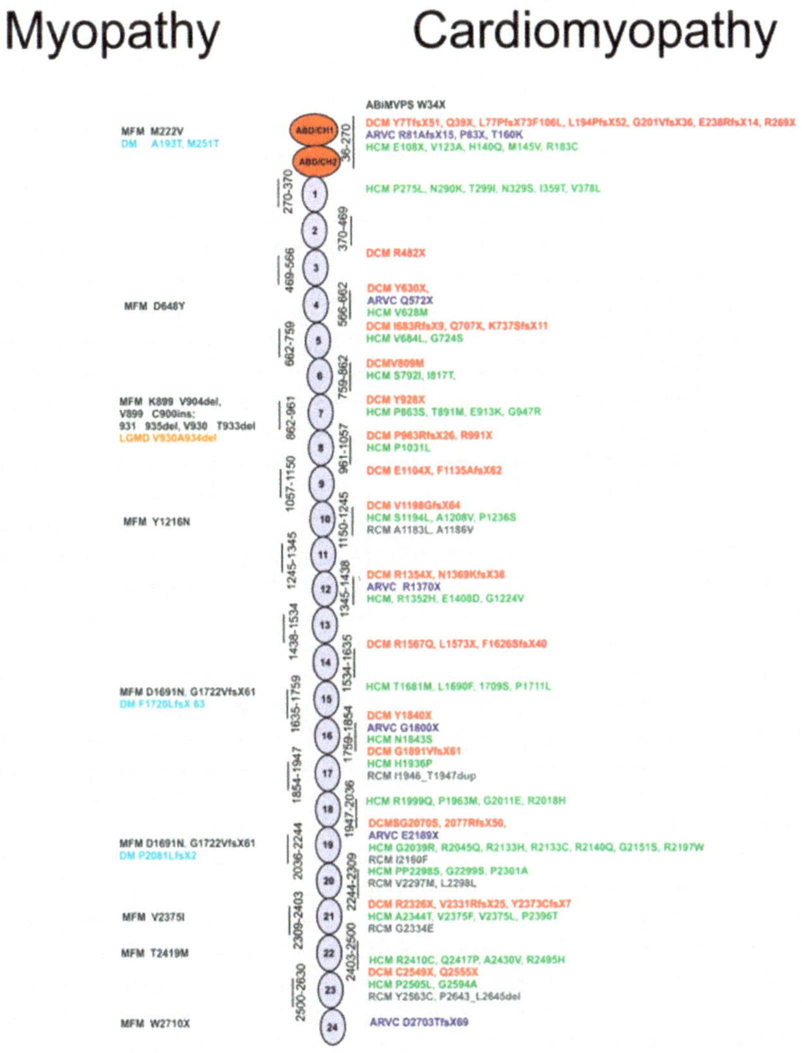

Figure 2. Summary of FLNC sequence variants in relation to disease phenotypes.

6. Filamin C Mutations in Mitral Valve Prolapse Syndrome

Very recently, a novel truncating mutation of FLNC (c201G > A; pTrp34) has also been linked to a special familiar form of arrhythmogenic bileaflet mitral valve prolapse syndrome (ABiMVPS) presenting with a combination of mitral-valve prolapse and associated electrophysiological alterations [43]. This finding, although it describes only one family pedigree, seems rather plausible since filamin A mutations have already been reported to cause similar mitral valve pathologies [7].

This illustration summarizes the structure of FLNC, showing its two calponin homology and actin binding domains (ABD/CH1 and ABD/CH2), Ig-like domains 1–24. Currently known mutations in FLNC gene are mapped to the protein structure and correlated to the phenotype of various skeletal muscle myopathies (MFM, distal myopathy (DM) and limb-girdle muscular dystrophy (LGMD)) on the left, whereas correlation with various forms of human cardiomyopathy (ABiMVPS, DCM, HCM, ARVC, RCM) phenotypes are displayed on the right (adapted from Mao et al. [7]).

7. Conclusions

Although it remains vague the precise mechanisms of how FLNC mutations and subsequent protein alterations affect different and partially overlapping cardiac phenotypes, it becomes increasingly clear that *FLNC* variants are found in and are associated with various forms of human cardiomyopathies. In particular in DCM, RCM, and ARVC cohorts, existing data suggests that *FLNC* mutations can affect cardiac phenotypes and even indicate patients at increased risk. Comparable to human laminopathies or desminopathies, filaminopathies seem to characterize a distinct group of electrically less stable cardiomyopathy patients. As *FLNC* mutations appear to predispose for arrhythmogenic events and sudden cardiac death in several cardiomyopathy entities, *FLNC* mutation might be an additional criteria for clinical decision making that favors early ICD implantation in cardiomyopathy. In particular, since truncating variants of *FLNC* seem to be more frequently found in patients with sudden cardiac death that *FLNC* variant carriers with missense mutations, this emphasizes a potential need for genetic testing of individuals and families [35]. This is further supported by the notion that the complex genetic heterogeneity, including resulting haploinsufficiency or loss of function variants, affects other phenotypic attributes like chamber hypertrophy and dilation.

For a final judgement if FLNC sequence variants play a clear role in hypertrophic cardiomyopathy, bigger cohorts have to be analyzed in detail and filaminopathies have to be further characterized mechanistically.

Author Contributions: Conceptualization, M.E. and N.F.; writing-original draft preparation M.E.; writing-review and editing M.E. and N.F.; supervision N.F. All authors have read and agreed to the published version of the manuscript.

Funding: This research received no external funding.

Institutional Review Board Statement: Not applicable.

Informed Consent Statement: Not applicable.

Data Availability Statement: Not applicable.

Conflicts of Interest: The authors declare no conflict of interest.

References

1. Burke, M.A.; Cook, S.A.; Seidman, J.G.; Seidman, C.E. Clinical and Mechanistic Insights into the Genetics of Cardiomyopathy. *J. Am. Coll. Cardiol.* **2016**, *68*, 2871–2886. [CrossRef]
2. Kamisago, M.; Sharma, S.D.; DePalma, S.R.; Solomon, S.; Sharma, P.; McDonough, B.; Smoot, L.; Mullen, M.P.; Woolf, P.K.; Wigle, E.D.; et al. Mutations in sarcomere protein genes as a cause of dilated cardiomyopathy. *N. Engl. J. Med.* **2000**, *343*, 1688–1696. [CrossRef]
3. Watkins, H.; Ashrafian, H.; Redwood, C. Inherited cardiomyopathies. *N. Engl. J. Med.* **2011**, *364*, 1643–1656. [CrossRef] [PubMed]

4. Elliott, P.; Andersson, B.; Arbustini, E.; Bilinska, Z.; Cecchi, F.; Charron, P.; Dubourg, O.; Kuhl, U.; Maisch, B.; McKenna, W.J.; et al. Classification of the cardiomyopathies: A position statement from the European Society of Cardiology Working Group on Myocardial and Pericardial Diseases. *Eur. Heart J.* **2008**, *29*, 270–276. [CrossRef] [PubMed]
5. Maron, B.J.; Towbin, J.A.; Thiene, G.; Antzelevitch, C.; Corrado, D.; Arnett, D.; Moss, A.J.; Seidman, C.E.; Young, J.B.; American Heart Association; et al. Contemporary definitions and classification of the cardiomyopathies: An American Heart Association Scientific Statement from the Council on Clinical Cardiology, Heart Failure and Transplantation Committee; Quality of Care and Outcomes Research and Functional Genomics and Translational Biology Interdisciplinary Working Groups; and Council on Epidemiology and Prevention. *Circulation* **2006**, *113*, 1807–1816. [PubMed]
6. Verdonschot, J.A.J.; Vanhoutte, E.K.; Claes, G.R.F.; Helderman-van den Enden, A.; Hoeijmakers, J.G.J.; Hellebrekers, D.; de Haan, A.; Christiaans, I.; Lekanne Deprez, R.H.; Boen, H.M.; et al. A mutation update for the FLNC gene in myopathies and cardiomyopathies. *Hum. Mutat.* **2020**, *41*, 1091–1111. [CrossRef]
7. Mao, Z.; Nakamura, F. Structure and Function of Filamin C in the Muscle Z-Disc. *Int. J. Mol. Sci.* **2020**, *21*, 2696. [CrossRef]
8. Modarres, H.P.; Mofradt, M.R. Filamin: A structural and functional biomolecule with important roles in cell biology, signaling and mechanics. *Mol. Cell. Biomech.* **2014**, *11*, 39–65.
9. Posch, M.G.; Thiemann, L.; Tomasov, P.; Veselka, J.; Cardim, N.; Garcia-Castro, M.; Coto, E.; Perrot, A.; Geier, C.; Dietz, R.; et al. Sequence analysis of myozenin 2 in 438 European patients with familial hypertrophic cardiomyopathy. *Med. Sci. Monit.* **2008**, *14*, CR372–CR374.
10. Frey, N.; Olson, E.N. Calsarcin-3, a novel skeletal muscle-specific member of the calsarcin family, interacts with multiple Z-disc proteins. *J. Biol. Chem.* **2002**, *277*, 13998–14004. [CrossRef]
11. Osio, A.; Tan, L.; Chen, S.N.; Lombardi, R.; Nagueh, S.F.; Shete, S.; Roberts, R.; Willerson, J.T.; Marian, A.J. Myozenin 2 is a novel gene for human hypertrophic cardiomyopathy. *Circ. Res.* **2007**, *100*, 766–768. [CrossRef]
12. Huby, A.C.; Mendsaikhan, U.; Takagi, K.; Martherus, R.; Wansapura, J.; Gong, N.; Osinska, H.; James, J.F.; Kramer, K.; Saito, K.; et al. Disturbance in Z-disk mechanosensitive proteins induced by a persistent mutant myopalladin causes familial restrictive cardiomyopathy. *J. Am. Coll. Cardiol.* **2014**, *64*, 2765–2776. [CrossRef]
13. Levitas, A.; Konstantino, Y.; Muhammad, E.; Afawi, Z.; Marc Weinstein, J.; Amit, G.; Etzion, Y.; Parvari, R. D117N in Cypher/ZASP may not be a causative mutation for dilated cardiomyopathy and ventricular arrhythmias. *Eur. J. Hum. Genet.* **2016**, *24*, 666–671. [CrossRef] [PubMed]
14. Takai, E.; Akita, H.; Shiga, N.; Kanazawa, K.; Yamada, S.; Terashima, M.; Matsuda, Y.; Iwai, C.; Kawai, K.; Yokota, Y.; et al. Mutational analysis of the cardiac actin gene in familial and sporadic dilated cardiomyopathy. *Am. J. Med. Genet.* **1999**, *86*, 325–327. [CrossRef]
15. Frank, D.; Frey, N. Cardiac Z-disc signaling network. *J. Biol. Chem.* **2011**, *286*, 9897–9904. [CrossRef]
16. Frank, D.; Kuhn, C.; Katus, H.A.; Frey, N. Role of the sarcomeric Z-disc in the pathogenesis of cardiomyopathy. *Future Cardiol.* **2007**, *3*, 611–622. [CrossRef]
17. Dalkilic, I.; Schienda, J.; Thompson, T.G.; Kunkel, L.M. Loss of FilaminC (FLNc) results in severe defects in myogenesis and myotube structure. *Mol. Cell. Biol.* **2006**, *26*, 6522–6534. [CrossRef]
18. Zhou, Y.; Chen, Z.; Zhang, L.; Zhu, M.; Tan, C.; Zhou, X.; Evans, S.M.; Fang, X.; Feng, W.; Chen, J. Loss of Filamin C Is Catastrophic for Heart Function. *Circulation* **2020**, *141*, 869–871. [CrossRef] [PubMed]
19. Ortiz-Genga, M.F.; Cuenca, S.; Dal Ferro, M.; Zorio, E.; Salgado-Aranda, R.; Climent, V.; Padron-Barthe, L.; Duro-Aguado, I.; Jimenez-Jaimez, J.; Hidalgo-Olivares, V.M.; et al. Truncating FLNC Mutations Are Associated with High-Risk Dilated and Arrhythmogenic Cardiomyopathies. *J. Am. Coll. Cardiol.* **2016**, *68*, 2440–2451. [CrossRef]
20. Fatkin, D.; MacRae, C.; Sasaki, T.; Wolff, M.R.; Porcu, M.; Frenneaux, M.; Atherton, J.; Vidaillet, H.J.; Spudich, S., Jr.; De Girolami, U.; et al. Missense mutations in the rod domain of the lamin A/C gene as causes of dilated cardiomyopathy and conduction-system disease. *N. Engl. J. Med.* **1999**, *341*, 1715–1724. [CrossRef]
21. Hasselberg, N.E.; Haland, T.F.; Saberniak, J.; Brekke, P.H.; Berge, K.E.; Leren, T.P.; Edvardsen, T.; Haugaa, K.H. Lamin A/C cardiomyopathy: Young onset, high penetrance, and frequent need for heart transplantation. *Eur. Heart J.* **2018**, *39*, 853–860. [CrossRef]
22. McLendon, P.M.; Robbins, J. Desmin-related cardiomyopathy: An unfolding story. *Am. J. Physiol. Heart Circ. Physiol.* **2011**, *301*, H1220–H1228. [CrossRef]
23. Li, D.; Tapscoft, T.; Gonzalez, O.; Burch, P.E.; Quinones, M.A.; Zoghbi, W.A.; Hill, R.; Bachinski, L.L.; Mann, D.L.; Roberts, R. Desmin mutation responsible for idiopathic dilated cardiomyopathy. *Circulation* **1999**, *100*, 461–464. [CrossRef]
24. Brodehl, A.; Pour Hakimi, S.A.; Stanasiuk, C.; Ratnavadivel, S.; Hendig, D.; Gaertner, A.; Gerull, B.; Gummert, J.; Paluszkiewicz, L.; Milting, H. Restrictive Cardiomyopathy is Caused by a Novel Homozygous Desmin (DES) Mutation p.Y122H Leading to a Severe Filament Assembly Defect. *Genes (Basel)* **2019**, *10*, 918. [CrossRef]
25. Oomen, A.; Jones, K.; Yeates, L.; Semsarian, C.; Ingles, J.; Sy, R.W. Rare desmin variant causing penetrant life-threatening arrhythmic cardiomyopathy. *Heart Rhythm. Case Rep.* **2018**, *4*, 318–323. [CrossRef] [PubMed]
26. Harada, H.; Hayashi, T.; Nishi, H.; Kusaba, K.; Koga, Y.; Koga, Y.; Nonaka, I.; Kimura, A. Phenotypic expression of a novel desmin gene mutation: Hypertrophic cardiomyopathy followed by systemic myopathy. *J. Hum. Genet.* **2018**, *63*, 249–254. [CrossRef]
27. Begay, R.L.; Tharp, C.A.; Martin, A.; Graw, S.L.; Sinagra, G.; Miani, D.; Sweet, M.E.; Slavov, D.B.; Stafford, N.; Zeller, M.J.; et al. FLNC Gene Splice Mutations Cause Dilated Cardiomyopathy. *JACC Basic Transl. Sci.* **2016**, *1*, 344–359. [CrossRef] [PubMed]

28. Reinstein, E.; Gutierrez-Fernandez, A.; Tzur, S.; Bormans, C.; Marcu, S.; Tayeb-Fligelman, E.; Vinkler, C.; Raas-Rothschild, A.; Irge, D.; Landau, M.; et al. Congenital dilated cardiomyopathy caused by biallelic mutations in Filamin C. *Eur. J. Hum. Genet.* **2016**, *24*, 1792–1796. [CrossRef]
29. Marcus, F.I.; McKenna, W.J.; Sherrill, D.; Basso, C.; Bauce, B.; Bluemke, D.A.; Calkins, H.; Corrado, D.; Cox, M.G.; Daubert, J.P.; et al. Diagnosis of arrhythmogenic right ventricular cardiomyopathy/dysplasia: Proposed modification of the Task Force Criteria. *Eur. Heart J.* **2010**, *31*, 806–814. [CrossRef]
30. Towbin, J.A.; McKenna, W.J.; Abrams, D.J.; Ackerman, M.J.; Calkins, H.; Darrieux, F.C.C.; Daubert, J.P.; de Chillou, C.; DePasquale, E.C.; Desai, M.Y.; et al. 2019 HRS expert consensus statement on evaluation, risk stratification, and management of arrhythmogenic cardiomyopathy: Executive summary. *Heart Rhythm* **2019**, *16*, e373–e407. [CrossRef]
31. Corrado, D.; Basso, C.; Judge, D.P. Arrhythmogenic Cardiomyopathy. *Circ. Res.* **2017**, *121*, 784–802. [CrossRef] [PubMed]
32. Mestroni, L.; Sbaizero, O. Arrhythmogenic Cardiomyopathy: Mechanotransduction Going Wrong. *Circulation* **2018**, *137*, 1611–1613. [CrossRef] [PubMed]
33. Begay, R.L.; Graw, S.L.; Sinagra, G.; Asimaki, A.; Rowland, T.J.; Slavov, D.B.; Gowan, K.; Jones, K.L.; Brun, F.; Merlo, M.; et al. Filamin C Truncation Mutations Are Associated with Arrhythmogenic Dilated Cardiomyopathy and Changes in the Cell-Cell Adhesion Structures. *JACC Clin. Electrophysiol.* **2018**, *4*, 504–514. [CrossRef]
34. Brun, F.; Gigli, M.; Graw, S.L.; Judge, D.P.; Merlo, M.; Murray, B.; Calkins, H.; Sinagra, G.; Taylor, M.R.; Mestroni, L.; et al. FLNC truncations cause arrhythmogenic right ventricular cardiomyopathy. *J. Med. Genet.* **2020**, *57*, 254–257. [CrossRef]
35. Ader, F.; De Groote, P.; Réant, P.; Rooryck-Thambo, C.; Dupin-Deguine, D.; Rambaud, C.; Khraiche, D.; Perret, C.; Pruny, J.F.; Mathieu-Dramard, M.; et al. FLNC pathogenic variants in patients with cardiomyopathies: Prevalence and genotype-phenotype correlations. *Clin. Genet.* **2019**, *96*, 317–329. [CrossRef] [PubMed]
36. Valdes-Mas, R.; Gutierrez-Fernandez, A.; Gomez, J.; Coto, E.; Astudillo, A.; Puente, D.A.; Reguero, J.R.; Alvarez, V.; Moris, C.; Leon, D.; et al. Mutations in filamin C cause a new form of familial hypertrophic cardiomyopathy. *Nat. Commun.* **2014**, *5*, 5326. [CrossRef] [PubMed]
37. Gómez, J.; Lorca, R.; Reguero, J.R.; Morís, C.; Martín, M.; Tranche, S.; Alonso, B.; Iglesias, S.; Alvarez, V.; Díaz-Molina, B.; et al. Screening of the Filamin C Gene in a Large Cohort of Hypertrophic Cardiomyopathy Patients. *Circ. Cardiovasc. Genet.* **2017**, *10*, e001584. [CrossRef] [PubMed]
38. Cui, H.; Wang, J.; Zhang, C.; Wu, G.; Zhu, C.; Tang, B.; Zou, Y.; Huang, X.; Hui, R.; Song, L.; et al. Mutation profile of FLNC gene and its prognostic relevance in patients with hypertrophic cardiomyopathy. *Mol. Genet. Genom. Med.* **2018**, *6*, 1104–1113. [CrossRef]
39. Walsh, R.; Buchan, R.; Wilk, A.; John, S.; Felkin, L.E.; Thomson, K.L.; Chiaw, T.H.; Loong, C.C.W.; Pua, C.J.; Raphael, C.; et al. Defining the genetic architecture of hypertrophic cardiomyopathy: Re-evaluating the role of non-sarcomeric genes. *Eur. Heart J.* **2017**, *38*, 3461–3468. [CrossRef] [PubMed]
40. Elliott, P.; Andersson, B.; Arbustini, E.; Bilinska, Z.; Cecchi, F.; Charron, P.; Dubourg, O.; Kuhl, U.; Maisch, B.; McKenna, W.J.; et al. Classification of the cardiomyopathies. *Kardiol. Pol.* **2008**, *66*, 533–540. [CrossRef]
41. Tucker, N.R.; McLellan, M.A.; Hu, D.; Ye, J.; Parsons, V.A.; Mills, R.W.; Clauss, S.; Dolmatova, E.; Shea, M.A.; Milan, D.J.; et al. Novel Mutation in FLNC (Filamin C) Causes Familial Restrictive Cardiomyopathy. *Circ. Cardiovasc. Genet.* **2017**, *10*, e001780. [CrossRef] [PubMed]
42. Xiao, F.; Wei, Q.; Wu, B.; Liu, X.; Mading, A.; Yang, L.; Li, Y.; Liu, F.; Pan, X.; Wang, H. Clinical exome sequencing revealed that FLNC variants contribute to the early diagnosis of cardiomyopathies in infant patients. *Transl. Pediatr.* **2020**, *9*, 21–43. [CrossRef] [PubMed]
43. Bains, S.; Tester, D.J.; Asirvatham, S.J.; Noseworthy, P.A.; Ackerman, M.J.; Giudicessi, J.R. A Novel Truncating Variant in FLNC-Encoded Filamin C May Serve as a Proarrhythmic Genetic Substrate for Arrhythmogenic Bileaflet Mitral Valve Prolapse Syndrome. *Mayo Clin. Proc.* **2019**, *94*, 906–913. [CrossRef] [PubMed]

Journal of
Clinical Medicine

MDPI

Article

Cardiac Arrhythmias in Muscular Dystrophies Associated with Emerinopathy and Laminopathy: A Cohort Study

Michał Marchel [1,*], Agnieszka Madej-Pilarczyk [2], Agata Tymińska [1], Roman Steckiewicz [1], Ewa Ostrowska [1], Julia Wysińska [1], Vincenzo Russo [3], Marcin Grabowski [1] and Grzegorz Opolski [1]

1 1st Department of Cardiology, Medical University of Warsaw, 02-097 Warsaw, Poland; tyminska.agata@gmail.com (A.T.); r.steckiewicz@pro.onet.pl (R.S.); ewa.ostrowska713@gmail.com (E.O.); julia.wysinska@gmail.com (J.W.); marcin.grabowski@wum.edu.pl (M.G.); grzegorz.opolski@wum.edu.pl (G.O.)

2 Department of Medical Genetics, The Children's Memorial Health Institute, 04-730 Warsaw, Poland; agamadpil@gmail.com

3 Department of Translational Medical Sciences, University of Campania "Luigi Vanvitelli"—Monaldi Hospital, 80131 Naples, Italy; v.p.russo@libero.it

* Correspondence: michal.marchel@wum.edu.pl; Tel.: +48-225992958

Abstract: Introduction: Cardiac involvement in patients with muscular dystrophy associated with Lamin A/C mutations (*LMNA*) is characterized by atrioventricular conduction abnormalities and life-threatening cardiac arrhythmias. Little is known about cardiac involvement in patients with emerin mutation (*EMD*). The aim of our study was to describe and compare the prevalence and time distribution of cardiac arrhythmias at extended follow-up. Patients and methods: 45 consecutive patients affected by muscular dystrophy associated to laminopathy or emerinopathy were examined. All patients underwent clinical evaluation, 12-lead surface electrocardiogram (ECG), 24 h electrocardiographic monitoring, and cardiac implanted device interrogation. Results: At the end of 11 (5.0–16.6) years of follow-up, 89% of the patients showed cardiac arrhythmias. The most prevalent was atrial standstill (AS) (31%), followed by atrial fibrillation/flutter (AF/Afl) (29%) and ventricular tachycardia (22%). *EMD* patients presented more frequently AF/AFl compared to *LMNA* (50% vs. 20%, $p = 0.06$). Half of the *EMD* patients presented with AS, whilst there was no occurrence of such in the *LMNA* ($p = 0.001$). Ventricular arrhythmias were found in 60% of patients with laminopathy compared to 3% in patients with emerinopathy ($p < 0.001$). The age of AVB occurrence was higher in the *LMNA* group (32.8 +/− 10.6 vs. 25.1 +/− 9.1, $p = 0.03$). Conclusions: Atrial arrhythmias are common findings in patients with muscular dystrophy associated with *EMD*/*LMNA* mutations; however, they occurred earlier in *EMD* patients. Ventricular arrhythmias were very common (60%) in *LMNA* and occurred definitely earlier compared to the *EMD* group.

Keywords: Emery–Dreifuss muscular dystrophy; *LMNA*; *EMD*; emerin; lamin A/C

Citation: Marchel, M.; Madej-Pilarczyk, A.; Tymińska, A.; Steckiewicz, R.; Ostrowska, E.; Wysińska, J.; Russo, V.; Grabowski, M.; Opolski, G. Cardiac Arrhythmias in Muscular Dystrophies Associated with Emerinopathy and Laminopathy: A Cohort Study. *J. Clin. Med.* **2021**, *10*, 732. https://doi.org/10.3390/jcm10040732

Academic Editor: Stefan Peters

Received: 10 January 2021
Accepted: 7 February 2021
Published: 12 February 2021

1. Introduction

Laminopathies and emerinopathies are genetic disorders caused by mutations in *LMNA* and *EMD* genes, respectively, encoding lamin A/C and emerin—ubiquitous proteins of the nuclear envelope. Both conditions show a heterogenous clinical presentation characterized by different neuromuscular and cardiac phenotypes. Cardiac involvement in patients with muscular dystrophy associated with laminopathy is typically characterized by atrioventricular conduction abnormalities, life-threatening cardiac arrhythmias, and heart remodeling towards dilated or restrictive cardiomyopathy [1]. Little is still known about cardiac involvement in patients with muscular dystrophy associated to emerinopathy. Additionally, data regarding timing of specific arrhythmias occurrence are still insufficient. The aim of our study was to describe and compare the prevalence and time distribution of cardiac arrhythmias in patients with muscular dystrophies associated with emerinopathy and laminopathy at extended follow-up.

2. Materials and Methods

2.1. Study Design and Population

This single-center prospective observational study included 45 consecutive patients affected by muscular dystrophy associated to laminopathy or emerinopathy admitted by and followed up at the 1st Department of Cardiology, Medical University of Warsaw. The study was approved by the Local Ethics Committee and was in accordance with the 1976 Declaration of Helsinki and its later amendments.

2.2. Study Protocol

Patients in the study underwent clinical evaluation, 12-lead surface electrocardiogram (ECG), 24 h electrocardiographic monitoring, cardiac implanted device interrogation at enrollment and every 12 months thereafter. Atrioventricular block (AVB) was assessed from a resting 12-lead electrocardiography (ECG) based on PR interval and P waves to QRS complexes relations. Atrial arrhythmias were collected from a resting ECG, Holter monitoring, pacemaker (PM), and implantable cardioverter-defibrillator (ICD) interrogation. Atrial arrhythmias were classified into supraventricular extra beats (SVEBs), atrial tachycardia (AT) with P wave of other than sinus morphology and rate 100–250/min, atrial flutter (AFl)—no P wave with F wave >250 min, and atrial fibrillation (AF)—no P wave with f wave >350/min. Atrial standstill (AS) or so-called atrial paralysis with no atrial activity was defined as no P, f, and F visible, confirmed by intracardiac electrograms. Nodal (junctional) rhythm (NR) was defined as a regular heart rate <50/min with narrow QRS complexes and no P waves preceding QRS complexes. Ventricular arrhythmias were classified as ventricular extra beats (VEBs), non-sustained ventricular tachycardia (nsVT), defined as ≥3 consecutive ventricular beats with a rate >120/min lasting <30 s, or sustained ventricular tachycardia (VT), defined as ventricular beats of a rate >120/min lasting >30 s.

2.3. Outcomes

The primary endpoint was the prevalence and the onset-time of cardiac arrhythmias among the study population.

2.4. Statistical Analysis

Distribution of continuous data was tested with the Kolmogorov–Smirnov and the Shapiro–Wilk test. Normally distributed variables were expressed as mean ± standard deviation (SD), whereas non-normal distributed ones as median (25th, 75th percentiles) and interquartile range (IQR). Categorical variables were reported as numbers and percentages. Differences between groups were compared using the Fisher exact test for categorical variables and the Mann–Whitney U test for continuous and ordinal variables. A two-sided *p*-value less than 0.05 was considered significant for all tests. All statistical analyses were performed using SPSS software, version 22 (IBM SPSS Statistics 22, New York, NY, USA).

3. Results

The baseline clinical, electrocardiographic, and echocardiographic characteristics of the study population are shown in Table 1. The study population included 30 patients with Emery–Dreifuss Muscular Dystrophy (EDMD1) (mutation in *EMD* gene encoding emerin) and 15 patients with muscular dystrophy associated with mutations in *LMNA* gene encoding lamin A/C: 12 patients with EDMD2, 2 with LGMD, and 1 with *LMNA*-related congenital muscular dystrophy (L-CMD). There were no significant differences in terms of baseline characteristics with the exception of gender, where 73% of *LMNA* patients were female and 80% of *EMD* were male ($p < 0.001$). All patients were free from other cardiovascular risk factors, which may be explained by their relatively young age. The median follow-up was 11 (5.0–16.6) years.

Table 1. Baseline characteristics of the study population.

	EMD Group *n* = 30	*LMNA* Group *n* = 15	*p*-Value
Age (years)	21.0 (15.25–30.0)	26.0 (18.0–33.0)	NS
Female (%)	20	73	<0.001
BMI (kg/m^2)	21.5 (19.4–25.2)	20.2 (17.3–25.1)	NS
Sporadic/familial	13/17	9/6	NS
LVEDV (mL)	119 (90–169)	103 (86–125)	NS
LAV (mL)	56.4 (47.8–73.3)	50.5 (38.5–63)	0.08
LVEF (%)	52 (48–58)	54 (48–58)	NS
NTpro-BNP (pg/mL)	70 (44–102)	109 (54–347)	NS
NYHA I-II (%)	0	20	0.08
NYHA III-IV	0	0	NS

BMI—body mass index; EMD—mutation in EMD gene; LAV—left atrial volume; LVEDV—left ventricle end-diastolic volume; LVEF—left ventricle ejection fraction; LMNA—mutation in LMNA gene; NS – not significant; NTpro-BNP—N-terminal pro hormone B-type natriuretic peptide; NYHA—New York Heart Association class.

3.1. Cardiac Arrhythmias at Inclusion

The mean age of the study population at first cardiac evaluation was 24.9 +/− 12 years. At the first electrocardiographic evaluation, 84% (*n*: 38) of patients showed sinus rhythm and 16% (*n*: 7) junctional rhythm. This was more common in the *EMD* group, although the difference was not statistically significant (20% vs. 6.7%; $p = 0.4$). Forty percent (*n*: 18) experienced AF or AFl at the first evaluation. An increasing trend in AF/AFl prevalence in the *EMD* group was shown (50% vs. 20%, $p = 0.06$). AS was shown in 7% of the study population (*n*: 3), and all of them were patients with emerinopathy. AVB were present in 58% of the study population, in particular the first-degree AVB in 11% (*n*: 5), second-degree AVB in 24% (*n*: 11), and third-degree in 22% (*n*: 10). No significant differences between *EMD* and *LMNA* were found (Table 2). In 13% of patients (6/45) VEBs were present in Holter monitoring, wherein 2/30 were from the *EMD* group and 4/15 from the *LMNA* group, respectively. No patients presented nsVT or VT at initial evaluation. The occurrence of different arrhythmias and conduction disturbances at first cardiac evaluation are presented in Table 2 and Figure 1.

Table 2. Differences in arrhythmias occurrence at initial evaluation.

	Total Group (*n* = 45)	*EMD* Group (*n* = 30)	*LMNA* Group (*n* = 15)	*p*-Value
SR, % (*n*)	84.4 (38)	80 (24)	93 (14)	0.40
NR, % (*n*)	15.6 (7)	20 (6)	6.7 (1)	0.40
AT, % (*n*)	24.4 (11)	16.7 (5)	40 (6)	0.14
AF, % (*n*)	28.9 (13)	33.3 (10)	20 (3)	0.49
AFl, % (*n*)	17.8 (8)	23.3 (7)	6.7 (1)	0.24
AS, % (*n*)	6.7 (3)	10 (3)	0 (0)	0.54
AVB 1st degree, % (*n*)	11.1 (5)	10 (3)	13.3 (2)	1.00
AVB 2nd degree, % (*n*)	24.4 (11)	20 (6)	33.3 (5)	0.46
AVB 3rd degree, % (*n*)	22.2 (10)	26.7 (8)	13.3 (2)	0.46
SVEBs, % (*n*)	37.8 (17)	36.7 (11)	40 (6)	1.00
VEBs, % (*n*)	13.3 (6)	6.7 (2)	26.7 (4)	0.16
nsVT, % (*n*)	0 (0)	0 (0)	0 (0)	-
VT, % (*n*)	0 (0)	0 (0)	0 (0)	-

AF—atrial fibrillation; AFl—atrial flutter; AS—atrial standstill; AT—atrial tachycardia; AVB—atrio-ventricular block; *EMD*—mutation in *EMD* gene; *LMNA*—mutation in *LMNA* gene; NR—nodal rhythm; nsVT—non-sustained ventricular tachycardia; SR—sinus rhythm; SVEBs—supraventricular extra beats; VEBs—ventricular extra beats; VT—ventricular tachycardia.

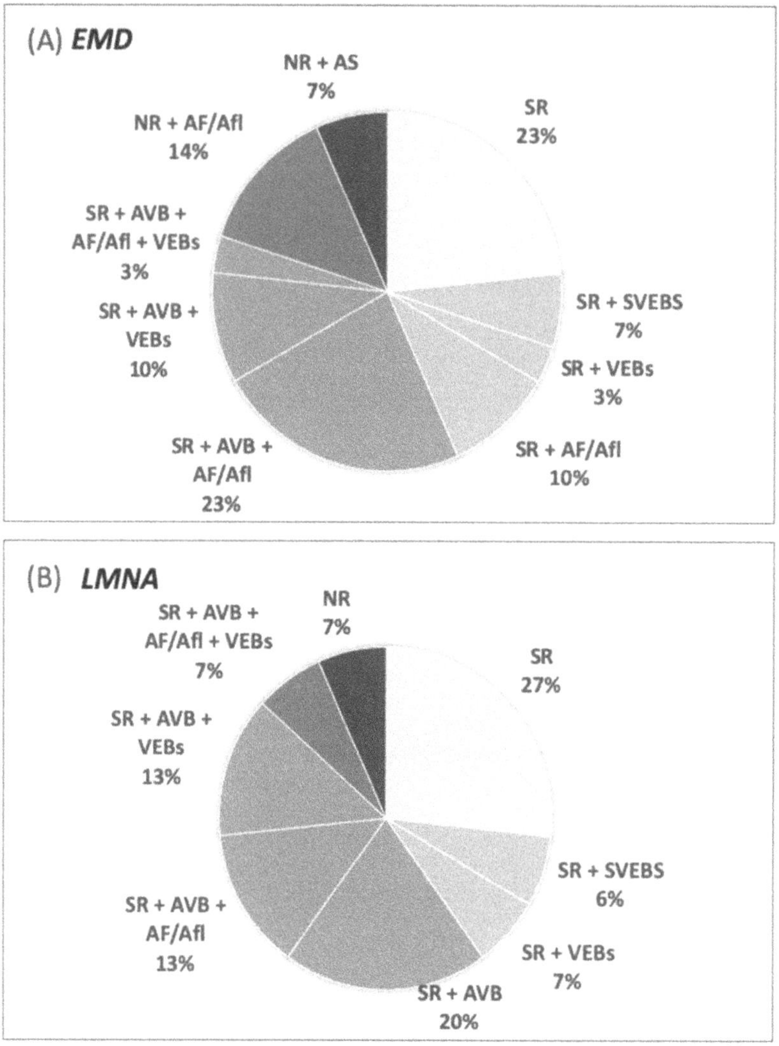

Figure 1. Cardiac arrhythmias at first evaluation. (**A**) Patients with mutation in *EMD* gene. (**B**) Patients with mutation in *LMNA* gene. AF—atrial fibrillation; AFl—A=atrial flutter; AS—atrial standstill; AVB—atrio-ventricular block; *EMD*—mutation in *EMD* gene; *LMNA*—mutation in *LMNA* gene; NR—noDAL RHYTHM; SR—SINUS rhythm; SVEBs—supraventricular extra beats; VEBs—ventricular extra beats.

3.2. Prevalence of Atrial Arrhythmias at Follow-Up

The mean age at the end of follow-up was 36.3 +/− 14.4 years. The prevalence of atrial arrhythmias at the end of follow-up is presented in Table 3. Only 22% of patients (*n*: 10) remained free from the sustained supraventricular arrhythmias or AS. One-third of patients with laminopathy and one-fourth with emerinopathy had AF/AFl. Almost half of the *EMD* group (*n*: 14) presented with AS, which did not occur in any patient from the *LMNA* group (*p* 0.001). Seventy-six percent of *EMD* patients needed PM implantation, while the percentage of PM implantation in the *LMNA* group was 47% (*p* 0.09). Half of the patients presented with SVEBS. The details are shown in Table 3.

Table 3. Occurrence of atrial and ventricular arrhythmias at the end of follow-up.

	Total Group (n = 45)	*EMD* (n = 30)	*LMNA* (n = 15)	p-Value
SVEBs, % (n)	48.9 (22)	46.7 (14)	53.3 (8)	0.76
AT only, % (n)	17.8 (8)	10 (3)	33.3 (5)	0.10
AF/Afl only, % (n)	28.9 (13)	26.7 (8)	33.3 (5)	0.73
AS only, % (n)	31.1 (14)	46.7 (14)	0 (0)	0.001
No AT/AF/AFl/AS, % (n)	22.2 (10)	16.7 (5)	33.3 (5)	0.26
VEBs, % (n)	40 (18)	30 (9)	60 (9)	0.11
VEBs couplets, % (n)	22.2 (10)	13.3 (4)	40 (6)	0.06
nsVT, % (n)	22.2 (10)	3.3 (1)	60 (9)	<0.001
VT, % (n)	8.9 (4)	6.7 (2)	13.3 (2)	0.59
nsVT/VT, % (n)	24.4 (11)	6.7 (2)	60 (9)	<0.001
PM implantation, % (n)	66.7 (30)	76.7 (23)	46.7 (7)	0.09
ICD implantation, % (n)	22,2 (10)	3,3 (1)	60 (9)	<0.001

AF—atrial fibrillation; AFl—atrial flutter; AS—atrial standstill; AT—atrial tachycardia; *EMD*—mutation in *EMD* gene; ICD—implantable cardioverter-defibrillator; *LMNA*—mutation in *LMNA* gene; nsVT—non-sustained ventricular tachycardia; PM—pacemaker; SVEBs—supraventricular extra beats; VEBs—ventricular extra beats; VT—ventricular tachycardia.

3.3. Prevalence of Ventricular Arrhythmias at Follow-Up

One-fourth of patients presented with nsVT—a potential risk factor for sudden cardiac death—and had an implantable cardioverter-defibrillator (ICD) implanted. Apart from ventricular arrhythmias being more frequent in laminopathies, more differences in terms of ventricular arrhythmias between patients from the *EMD* and *LMNA* groups were observed. nsVT was present in as much as 60% (n: 9) of *LMNA* patients, while only 3% of *EMD* patients (n: 1) had nsVT ($p < 0.001$). Moreover, premature ventricular complexes (PVCs) or PVC couplets (considered as more benign arrhythmias), already present at initial evaluation, finally occurred in 60% (n: 9) of patients with laminopathy and in 30% (n: 9) of patients with emerinopathy. Since ventricular arrhythmias occurred more frequently in the *LMNA* group, the number of implanted ICD devices was accordingly higher in these patients ($p < 0.001$). Ventricular arrhythmias occurrence is shown in Table 3.

3.4. Timing of Arrhythmia's Occurrence

Furthermore, the time of the arrhythmia's occurrence was analyzed, including the evaluation on the differences between *EMD* and *LMNA* cohorts, and are depicted in Figures 2 and 3. In our group, the age of AVB occurrence was relatively higher in patients with laminopathy (32.8 +/− 10.6 vs. 25.1 +/− 9.1, $p = 0.03$). Difference in the age of AF/AFl onset (31.8 +/− 3.9 vs. 24.2 +/− 10.4, $p = 0.053$) for *LMNA* and *EMD* patients, respectively, was close to significant. As for ventricular arrhythmias, patients with emerinopathy were generally older at the time of first occurrence, although the differences did not reach statistical significance.

In all patients with emerinopathy evident clinical signs of skeletal muscle involvement, typically seen in the first decade of life, preceded cardiac symptoms, which occurred at the end of the second decade or slightly later. However, this was not true for patients with laminopathy, as in some of them cardiac arrhythmia was the first health problem, being the reason to seek medical advice. Only further detailed neurological assessment led to final diagnosis of skeletal muscle laminopathy.

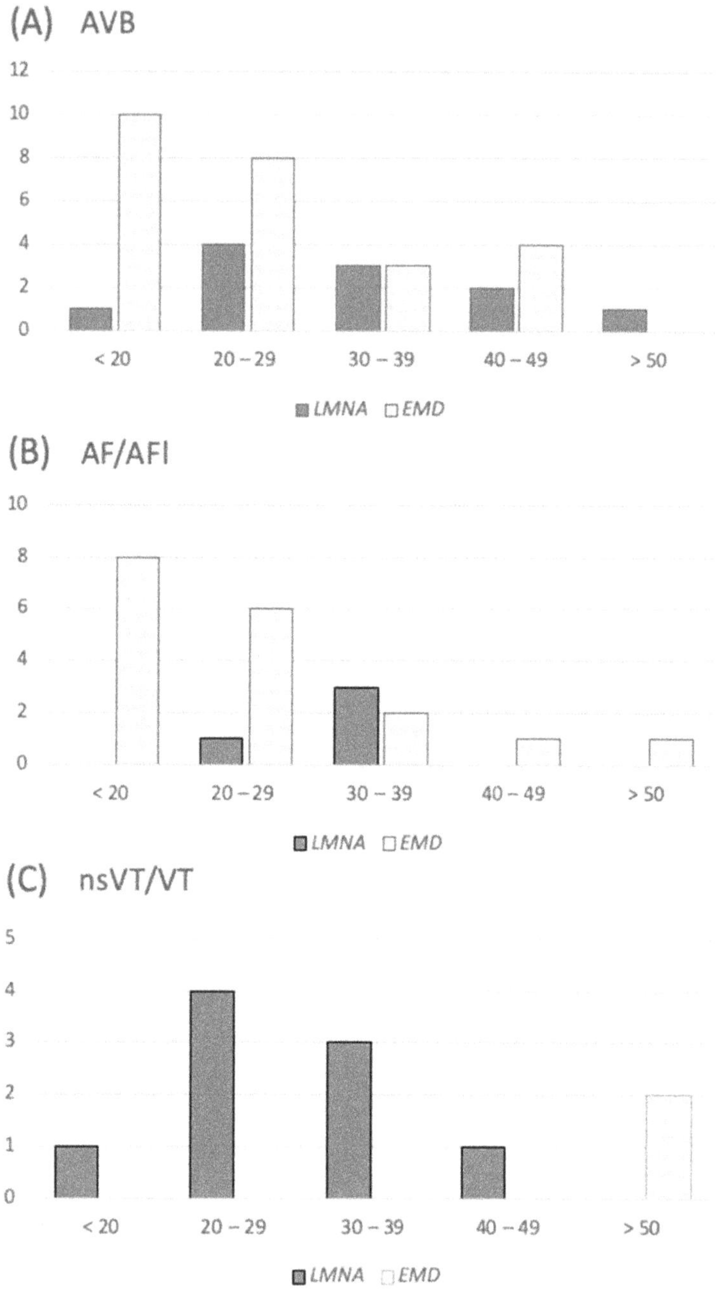

Figure 2. Age distribution of the occurrence of cardiac arrhythmias. (**A**) AVB – atrio-ventricular block. (**B**) AF/AFl Atrial fibrillation and atrial flutter. (**C**) nsVT/VT Non-sustained ventricular tachycardia and ventricular tachycardia. AF—atrial fibrillation; AFl—atrial flutter; AVB—atrio-ventricular block; EMD—mutation in EMD gene; LMNA—mutation in LMNA gene; nsVT—non-sustained ventricular tachycardia; VT—ventricular tachycardia.

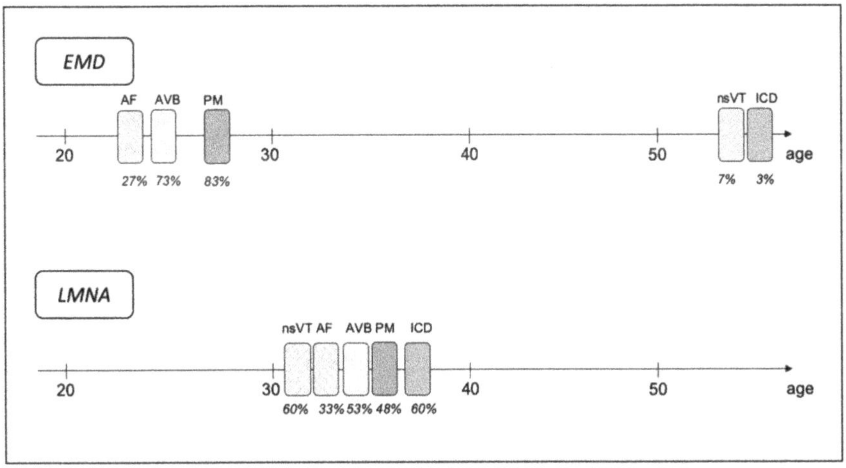

Figure 3. Timeline of arrhythmic events and interventions for both *EMD* and *LMNA* patients. The position of the bar on the line corresponds to the mean age of event occurrence. The percentage below shows the frequency of the event. AF—atrial fibrillation; AVB—atrio-ventricular block; *EMD*—mutation in *EMD* gene; ICD—implantable cardioverter-defibrillator; *LMNA*—mutation in *LMNA* gene; nsVT—non-sustained ventricular tachycardia; PM—pacemaker.

4. Discussion

Several muscular dystrophies manifest in cardiac involvement. Knowledge of the incidence and timeline of occurrence of different arrhythmias may be crucial for cardiac screening, as well as thromboembolic and SCD risk assessment. In the most common X-linked muscular dystrophinopathies, Duchenne (DMD) and Becker (BMD) muscular dystrophy, dilated cardiomyopathy (DCM) precedes appearance of severe cardiac arrhythmias in a typical scenario. The time course of cardiac dysfunction in DMD is fairly well predictable [2]. Muscular dystrophies associated with laminopathies belong to the group of ultra-rare diseases (incidence of 0.39 per 100,000) [3]. Thus, the natural course of arrhythmias is more difficult to establish due to smaller groups of patients available for observation. More and more studies concerning *LMNA*-positive patients are being conducted [4,5]. In the muscular dystrophies due to laminopathies the risk of arrhythmias increases with age (the penetrance of *LMNA* mutations is almost complete for cardiac phenotype), but their occurrence may be different in patients with emerinopathy and laminopathy. Early cardiac involvement in laminopathies is usually characterized by a prolonged PR interval, which may progress to advanced AVB and is explained by gradual replacement of myocardium by fibrous and adipose tissue [6,7]. Several hypotheses have been proposed to explain the problem of cardiac phenotype variability in patients with mutated *LMNA* or *EMD* genes [8,9]. It has been suggested that in *EMD* peripheral muscle manifestation usually occurs before cardiac symptoms [9]. There is a fair amount of data concerning differences in peripheral muscle involvement including the results from microscopic examinations of the muscle biopsies [10,11]. In addition, previous papers suggested that patients with laminopathy and neuromuscular presentation had an earlier and more advanced cardiac involvement [12,13]. However, none provided a direct comparison of cardiac involvement in *EMD* and *LMNA* in a considerable cohort and extended follow-up yet.

In our study atrioventricular conduction abnormalities typical for laminopathies were already present at the first cardiac screening. As many as 14% of patients had junctional escape rhythm in ECG tracings. According to guidelines, in patients with muscular dystrophy associated with *EMD* mutations, early implantation of the PM may be justified, while in laminopathy, primary prevention of SCD should be realized by ICD implantation [14]. In 44% of our cohort first cardiac evaluation ends up with the decision of PM implantation. Interestingly, during follow-up, AVB occurred significantly earlier in patients with emerinopathy (usually in the second or third decade of life), while the time of its distribution in laminopathy was more spread over the decades (Figures 2 and 3). This discovery might be consistent with the findings of Hong et al. [15]. They described three cases, among them two *EMD* and one *LMNA* patient presented with AS and junctional nodal rhythm, although the *LMNA* patient was in the fourth decade, while *EMD* patients were in the second decade of their lives. In a cohort of 79 Norwegian *LMNA* DCM patients and asymptomatic family members, 72% presented with AVB and 37% were PM-dependent at the end of the follow-up [16]. The need for pacing in EDMD patients was previously described in a paper by Steckiewicz et al. [17], where most of the patients were implanted with a PM and one with an ICD. Of 41 of patients with laminopathy and skeletal muscle involvement described in the paper by Bonne et al., 23 had arrhythmias, 6 were implanted with a PM, and 1 with an ICD, but no more details were provided [10]. In van Berlo's meta-analysis 28% of patients with laminopathy received a PM [4]. Little is known about cardiac resynchronization therapy (CRT) applied in EDMD patients. In one of the biggest cohorts of *LMNA* patients with a neuromuscular onset [12] only two patients were implanted with CRT-D in primary prevention. In our group only one patient with *LMNA*, low ejection fraction, and symptomatic heart failure was implanted with CRT-D. These low numbers are probably due to preserved systolic function and no signs of heart failure at the time of the occurrence of severe atrio-ventricular conduction disturbances. This is particularly true for *EMD*. In *LMNA* there is probably more room for CRT, which should be considered in patients with signs of cardiomyopathy, especially when ICD is needed for SCD prevention and the CRT-D device may be implanted.

Several longitudinal studies suggested that AF and AFl are the most frequent cardiac arrhythmias in laminopathies [18]. Many patients at first cardiac evaluation already had supraventricular arrythmias present, which may suggest that they are low-symptomatic at early stage of the disease [17]. On the contrary, especially in case of AF and AFl, young patients in the general population usually develop symptoms of arrhythmia. In the *EMD* group the onset of AF and AFl occurred in the second or third decade of life in the majority of patients. This is uncommon for any other muscular dystrophy. In the *LMNA* group the prevalence of this arrhythmia was less frequent yet still significant, and the mean age of the occurrence was higher in comparison to the *EMD* group. Nevertheless, the patients were relatively young (mean age 32). Realizing the early occurrence of asymptomatic AF patients with emerinopathy and laminopathy may be of great importance due to elevated thromboembolic risk (even without symptoms of AF) and emphasizes the necessity of early cardiac screening. The AS phenomenon, described as pathognomonic for *EMD* patients [18,19], was present at the first screening in only 7% of our patients. Interestingly, at the end of follow-up one-third of patients from the *LMNA* group developed AF, one-third AT, yet no patient had AS. In the *EDM* group the prevalence of supraventricular arrhythmias was even higher with half of the patients with AS and one-fourth with AF/AFl, all together 10% presented with AT. The mean age when AS had been confirmed was 34 years. The third and fourth decade of life used to be considered typical for the onset of atrial arrythmias in EDMD. In a paper by Bialer et al. affected patients younger than 20 years old did not present any ECG changes, while all affected men at the age of 35 years or older already had arrhythmias [20]. Boriani et al. [21] described 18 EDMD patients, both with emerinopathy (10) and laminopathy (8). Sixty-one percent (*n*: 11) experienced AF/Afl during follow-up. Forty-five percent (*n*: 5) of those who had AF/AFl subsequently developed AS. AF/AFl were present in both *EMD* and *LMNA* groups, irrespectively of severity of muscle involvement. In our group 78% of all EDMD patients presented either AF, AFl, AT, or AS at the end of follow-up. Our research suggests a significant difference in the time of occurrence of atrial arrhythmias in laminopathic patients with different genetic background.

Patients with laminopathies are at risk of SCD. This phenomenon is present in *LMNA* patients with both EDMD2, LGMD, and pure DCM without any peripheral muscle involvement [1,22,23]. There are dedicated risk calculators to assess the SCD risk in *LMNA*-positive subjects [24,25]. Several risk factors for malignant ventricular arrhythmias have also been identified. According to van Rijsingen et al. [26] the following four are the most important ones: male gender, nonsense mutation (ins- del/truncating or mutations affecting splicing), left ventricle ejection fraction (LVEF) <45% at first medical contact, and presence of nsVT. Among our cohort of 15 *LMNA* patients there were 4 male patients, 2 with non-sense mutation, 5 with decreased LVEF (<45%), and 9 patients presented with nsVT. This translates into five *LMNA* patients with no risk factors, four with one, and six with two or more. One *LMNA* and one *EMD* patient were implanted with ICD in secondary prevention, while the other eight *LMNA* in primary prevention. Although VT in patients with *EMD* mutation who had ICD implanted was previously described [27,28], the frequency of this form of arrhythmia in emerinopathy is not fully defined. The only one *EMD* patient implanted with ICD in our cohort had a reduced LVEF, while in *LMNA* ventricular arrythmias were present in patients with both reduced (5/15) and preserved LVEF (4/15). This may be an argument for a thesis that ventricular arrhythmias may precede systolic dysfunction in the *LMNA* group, which was not described in the *EMD* group. In patients from the *LMNA* group ventricular arrhythmias occurred in the third and fourth decade of life, while in the *EMD* group it was postponed above age fifty. One-fourth of all *LMNA* patients with muscular involvement presented significant ventricular arrhythmias, although in the laminopathy subgroup its prevalence was as high as 60%.

Limitation of the study. Follow-up depended on patients' age at first presentation. Some patients have been available since childhood, while others had their first consultation in adulthood. Therefore, the precise determination of the onset, type and severity of skeletal muscle symptoms, and sequence of cardiac and muscle involvement were difficult to establish. Frequency of the follow-up was not the same in all patients due to various adherence to medical recommendations resulting from disability and social circumstances.

The purpose of the current study was to analyze the occurrence of arrythmias in a Polish cohort of patients with laminopathy and emerinopathy, both coexisting with peripheral muscle involvement. Atrial arrhythmias were the most common arrhythmia in this group. In the *EMD* group it occurred first usually in the second or third decade of life. In the *LMNA* group it seemed to occur later. At the end of follow-up only 22% of patients were free of either AF, Afl, AT, or AS. AS did not occur in the patients with *LMNA* mutation from our cohort. Many patients with laminopathies presented with AVB early in the course of the disease. In *EMD* patients it occurred significantly earlier than in *LMNA* patients, in whom time distribution was more spread over the years. Two-thirds of patients ended up with a pacemaker at the end of follow-up. Ventricular arrhythmias were very common among patients from the *LMNA* group and occurred definitely earlier compared to the patients from the *EMD* group, whereas no significant ventricular arrhythmias occurred before the age of 50. The difference in cardiac arrhythmias occurrence in *LMNA* and *EMD* groups indicates a need for precise genetic diagnosis amongst patients with muscular dystrophy. On the other hand, atrioventricular conduction abnormalities and/or early onset of atrial arrhythmia may be a red flag to search for laminopathy in otherwise healthy young patients without any known previous neurologic diagnosis [29,30]. Does arrythmia burden in neuromuscular dystrophies contribute to the risk of clinical events? This is a question for future research.

Author Contributions: M.M. was responsible for conceptualization, design of the research, data collection, formal analysis, investigation, methodology, and writing of the original draft. A.M.-P. was responsible for investigation, data collection, review and editing. A.T. was responsible for statistical analysis, review and editing. R.S. was responsible for investigation and data collection. E.O. was responsible for data analysis, writing, review and editing. J.W. was responsible for data analysis, writing review and editing. V.R. was responsible for conceptualization, writing, review and editing. M.G. was responsible for investigation and supervision. G.O. was responsible for investigation and supervision. All authors have read and agreed to the published version of the manuscript.

Funding: This research received no external funding.

Institutional Review Board Statement: The study was approved by the Local Ethics Committee (KB/2/2005) and was in accordance with the 1976 Declaration of Helsinki and its later amendments.

Informed Consent Statement: Informed consent was obtained from all subjects involved in the study.

Data Availability Statement: The data presented in this study are available on request from the corresponding author. The data are not publicly available in order to protect patient privacy.

Conflicts of Interest: The authors declare no conflict of interest.

References

1. Captur, G.; Arbustini, E.; Bonne, G.; Syrris, P.; Mills, K.; Wahbi, K.; Mohiddin, S.A.; McKenna, S.; Pettit, S.; Ho, C.Y.; et al. Lamin and the heart. *Heart* **2017**, *104*, 468–479. [CrossRef] [PubMed]
2. Birnkrant, D.J.; Bushby, K.; Bann, C.M.; Alman, B.A.; Apkon, S.D.; Blackwell, A.; Case, L.E.; Cripe, L.; Hadjiyannakis, S.; Olson, A.K.; et al. Diagnosis and management of Duchenne muscular dystrophy, part 2: Respiratory, cardiac, bone health, and orthopaedic management. *Lancet Neurol.* **2018**, *17*, 347–361. [CrossRef]
3. Mah, J.K.; Korngut, L.; Fiest, K.M.; Dykeman, J.; Day, L.J.; Pringsheim, T.; Jette, N. A Systematic Review and Meta-analysis on the Epi-demiology of the Muscular Dystrophies. *Can. J. Neurol. Sci.* **2016**, *43*, 163–177. [CrossRef] [PubMed]
4. Van Berlo, J.H.; de Voogt, W.G.; van der Kooi, A.J.; van Tintelen, J.P.; Bonne, G.; Yaou, R.B.; Duboc, D.; Rossenbacker, T.; Heidbüchel, H.; de Visser, M.; et al. Meta-analysis of clinical characteristics of 299 carriers of LMNA gene mutations: Do lamin A/C mutations portend a high risk of sudden death? *J. Mol. Med.* **2005**, *83*, 79–83. [CrossRef]
5. Sanna, T.; Russo, A.D.; Toniolo, D.; Vytopil, M.; Pelargonio, G.; De Martino, G.; Ricci, E.; Silvestri, G.; Giglio, V.; Messano, L.; et al. Cardiac features of Emery-Dreifuss muscular dystrophy caused by lamin A/C gene mutations. *Eur. Heart J.* **2003**, *24*, 2227–2236. [CrossRef]
6. Wang, S.; Peng, D. Cardiac Involvement in Emery-Dreifuss Muscular Dystrophy and Related Management Strategies. *Int. Heart J.* **2019**, *60*, 12–18. [CrossRef]
7. Fishbein, M.C.; Siegel, R.J.; Thompson, C.E.; Hopkins, L.C. Sudden Death of a Carrier of X-Linked Emery-Dreifuss Muscular Dystrophy. *Ann. Intern. Med.* **1993**, *119*, 900. [CrossRef] [PubMed]
8. Tesson, F.; Saj, M.; Uvaize, M.M.; Nicolas, H.; Płoski, R.; Bilińska, Z. Lamin A/C mutations in dilated cardiomyopathy. *Cardiol. J.* **2014**, *21*, 331–342. [CrossRef] [PubMed]
9. Heller, S.A.; Shih, R.; Kalra, R.; Kang, P.B. Emery-Dreifuss muscular dystrophy. *Muscle Nerve* **2020**, *61*, 436–448. [CrossRef] [PubMed]
10. Bonne, G.; Mercuri, E.; Muchir, A.; Urtizberea, A.; Becane, H.M.; Recan, D.; Merlini, L.; WEhnert, M.; Boor, R.; Reuner, U. Clinical and molecular genetic spectrum of autosomal dominant Emery-Dreifuss muscular dystrophy due to mutations of the lamin A/C gene. *Ann. Neurol.* **2000**, *48*, 70–80. [CrossRef]
11. Emery, A.E.; Dreifuss, F.E. Unusual type of benign x-linked muscular dystrophy. *J. Neurol. Neurosurg. Psychiatry* **1966**, *29*, 338–342. [CrossRef] [PubMed]
12. Ditaranto, R.; Boriani, G.; Biffi, M.; Lorenzini, M.; Graziosi, M.; Ziacchi, M.; Pasquale, F.; Vitale, G.; Berardini, A.; Rinaldi, R.; et al. Differences in cardiac phenotype and natural history of laminopathies with and without neuromuscular onset. *Orphanet J. Rare Dis.* **2019**, *14*, 263. [CrossRef]
13. Peretto, G.; Di Resta, C.; Perversi, J.; Forleo, C.; Maggi, L.; Politano, L.; Barison, A.; Previtali, S.C.; Carboni, N.; Brun, F.; et al. Cardiac and Neuromuscular Features of Patients WithLMNA-Related Cardiomyopathy. *Ann. Intern. Med.* **2019**, *171*, 458. [CrossRef]
14. Priori, S.G.; Blomström-Lundqvist, C.; Mazzanti, A.; Blom, N.; Borggrefe, M.; Camm, J.; Elliott, P.M.; Fitzsimons, D.; Hatala, R.; Hindricks, G.; et al. 2015 ESC Guidelines for the management of patients with ventricular arrhythmias and the prevention of sudden cardiac Death. The Task Force for the Management of Patients with Ventricular Arrhythmias and the Prevention of Sudden Cardiac Death of the European Society of Cardiology (ESC). *G. Ital. Cardiol.* **2016**, *17*. [CrossRef]
15. Hong, J.-S.; Ki, C.-S.; Kim, J.-W.; Suh, Y.-L.; Kim, J.S.; Baek, K.K.; Kim, B.J.; Ahn, K.J.; Kim, D.-K. Cardiac Dysrhythmias, Cardiomyopathy and Muscular Dystrophy in Patients with Emery-Dreifuss Muscular Dystrophy and Limb-Girdle Muscular Dystrophy Type 1B. *J. Korean Med. Sci.* **2005**, *20*, 283–290. [CrossRef] [PubMed]
16. Hasselberg, N.E.; Haland, T.F.; Saberniak, J.; Brekke, P.H.; Berge, K.E.; Leren, T.P.; Edvardsen, T.; Haugaa, K.H. Lamin A/C cardiomyopathy: Young onset, high penetrance, and frequent need for heart transplantation. *Eur. Heart J.* **2017**, *39*, 853–860. [CrossRef]
17. Steckiewicz, R.; Stolarz, P.; Świętoń, E.; Madej-Pilarczyk, A.; Grabowski, M.; Marchel, M.; Pieniak, M.; Filipiak, K.J.; Hausmanowa-Petrusewicz, I.; Opolski, G. Cardiac pacing in 21 patients with Emery-Dreifuss muscular dystrophy: A single-centre study with a 39-year follow-up. *Kardiol. Polska* **2015**, 576–583. [CrossRef]
18. Buckley, A.E.; Dean, J.; Mahy, I.R. Cardiac involvement in Emery Dreifuss muscular dystrophy: A case series. *Heart* **1999**, *82*, 105–108. [CrossRef]

19. Steckiewicz, R.; Stolarz, P.; Kosior, D.A.; Marchel, M.; Pieniak, M.; Świętoń, E.; Piotrowska-Kownacka, E.; Grabowski, M. Atrial mechanical and electrical dysfunction in patient with Emery-Dreifuss muscular dystrophy reason of change in electrotherapeutical approach: Frequent result of rare disease. *Kardiol. Pol.* **2013**, *71*, 406–409. [CrossRef] [PubMed]
20. Bialer, M.G.; McDaniel, N.L.; E Kelly, T. Progression of cardiac disease in Emery-Dreifuss muscular dystrophy. *Clin. Cardiol.* **1991**, *14*, 411–416. [CrossRef]
21. Boriani, G.; Gallina, M.; Merlini, L.; Bonne, G.; Toniolo, D.; Amati, S.; Biffi, M.; Martignani, C.; Frabetti, L.; Bonvicini, M.; et al. Clinical relevance of atrial fibrillation/flutter, stroke, pacemaker implant, and heart failure in Emery-Dreifuss muscular dystrophy: A long-term longitudinal study. *Stroke* **2003**, *34*, 901–908. [CrossRef]
22. Sakata, K.; Shimizu, M.; Ino, H.; Yamaguchi, M.; Terai, H.; Fujino, N.; Hayashi, K.; Kaneda, T.; Inoue, M.; Oda, Y.; et al. High Incidence of Sudden Cardiac Death With Conduction Disturbances and Atrial Cardiomyopathy Caused by a Nonsense Mutation in the STA Gene. *Circulation* **2005**, *111*, 3352–3358. [CrossRef] [PubMed]
23. Madej-Pilarczyk, A.; Marchel, M.; Fidziańska, A.; Opolski, G.; Hausmanowa-Petrusewicz, I. Low symptomatic malignant cardiac arrhythmia in a patient with lamin-related congenital muscular dystrophy. *Kardiol. Polska* **2015**, *73*, 942. [CrossRef]
24. Pasotti, M.; Klersy, C.; Pilotto, A.; Marziliano, N.; Rapezzi, C.; Serio, A.; Mannarino, S.; Gambarin, F.; Favalli, V.; Grasso, M.; et al. Long-Term Outcome and Risk Stratification in Dilated Cardiolaminopathies. *J. Am. Coll. Cardiol.* **2008**, *52*, 1250–1260. [CrossRef]
25. Wahbi, K.; Ben Yaou, R.; Gandjbakhch, E.; Anselme, F.; Gossios, T.; Lakdawala, N.K.; Stalens, C.; Sacher, F.; Babuty, D.; Trochu, J.-N.; et al. Development and Validation of a New Risk Prediction Score for Life-Threatening Ventricular Tachyarrhythmias in Laminopathies. *Circulation* **2019**, *140*, 293–302. [CrossRef] [PubMed]
26. Van Rijsingen, I.A.; Arbustini, E.; Elliott, P.M.; Mogensen, J.; Hermans-van Ast, J.F.; van der Kooi, A.J.; van Tintele, J.P.; van den Berg, M.P.; Pilotto, A.; Pasotti, M.; et al. Risk factors for malignant ventricular arrhythmias in lamin a/c mutation carriers a European cohort study. *J. Am. Coll. Cardiol.* **2012**, *59*, 493–500. [CrossRef] [PubMed]
27. Carboni, N.; Mura, M.; Mercuri, E.; Marrosu, G.; Manzi, R.C.; Cocco, E.; Nissardi, V.; Isola, F.; Mateddu, A.; Solla, E.; et al. Cardiac and muscle imaging findings in a family with X-linked Emery–Dreifuss muscular dystrophy. *Neuromuscul. Disord.* **2012**, *22*, 152–158. [CrossRef]
28. Nigro, G.; Russo, V.; Ventriglia, V.M.; Della Cioppa, N.; Palladino, A.; Nigro, V.; Calabrò, R.; Nigro, G.; Politano, L. Early onset of cardiomyopathy and primary prevention of sudden death in X-linked Emery–Dreifuss muscular dystrophy. *Neuromuscul. Disord.* **2010**, *20*, 174–177. [CrossRef]
29. Madej-Pilarczyk, A.; Marchel, M.; Ochman, K.; Cegielska, J.; Steckiewicz, R. Low-symptomatic skeletal muscle disease in patients with a cardiac disease—Diagnostic approach in skeletal muscle laminopathies. *Neurol. Neurochir. Polska* **2018**, *52*, 174–180. [CrossRef]
30. Kalin, K.; Oreziak, A.; Franaszczyk, M.; Bilinska, Z.T.; Ploski, R.; Bilinska, M. Genetic muscle disorder mimicking atrial arrhythmias with conduction defects requiring pacemaker implantation. *Pol. Arch. Intern. Med.* **2019**, *129*, 627–629. [PubMed]

Journal of
Clinical Medicine

MDPI

Review

Role of Provocable Brugada ECG Pattern in The Correct Risk Stratification for Major Arrhythmic Events

Nicolò Martini [1], Martina Testolina [2], Gian Luca Toffanin [2], Rocco Arancio [3], Luca De Mattia [4], Sergio Cannas [2], Giovanni Morani [2] and Bortolo Martini [2,*]

[1] Department of Cardio-Thoraco-Vascular Sciences and Public Health, University of Padua, 35128 Padua, Italy; nicolo.martini2@gmail.com
[2] Cardiac Unit, Alto Vicentino Hospital, 36014 Santorso, Italy; martina.testolina@aulss7.veneto.it (M.T.); gianluca.toffanin@aulss7.veneto.it (G.L.T.); sergio.cannas64@gmail.com (S.C.); giovanni.morani@aulss7.veneto.it (G.M.)
[3] Cardiac Unit, Ospedale Umberto Primo, 96100 Siracusa, Italy; arancior@tiscali.it
[4] Cardiac Unit, Treviso Hospital, 32111 Treviso, Italy; dmluca.it@gmail.com
* Correspondence: bortolo.martini@gmail.com

Abstract: The so-called Brugada syndrome (BS), first called precordial early repolarization syndrome (PERS), is characterized by the association of a fascinating electrocardiographic pattern, namely an aspect resembling right bundle branch block with a coved and sometime upsloping ST segment elevation in the precordial leads, and major ventricular arrhythmic events that could rarely lead to sudden death. Its electrogenesis has been related to a conduction delay mostly, but not only, located on the right ventricular outflow tract (RVOT), probably due to a progressive fibrosis of the conduction system. Many tests have been proposed to identify people at risk of sudden death and, among all, ajmaline challenge, thanks to its ability to enhance latent conduction defects, became so popular, even if its role is still controversial as it is neither specific nor sensitive enough to guide further invasive investigations and managements. Interestingly, a type 1 pattern has also been induced in many other cardiac diseases or systemic diseases with a cardiac involvement, such as long QT syndrome (LQTS), arrhythmogenic right ventricular cardiomyopathy (ARVC), hypertrophic cardiomyopathy (HCM) and myotonic dystrophy, without any clear arrhythmic risk profile. Evidence-based studies clearly showed that a positive ajmaline test does not provide any additional information on the risk stratification for major ventricular arrhythmic events on asymptomatic individuals with a non-diagnostic Brugada ECG pattern.

Keywords: ajmaline challenge; Brugada syndrome; early repolarization syndrome; arrhythmogenic right ventricular cardiomyopathy; long QT syndrome; hypertrophic cardiomyopathy

Citation: Martini, N.; Testolina, M.; Toffanin, G.L.; Arancio, R.; De Mattia, L.; Cannas, S.; Morani, G.; Martini, B. Role of Provocable Brugada ECG Pattern in The Correct Risk Stratification for Major Arrhythmic Events. *J. Clin. Med.* **2021**, *10*, 1025. https://doi.org/10.3390/jcm10051025

Academic Editors: Gani Bajraktari and Stefan Peters

Received: 11 January 2021
Accepted: 23 February 2021
Published: 2 March 2021

1. Introduction

The so-called Brugada syndrome (BS), initially called precordial early repolarization syndrome (PERS) [1,2], is mainly characterized by an aspect resembling right bundle branch block, with a coved and sometime upsloping ST segment elevation in the precordial leads (defined as type 1 and 2 patterns) (Figure 1). This electrocardiogram (ECG) has a frequent dynamic behavior, changing from a normal trace to the two types. This ECG pattern that has historically been described as a benign entity [3] has been later rarely associated with arrhythmic cardiac death, and this association has become a popular syndrome nowadays described in more than 5000 papers. The first reports of PERS in a healthy young man [1,2], resuscitated from sudden cardiac death (SCD), was published early in 1988–1989 by Andrea Nava and Bortolo Martini, but became popular a few years later with a different name [4]. Since those old years, many efforts have been made to understand the pathophysiology of this strange ECG (depolarization or repolarization abnormality?), and to identify a correct risk stratification for the affected population. There is robust evidence that the true syndrome, namely the association of a major arrhythmic event and the mentioned ECG pattern, is so rare, but the same cannot be said for the ECG pattern alone. It is noteworthy that many other cardiac or extracardiac conditions, called phenocopies, may share this electrocardiographic pattern [5] but their arrhythmic risk is still unknown, also if they often induce a lot of fear (Brugadaphobia), and an unjustified complex diagnostic and therapeutic management. There has been a rush in medical literature to publish additional patterns to the spontaneous ECG, which could indicate and multiplicate people at risk, but unfortunately at present time, nobody has identified the gold standard, and all this literature is probably nothing more than an anecdotal collection. This paper will discuss, among all the available diagnostic tools, the drug inducible type 1 pattern whose specificity and role in the risk stratification are so controversial, with more doubts than confidences.

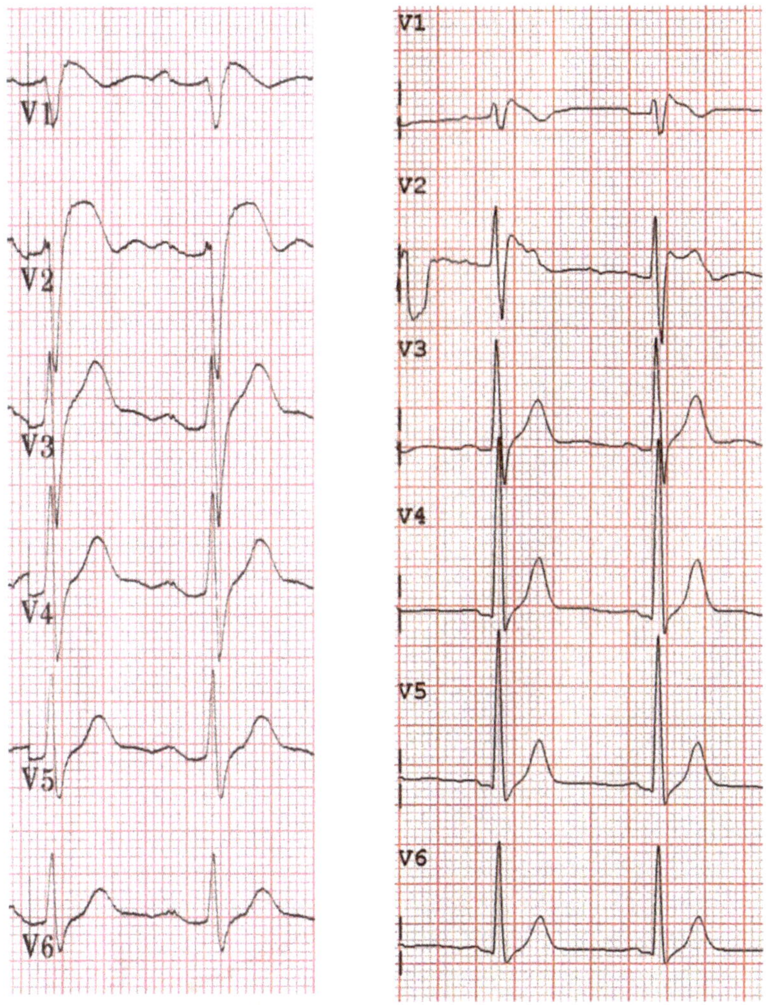

(**a**) (**b**)

Figure 1. Electrocardiograms (ECGs) showing the precordial leads (V1–V6) of two different patients respectively with a predominant spontaneous type 1 pattern and terminal QRS fragmentations (**a**) and a type 2 pattern (**b**).

2. The ECG Patterns

In the worldwide literature, there is an insistent confusion between a syndrome and an ECG pattern alone. A syndrome is the association between symptoms and signs, but the isolated detection of an abnormal ECG does not authorize anybody to make a diagnosis of a lethal condition that is an act that may only induce a severe psychiatric illness in many healthy young people. The true syndrome is so rare, while the isolated type 1 ECG pattern can probably be found in 1 out of thousand people, with the highest prevalence among the Asian population, and type 2 and 3 in up to 3% of healthy people in many reports (Figure 1). A major event can however yearly occur respectively in 0.38 and 0.06% of spontaneous and drug-induced type 1 pattern [6], values like the yearly rate of sudden death in the general population (0.1%).

There is not a typical ECG of the syndrome, that can vary over time, but there is an ECG pattern (defined as type 1), which is more frequent in the true cases of the syndrome. A popular classification in three types, however, does not have a scientific basis as it was only the description of the dynamic behaviour in one single patient [7]. This classification (whence type 3 has now been erased), and the recording of the precordial leads in the upper intercostal spaces has been severely abused. Asymptomatic healthy individuals incidentally found (both spontaneously or drug related) to have one of these three patterns have (and are) been submitted to invasive studies and therapies. Type 1 ECG is indeed a fascinating pattern, that in the true syndromes is more frequently associated to other features, such as a major familial incidence, genetic abnormalities, QRS fractioning, PR interval prolongation, left axis deviation, abnormal electrophysiological investigations, and presence of late potentials, are frequently found in patients with the syndrome [8], but all these findings do not reach enough statistic power to establish any serious evidence-based guideline.

3. The Pathophysiological Basis of the Coved Type ECG Pattern

This topic has been the subject of a heavy debate as this pattern, whether inducible or spontaneous, is still poorly understood as well as its prognostic value. Many theories have been proposed, but two major hypotheses have been debated: an organic disease [1,2] vs. a functional abnormality [4]. The first one suggested a conduction delay at the right ventricular outflow tract (RVOT) level as the origin of the ECG pattern and this was retained part of some right ventricular cardiomyopathy as demonstrated by old necropsy study and confirmed by different authors [8–11]. The disease mainly involves the conduction system (that explains the right bundle branch block (RBBB) pattern, the PR prolongation, the left axis deviation, and the presence of late potentials), and is probably closer to Lev-Lenegre disease (same *SCN5A* genetic abnormality and fibrosis of the conduction system) than to the typical right ventricular cardiomyopathy (ARVC), that has usually different clinical and genetic findings. The ST elevation is a depolarization, rather than a repolarization abnormality, probably reflecting a lesion of the Purkinje network at the RVOT that could also have some embryologic origin [12]. The functional theory instead, proposed that a difference in the action potentials between epicardium and endocardium, (due to ionic channels abnormalities) gives origin to the ECG [13,14]. The organic theory was initially refused [15] and a greater attention was devoted to the functional one that has recently almost been abandoned [16,17]. A re-writing of the controversial history of this syndrome has then been re-proposed [18].

4. The Drug Inducible "Brugadophobic" ECG

The syndrome is still retained as one of the leading causes of sudden death and many efforts are made to identify latent asymptomatic carriers at risk. Many tests have been proposed including high precordial recordings, full stomach test, genetic research, signal averaged ECG, vectorcardiography, t-wave alternans, echocardiogram, cardiac magnetic resonance imaging, electrophysiological study, and electroanatomic mapping, but no-one reached enough statistical relevance. Over time, many drug tests have become extremely popular, even if after the occasional identification of a spontaneous type 1 ECG, or maybe a doubtful type 2 or even 3, converted to a type 1 with a pharmacological challenge, a Pandora's box is sometimes opened. Nowadays, up to 70% of people (mostly asymptomatic) in whom a diagnosis of BS or pattern is made, have been diagnosed by a drug test, performed after a suspicious basal ECG, which only contribute to the creation of the "Brugadophobia", proposed by Sami Viskin.

Ajmaline is an alkaloid derived from Rauwolfia Serpentina and its effect on cardiac electrogenesis is mediated by the class 1a anti-arrhythmic properties and the ability to induce or enhance a conduction delay [19]. Specifically, an intravenous administration of ajmaline could induce a prolongation of AH and HV intervals, a widening of QRS duration and transient AV blocks [20,21]. Like ajmaline, other antiarrhythmic drugs, particularly class 1c Flecainide, could induce similar abnormalities and are widely used when ajmaline is not available. A similar pattern could also be induced by other cardiological and non-cardiological drugs [22], but this effect is usually due to high or toxic dosages and, at present time, the popular classification of drugs to be avoided is mostly based on their toxic effects and not on a dangerous use of common dosages [23].

The problem is why ajmaline, flecainide, and the others induce a RVOT delay in many subjects either asymptomatic (up to 5% of normal population treated with flecainide for supraventricular tachycardia, in our experience), or symptomatic with a normal o mildly abnormal ECG. According to Durrer, if we consider the normal activation of the heart, the latest activated portion of the myocardium is the posterior-basal region and the pulmonary conus (RVOT) with different degrees among individuals [24] (Figure 2). Thus, the administration of these drugs could induce or enhance three major conduction delays: a prolongation of HV interval, a right bundle branch block, and a delay at the RVOT-Purkinje system, with the effect of creating an upsloping coved ST segment on the right precordial leads (Type 1) and a vectorcardiographic pattern of upper-posterior terminal QRS delay (Figure 3). The widespread use of these tests is however not totally safe and major ventricular arrhythmias and electromechanical dissociation have been described.

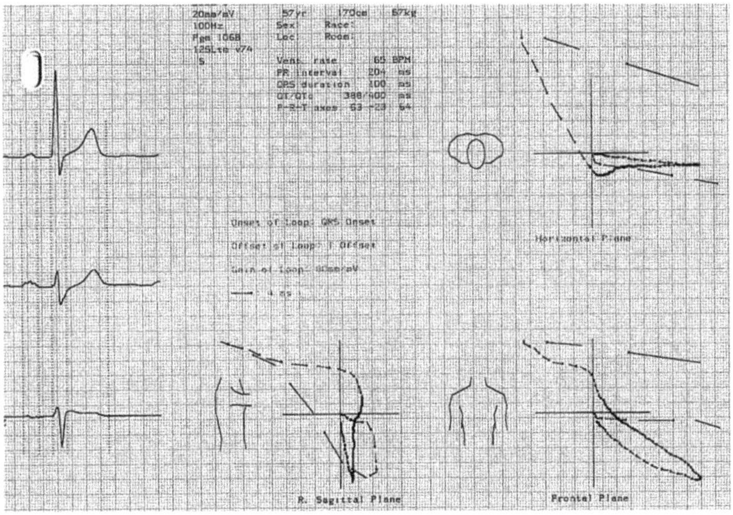

Figure 2. The vectorcardiographic trace of a patient with a spontaneous type 1 pattern. Here, are represented three main loops that indicate the direction of the ventricular activation along three different planes (sagittal, frontal, and horizontal). A right upper-posterior delay is showed, which denotes a late activated portion of the myocardium is the posterior-basal region and the pulmonary conus consistent with a right end conduction disturbance at the right ventricular outflow tract (RVOT).

The use of ajmaline introduced by Brugada [25], the flecainide test, and other drugs challenges have different protocols. In Western countries, ajmaline (0.7 mg/kg in 5 min), flecainide (2 mg/kg over 10 min), procainamide (10 mg/kg over 10 min), and propafenone are used. In Japan, pilsicainide, which is a pure Na^+-channel blocker and a class Ic drug in the Vaughan Williams classification, is usually administrated intravenously at 0.1–1 mg/kg over 10 min. (total 1 mg/kg). No evidence-based differences have been clearly documented between them [26]. Ajmaline was associated to more inducibility of the type 1 pattern compared to procainamide, but no additional prognostic information has been provided, while the pilsicainide challenge showed a major incidence of ventricular arrhythmias, without benefits [27,28]. Despite their diffuse availability and relatively safe profile, major ventricular arrhythmias and electromechanical dissociation have been described as compliances [28–30].

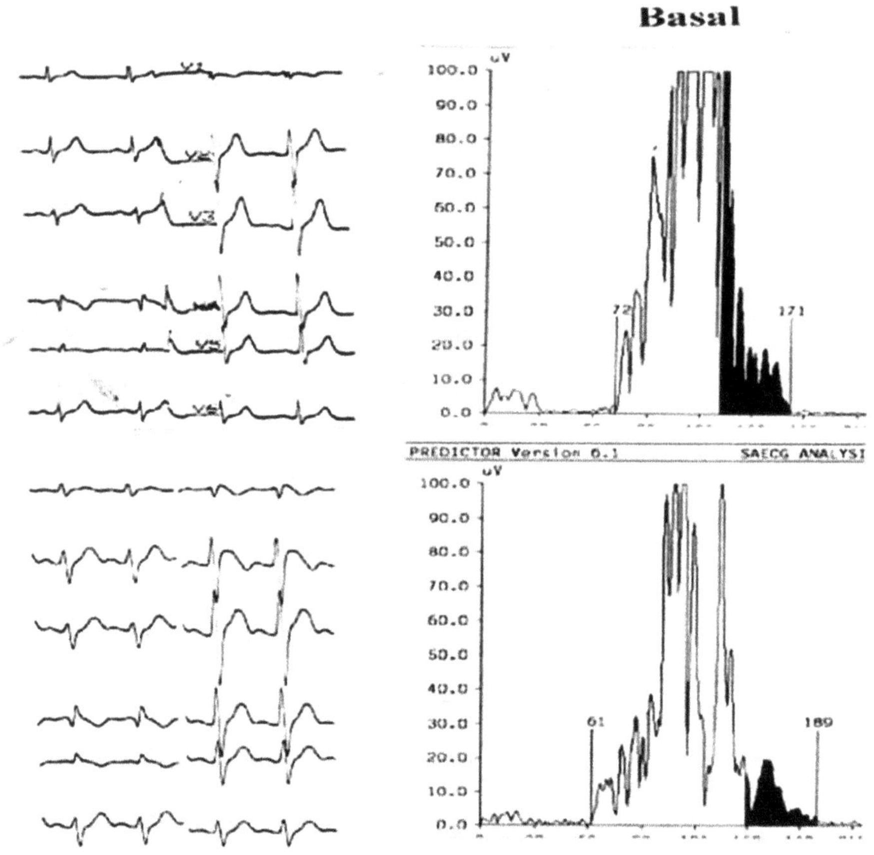

Figure 3. Signal-averaged electrocardiogram (SAECG) of a patient before and after the administration of flecainide. The upper part of the figure shows the baseline ECG and its SAECG trace and no late potentials can be seen. The lower part of the figure belongs to the same patient after the infusion of flecainide: a coved type pattern appears and positive late potentials are induced.

Their use to elicit the type 1 ECG pattern is quite sensitive in people with some precordial r1-ST abnormalities but so poorly specific for a clinical syndrome, with a limited predictive value. Unfortunately, the recognition that sodium channel blockers temporarily induce type 1 pattern has let the uncontrolled use of these drugs to unravel the diagnostic ECG; the medical community embraced these new diagnostic tests and at present time, most of the clinical series include asymptomatic people with a drug inducible type 1 ECG, who do not have any syndrome unless proven [31]. As reported by Viskin et al., in Europe, 70% of asymptomatic patients have been diagnosed after a positive ajmaline test, while one of the major reasons for Implantable Cardioverter Defibrillator (ICD) implantation for BS is a positive ajmaline test followed by an inducible ventricular fibrillation (VF) on electrophysiologic studies [31].

The worldwide prevalence of a drug induced type 1 ECG is quite high. It could be elicited in up to 50% of Italian and in 85% of German and French healthy asymptomatic individuals with a type 2 or 3 pattern [32–34]. Other series reported a positive response to the Na^+-channel blocker in 28% of healthy people with a normal baseline ECG and in 2% of people evaluated solely for syncope of unknown origin [35].

The drug induced coved type pattern also showed a good prognosis, as Shimitzu calculated a yearly risk of lethal events of 0.2% [35]. In another analysis performed by Viskin, the risk of a spontaneous VF on asymptomatic patients was only 0.3% per year [36]. A low rate of arrhythmic events was also reported by many other series [37,38], while only a spontaneous coved type pattern seemed to be linked to an increased risk profile [39]. In a more recent metanalysis, Delise calculated a 0.06% annual incidence of lethal events [6].

Other different studies evaluated the role of these drug challenges on the screening of families affected by the syndrome, reporting a low correlation with Sodium Voltage-gated Channel Alpha Subunit 5 (*SCN5A*) gene abnormalities. It is noteworthy that there were more positive tests in asymptomatic subjects than in symptomatic or familial cases, which raises scientific, ethical, and legal questions on these, sometime unsafe, challenges [40–43]. In these and other published studies, severe limitations were noted because of the low prevalence of the true syndrome, the low event rate, and the short follow up period. The linkage with genetic abnormalities has now been retracted: Brugada initially proposed a 100% correlation between *SCN5A* carriers and the spontaneous or drug inducible ECG pattern, but this assumption was not confirmed, and Priori demonstrated that the test might be negative in as many as 80% of asymptomatic gene carriers [44]. Nobody denied that patients with a drug-induced Brugada-type ECG have a poor prognosis if they also have a history of VF or aborted sudden cardiac death, because the risk of a drug induced Brugada-type ECG is the same as that of a spontaneous Brugada-type ECG [45].

Many concerns raised regarding the invasive electrophysiological study with cardiac stimulation following intra venous injection of the above-mentioned drugs; this can surely increase the number of positive subjects but with a lack in specificity. In recent years, ajmaline has been widely used during epicardial ablation to identify all the areas with a latent conduction disturbance, where to perform extensive ablation. This experimental procedure deserves cautions as there is not consensus in its wide implementation especially in the asymptomatic people submitted to this major invasive procedure.

Ajmaline is not specific for BS, and the type 1 pattern was sometimes induced in patients with long QT syndrome (LQT3), but no prognostic values were detected [46]. Patients with ARVC may have similar features (Figure 4). Peters et al. performed the ajmaline challenge on 55 people with a definite diagnosis of ARVC, and 9 of them showed a type 1 pattern [47]. The same author performed the ajmaline test again on 106 patients, 17 of which showed a coved type feature; they were older, mostly of female gender, and symptomatic for syncope [48]. It is of interest that the group of people with a provokable Brugada phenomenon had a low risk of ventricular arrhythmias on follow up, but a higher risk of developing a conduction disease (high degree of atrioventricular block and sinoatrial block) [49].

Ajmaline may disclose the presence of epsilon waves and QRS fragmentation [50,51], like ECG traces in ARVC. This does not mean that BS and ARVC are the same entity but that both can share some RVOT structural abnormalities and consequent similar ECG abnormalities [51].

A positive flecainide testing was also provided in a family (seven members) with an alpha-tropomyosin-induced hypertrophic cardiomyopathy with a very high risk of sudden cardiac death and in 18% of patients affected by myotonic dystrophy and minor ECG anomalies [52–54]. Nevertheless, caution should be taken that alpha-tropomyosin gene missense mutation is for certain the cause of a novel overlapping entity with hypertrophic cardiomyopathy and BS. It must be stated that BS may not always be an ion channel dysfunction but may also originate from a myofilament dysfunction that alters Ca^{2+} signaling [53].

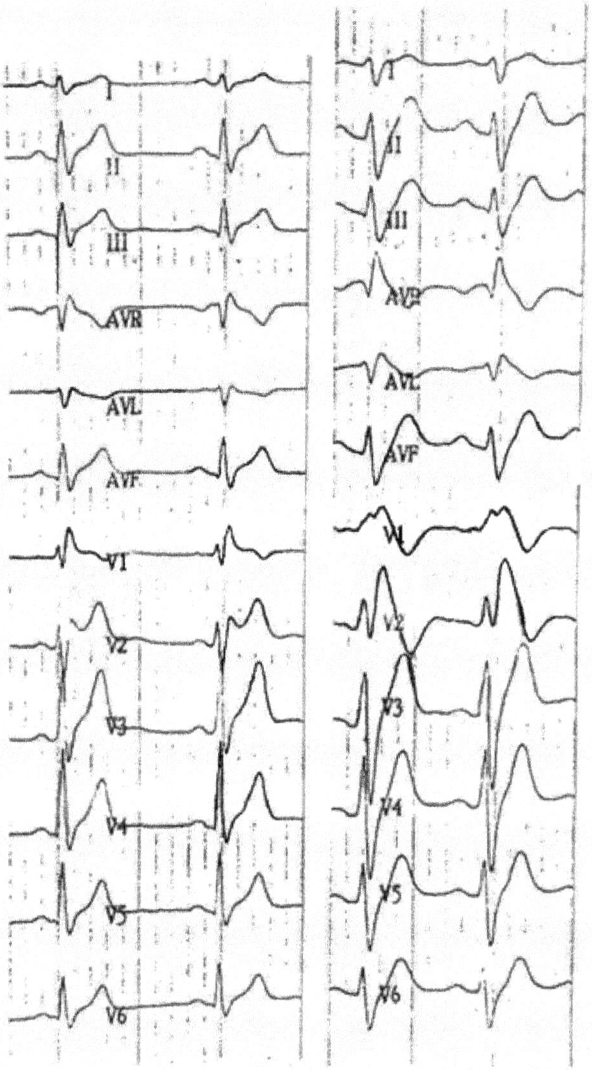

Figure 4. Two 12 leads ECGs of a patient with a familial form of ARVC before (on the left) and after the flecainide challenge (on the right). A massive type 1 pattern appears after the drug administration.

5. Conclusions

Ajmaline is a drug that has been extensively used throughout the electrophysiological world. Its main role is to enhance various degree of conduction defects [55]. What we can derive from evidence-based study, is that a positive ajmaline test, nowadays, does not provide any clear additional information on the risk stratification for major ventricular arrhythmic events on asymptomatic individuals with a non-diagnostic Brugada ECG pattern, but surely those individuals have a low risk arrhythmic profile. This conclusion reaffirms the wise statements of Sami Viskin: "To conclude, a note of caution: in a recent study simulating screening for Brugada syndrome, as many as 45% of healthy control subjects had minor imperfections in the right precordial leads that could be interpreted as type 2/3 Brugada ECG. We are forced to wonder how often asymptomatic individuals enter a path to rule out BS for the wrong reasons, have a false positive ajmaline test followed by a positive EP study, and faced with the alternative of facing sudden death, end up with an unjustified ICD implantation. Considering the imperfections of the ajmaline test, the study by Tadros has a clear message: A positive ajmaline test does not always mean you have Brugada syndrome" [56].

Author Contributions: Draft preparation, N.M. and B.M.; Supervision, M.T., L.D.M., G.L.T., S.C., R.A., G.M. All authors have read and agreed to the published version of the manuscript.

Funding: This research received no external funding.

Institutional Review Board Statement: Not applicable.

Informed Consent Statement: Not applicable.

Data Availability Statement: No new data were created or analyzed in this study. Data sharing is not applicable to this article.

Conflicts of Interest: The authors declare no conflict of interest.

References

1. Nava, A.; Canciani, B.; Schiavinato, M.L.; Martini, B.; Buja, G. La repolarisation precoce dans le precordiales droites: Trouble de la conduction intraventriculaire droite? Correlations de l'electrocardiographie-vectorcardiographie avec l'electro-physiologie. *Mises J. Cardiol.* **1988**, *17*, 157–159.
2. Martini, B.; Nava, A.; Thiene, G.; Buja, G.F.; Canciani, B.; Scognamiglio, R.; Daliento, L.; Volta, S.D. Ventricular fibrillation without apparent heart disease: Description of six cases. *Am. Hearth J.* **1989**, *118*, 1203–1209. [CrossRef]
3. Osher, H.; Wolff, L. Electrocardiographic pattern simulating acute myocardial injury. *Am. J. Med. Sci.* **1953**, *226*, 541–545. [CrossRef] [PubMed]
4. Brugada, P.; Brugada, J. Right bundle branch block, persistent ST segment elevation and sudden cardiac death: A distinct clinical and electrocardiographic syndrome. *J. Am. Coll. Cardiol.* **1992**, *20*, 1391–1396. [CrossRef]
5. Baranchuk, A.; Nguyen, T.; Ryu, M.H.; Femenía, F.; Zareba, W.; Wilde, A.A.M.; Shimizu, W.; Brugada, P.; Pérez-Riera, A.R. Brugada Phenocopy: New Terminology and Proposed Classification. *Ann. Noninvasive Electrocardiol.* **2012**, *17*, 299–314. [CrossRef] [PubMed]
6. Delise, P.; Probst, V.; Allocca, G.; Sitta, N.; Sciarra, L.; Brugada, J.; Kamakura, S.; Takagi, M.; Giustetto, C.; Calò, L. Clinical outcome of patients with the Brugada type 1 electrocardiogram without prophylactic implantable cardioverter defibrillator in primary prevention: A cumulative analysis of seven large prospective studies. *Europace* **2017**, *20*, f77–f85. [CrossRef] [PubMed]
7. Wilde, A.A.M.; Antzelevitch, C.; Borggrefe, M.; Borggrefe, M.; Brugada, J.; Brugada, R.; Brugada, P.; Corrado, D.; Hauer, R.N.W.; Kass, R.S.; et al. Proposed diagnostic criteria for the Brugada syndrome. *Eur. Heart J.* **2002**, *23*, 1648–1654. [CrossRef] [PubMed]
8. Martini, B.; Martini, N.; Dorantes Sánchez, M.; Márquez, M.F.; Zhang, L.; Fontaine, G.; Nava, A. Pistas de una enfermedad orgánica subyacente en el síndrome de Brugada. *Archivos De Cardiología De México* **2017**, *87*, 49–60. [CrossRef]
9. Martini, B.; Corrado, D.; Nava, A.; Thiene, G. Syndrome of Right bundle branch block, ST segment elevation and sudden death. Evidence of an organic substrate. In *Arrhythmogenic Right Ventricular Cardiomyopathy/Dysplasia*; Nava, A., Rossi, L., Thiene, G., Eds.; Elsevier: Amsterdam, The Netherlands, 1997; pp. 438–453.
10. Corrado, D.; Nava, A.; Buja, G.; Martini, B.; Fasoli, G.; Oselladore, L.; Turrini, P.; Thiene, G. Familial cardiomyopathy underlies syndrome of right bundle branch block, ST segment elevation and sudden death. *J. Am. Coll. Cardiol.* **1996**, *27*, 443–448. [CrossRef]
11. Corrado, D.; Basso, C.; Buja, G.; Nava, A.; Rossi, L.; Thiene, G. Right bundle branch block, right precordial st-segment elevation, and sudden death in young people. *Circulation* **2001**, *103*, 710–717. [CrossRef]

12. Elizari, M.V.; Levi, R.; Acunzo, R.S.; Chiale, P.A.; Civetta, M.M.; Ferreiro, M.; Sicouri, S. Abnormal expression of cardiac neural crest cells in heart development: A different hypothesis for the etiopathogenesis of Brugada syndrome. *Hearth Rhythm.* **2007**, *4*, 359–365. [CrossRef]
13. Szél, T.; Antzelevitch, C. Abnormal Repolarization as the Basis for Late Potentials and Fractionated Electrograms Recorded from Epicardium in Experimental Models of Brugada Syndrome. *J. Am. Coll. Cardiol.* **2014**, *63*, 2037–2045. [CrossRef]
14. Patocskai, B.; Yoon, N.; Antzelevitch, C. Mechanisms Underlying Epicardial Radiofrequency Ablation to Suppress Arrhythmogenesis in Experimental Models of Brugada Syndrome. *JACC Clin. Electrophysiol.* **2017**, *3*, 353–363. [CrossRef] [PubMed]
15. Brugada, P.; Brugada, J. Let us do not get confused, please! *G. Ital. Cardiol.* **1994**, *24*, 797–799.
16. Nademanee, K.; Veerakul, G.; Chandanamattha, P.; Chaothawee, L.; Ariyachaipanich, A.; Jirasirirojanakorn, K.; Likittanasombat, K.; Bhuripanyo, K.; Ngarmukos, T. Prevention of Ventricular Fibrillation Episodes in Brugada Syndrome by Catheter Ablation Over the Anterior Right Ventricular Outflow Tract Epicardium. *Circulation* **2011**, *123*, 1270–1279. [CrossRef]
17. Scheirlynck, E.; Chivulescu, M.; Lie, Ø.H.; Scheirlynck, E.; Chivulescu, M.; Øyvind, L.; Motoc, A.; Koulalis, J.; de Asmundis, C.; Sieira, J.; et al. Worse Prognosis in Brugada Syndrome Patients with Arrhythmogenic Cardiomyopathy Features. *J. Am. Coll. Cardiol. Electophysiol.* **2020**, *6*, 1353–1363. [CrossRef] [PubMed]
18. Havakuk, O.; Viskin, S. A Tale of 2 Diseases: The History of Long-QT Syndrome and Brugada Syndrome. *J. Am. Coll. Cardiol.* **2016**, *67*, 100–108. [CrossRef]
19. Obayashi, K.; Nagasawa, K.; Mandel, W.J.; Vyden, J.K.; Parmley, W.W. Cardiovascular effects of ajmaline. *Am. Hearth J.* **1976**, *92*, 487–496. [CrossRef]
20. Padrini, R.; Piovan, D.; Javarnaro, A.; Cucchini, F.; Ferrari, M. Pharmacokinetics and Electrophysiological Effects of Intravenous Ajmaline. *Clin. Pharmacokinet.* **1993**, *25*, 408–414. [CrossRef] [PubMed]
21. Conte, G.; Levinstein, M.; Sarkozy, A.; Sieira, J.; De Asmundis, C.; Chierchia, G.-B.; Di Giovanni, G.; Baltogiannis, G.; Ciconte, G.; Wauters, K.; et al. The clinical impact of ajmaline challenge in elderly patients with suspected atrioventricular conduction disease. *Int. J. Cardiol.* **2014**, *172*, 423–427. [CrossRef] [PubMed]
22. Letsas, K.P.; Kavvouras, C.; Kollias, G.; Tsikrikas, S.; Korantzopoulos, P.; Efremidis, M.; Sideris, A. Drug-Induced Brugada Syndrome by Noncardiac Agents. *Pacing Clin. Electrophysiol.* **2013**, *36*, 1570–1577. [CrossRef] [PubMed]
23. Postema, P.G.; Wolpert, C.; Amin, A.S.; Probst, V.; Borggrefe, M.; Roden, D.M.; Priori, S.G.; Tan, H.L.; Hiraoka, M.; Brugada, J.; et al. Drugs and Brugada syndrome patients: Review of the literature, recommendations, and an up-to-date website (www.brugadadrugs.org). *Hearth Rhythm* **2009**, *6*, 1335–1341. [CrossRef] [PubMed]
24. Durrer, D.; Van Dam, R.T.; Freud, G.E.; Janse, M.J.; Meijler, F.L.; Arzbaecher, R.C. Total Excitation of the Isolated Human Heart. *Circulation* **1970**, *41*, 899–912. [CrossRef] [PubMed]
25. Brugada, J.; Brugada, P.; Brugada, R. Ajmaline unmasks right bundle branch block-like and ST segment elevation in V1-V3 in patients with idiopathic ventricular fibrillation. *PACE* **1996**, *19*, 59911.
26. Tadros, R.; Wilde, A.A. Revisiting the sensitivity of sodium channel blocker testing in Brugada syndrome using obligate transmittance. *Int. J. Cardiol.* **2017**, *245*, 183–184. [CrossRef] [PubMed]
27. Cheung, C.C.; Mellor, G.; Deyell, M.W.; Ensam, B.; Batchvarov, V.; Papadakis, M.; Roberts, J.D.; Leather, R.; Sanatani, S.; Healey, J.S.; et al. Comparison of Ajmaline and Procainamide Provocation Tests in the Diagnosis of Brugada Syndrome. *JACC: Clin. Electrophysiol.* **2019**, *5*, 504–512. [CrossRef] [PubMed]
28. Chinushi, M.; Komura, S.; Izumi, D.; Furushima, H.; Tanabe, Y.; Washizuka, T.; Aizawa, Y. Incidence and Initial Characteristics of Pilsicainide-Induced Ventricular Arrhythmias in Patients with Brugada Syndrome. *Pacing Clin. Electrophysiol.* **2007**, *30*, 662–671. [CrossRef] [PubMed]
29. Conte, G.; Sieira, J.; Sarkozy, A.; De Asmundis, C.; Di Giovanni, G.; Chierchia, G.-B.; Ciconte, G.; Levinstein, M.; Casado-Arroyo, R.; Baltogiannis, G.; et al. Life-threatening ventricular arrhythmias during ajmaline challenge in patients with Brugada syndrome: Incidence, clinical features, and prognosis. *Hearth Rhythm* **2013**, *10*, 1869–1874. [CrossRef]
30. Moreno, J.; Magaldi, M.; Fontanals, J.; Gómez, L.; Berne, P.; Berruezo, A.; Brugada, J. Use of therapeutic hypothermia and extracorporeal life support after an unusual response to the ajmaline challenge in a patient with Brugada syndrome. *J. Cardiol. Cases* **2014**, *10*, 34–38. [CrossRef]
31. Viskin, S.; Rosso, R.; Friedensohn, L.; Havakuk, O.; Wilde, A.A.M. Everybody has Brugada syndrome until proven otherwise? *Hearth Rhythm* **2015**, *12*, 1595–1598. [CrossRef]
32. Veltmann, C.; Wolpert, C.; Sacher, F.; Mabo, P.; Schimpf, R.; Streitner, F.; Brade, J.; Kyndt, F.; Kuschyk, J.; Le Marec, H.; et al. Response to intravenous ajmaline: A retrospective analysis of 677 ajmaline challenges. *Eurospace* **2009**, *11*, 1345–1352. [CrossRef] [PubMed]
33. Zorzi, A.; Migliore, F.; Marras, E.; Marinelli, A.; Baritussio, A.; Allocca, G.; Leoni, L.; Perazollo Marra, M.; Basso, C.; Buja, G.; et al. Should all individuals with a no diagnostic Brugada-electrocardiogram undergo sodium-channel block test? *Heart Rhythm* **2012**, *9*, 909–916. [CrossRef]
34. Gasparini, M.; Priori, S.G.; Mantica, M.; Napolitano, C.; Galimberti, P.; Ceriotti, C.; Simonini, S. Flecainide Test in Brugada Syndrome: A Reproducible but Risky Tool. *Pacing Clin. Electrophysiol.* **2003**, *26*, 338–341. [CrossRef] [PubMed]
35. Shimizu, W. Is This a Philosophic Issue?—Do Patients with Drug-Induced Brugada Type ECG Have Poor Prognosis? *(Pro) Circ. J.* **2010**, *74*, 2455–2463. [CrossRef] [PubMed]

36. Viskin, S.; Rosso, M. Read My Lips A Positive Ajmaline Test Does Not Always Mean You Have Brugada Syndrome. *JACC* **2017**, *3*, 1409–1411.
37. Sieira, J.; Ciconte, G.; Conte, G.; De Asmundis, C.; Chierchia, G.-B.; Baltogiannis, G.; Di Giovanni, G.; Saitoh, Y.; Casado-Arroyo, R.; Juliá, J.; et al. Long-term prognosis of drug-induced Brugada syndrome. *Hearth Rhythm* **2017**, *14*, 1427–1433. [CrossRef] [PubMed]
38. Nishizaki, M.; Sakurada, H.; Yamawake, N.; Ueda-Tatsumoto, A.; Hiraoka, M. Low risk for arrhythmic events in asymptomatic patients with drug-induced type 1 ECG. Do patients with drug-induced Brugada type ECG have poor prognosis? *(Con). Circ. J.* **2010**, *74*, 2464–2473. [CrossRef] [PubMed]
39. Okamura, H.; Kamakura, T.; Morita, H.; Tokioka, K.; Nakajima, I.; Wada, M.; Ishibashi, K.; Miyamoto, K.; Noda, T.; Aiba, T.; et al. Risk Stratification in Patients with Brugada Syndrome Without Previous Cardiac Arrest. *Circ. J.* **2015**, *79*, 310–317. [CrossRef] [PubMed]
40. Joshi, S.; Raiszadeh, F.; Pierce, W.; Steinberg, J.S. Antiarrhythmic Induced Electrical Storm in Brugada Syndrome: A Case Report. *Ann. Noninvasive Electrocardiol.* **2007**, *12*, 274–278. [CrossRef]
41. Morita, H.; Morita, S.T.; Nagase, S.; Banba, K.; Nishii, N.; Tani, Y.; Watanabe, A.; Nakamura, K.; Kusano, K.F.; Emori, T.; et al. Ventricular arrhythmia induced by sodium channel blocker in patients with Brugada syndrome. *J. Am. Coll. Cardiol.* **2003**, *42*, 1624–1631. [CrossRef]
42. Antzelevitch, C.; Brugada, P.; Brugada, J.; Brugada, R.; Towbin, J.A.; Nademanee, K. Brugada syndrome: 1992-2002: A historical perspective. *J. Am. Coll. Cardiol.* **2003**, *41*, 1665–1671. [CrossRef]
43. Priori, S.G.; Napolitano, C.; Schwartz, P.J.; Bloise, R.; Crotti, L.; Ronchetti, E. The Elusive Link between LQT3 and Brugada Syndrome. *Circulation* **2000**, *102*, 945–947. [CrossRef]
44. Priori, S.G.; Napolitano, C.; Gasparini, M.; Pappone, C.; Della Bella, P.; Giordano, U.; Bloise, R.; Giustetto, C.; De Nardis, R.; Grillo, M.; et al. Natural History of Brugada Syndrome: Insights for risk stratification and management. *Circulation* **2002**, *105*, 1342–1347. [CrossRef]
45. Martini, B.; Zolla, C.; Guglielmi, F.; Toffanin, G.L.; Cannas, S.; Martini, N.; Arancio, R. Who is the guilty among these two silent killers? *Heart Rhythm Case Rep.* **2017**, *3*, 33–35. [CrossRef]
46. Hohmann, S.; Rudic, B.; Konrad, T.; Duncker, D.; König, T.; Tülümen, E.; Rostock, T.; Borggrefe, M.; Veltmann, C. Systematic ajmaline challenge in patients with long QT 3 syndrome caused by the most common mutation: A multicentre study. *Eurospace* **2016**, *19*, 1723–1729. [CrossRef]
47. Peters, S.; Trümmel, M.; Denecke, S.; Koehler, B. Results of ajmaline testing in patients with arrhythmogenic right ventricular dysplasia–cardiomyopathy. *Int. J. Cardiol.* **2004**, *95*, 207–210. [CrossRef] [PubMed]
48. Peters, S. Arrhythmogenic right ventricular dysplasia-cardiomyopathy and provocable coved-type ST-segment elevation in right precordial leads: Clues from long-term follow-up. *Eurospace* **2008**, *10*, 816–820. [CrossRef] [PubMed]
49. Aras, D.; Ozeke, O.; Çay, S.; Ozcan, F.; Acar, B.; Topaloglu, S. Ajmaline-induced epsilon wave: As a potential interim risk factor between the spontaneous- and drug-induced type 1 Brugada electrogram? *Europace* **2018**, *20*, 1225–1226. [CrossRef] [PubMed]
50. Martini, B.; Nava, A. A long-lasting electrocardiographic story. *Heart Rhythm* **2010**, *7*, 1521. [CrossRef] [PubMed]
51. Corrado, D.; Zorzi, A.; Cerrone, M.; Rigato, I.; Mongillo, M.; Bauce, B.; Delmar, M. Relationship Between Arrhythmogenic Right Ventricular Cardiomyopathy and Brugada Syndrome. *Circ. Arrhythmia Electrophysiol.* **2016**, *9*, e003631. [CrossRef] [PubMed]
52. Mango, R.; Luchetti, A.; Sangiuolo, R.; Ferradini, V.; Briglia, N.; Giardina, E.; Ferre, F.; Helmer Citterich, M.; Romeo, F.; Novelli, G.; et al. Next generation sequencing and linkage analysis for the molecular diagnosis of a novel overlapping syndrome charactrized by hypertrophic Cardiomyopathy and typical electrical instability of Brugada syndrome. *Circ. J.* **2016**, *80*, 938–949. [CrossRef] [PubMed]
53. Monasky, M.M.; Ciconte, G.; Anastasia, L.; Pappone, C. Commentary: Next Generation Sequencing and Linkage Analysis for the Molecular Diagnosis of a Novel Overlapping Syndrome Characterized by Hypertrophic Cardiomyopathy and Typical Electrical Instability of Brugada Syndrome. *Front. Physiol.* **2017**, *8*, 1056. [CrossRef] [PubMed]
54. Maury, P.; Audoubert, M.; Cintas, P.; Rollin, A.; Duparc, A.; Mondoly, P.; Chiriac, A.-M.; Acket, B.; Zhao, X.; Pasquié, J.L.; et al. Prevalence of type 1 Brugada ECG pattern after administration of Class 1C drugs in patients with type 1 myotonic dystrophy: Myotonic dystrophy as a part of the Brugada syndrome. *Hearth Rhythm* **2014**, *11*, 1721–1727. [CrossRef]
55. Migliore, F.; Testolina, M.; Zorzi, A.; Bertaglia, E.; Silvano, M.; Leoni, L.; Bellin, A.; Basso, C.; Thiene, G.; Allocca, G.; et al. First-degree atrioventricular block on basal electrocardiogram predicts future arrhythmic events in patients with Brugada syndrome: A long-term follow-up study from the Veneto region of North-eastern Italy. *Europace* **2019**, *21*, 322–333. [CrossRef] [PubMed]
56. Viskin, S.; Rosso, R. Read My Lips. *JACC Clin. Electrophysiol.* **2017**, *3*, 1409–1411. [CrossRef] [PubMed]

Journal of
Clinical Medicine

MDPI

Article

Nucleoside Analogue Reverse Transcriptase Inhibitors Improve Clinical Outcome in Transcriptional Active Human Parvovirus B19-Positive Patients

Heinz-Peter Schultheiss [1,2,*], Thomas Bock [1,3], Heiko Pietsch [1,4,5], Ganna Aleshcheva [1], Christian Baumeier [1], Friedrich Fruhwald [6] and Felicitas Escher [1,4,5]

1 Institute of Cardiac Diagnostics and Therapy, 12203 Berlin, Germany; BockC@rki.de (T.B.); heiko.pietsch@ikdt.de (H.P.); ganna.aleshcheva@ikdt.de (G.A.); christian.baumeier@ikdt.de (C.B.); felicitas.escher@charite.de (F.E.)
2 Department of Cardiology, Campus Benjamin Franklin, Charité-Universitätsmedizin Berlin, 12200 Berlin, Germany
3 Institute of Tropical Medicine, University of Tübingen, 72074 Tübingen, Germany
4 Department of Internal Medicine and Cardiology, Campus Virchow Klinikum, Charité-Universitätsmedizin Berlin, 13353 Berlin, Germany
5 DZHK (German Centre for Cardiovascular Research), Berlin, Germany
6 Department of Cardiology, Medical University Graz, 8036 Graz, Austria; friedrich.fruhwald@medunigraz.at
* Correspondence: heinz-peter.schultheiss@ikdt.de; Tel.: +49-30-84415540

Abstract: Human parvovirus B19 (B19V) is the predominant cardiotropic virus associated with dilated inflammatory cardiomyopathy (DCMi). Transcriptionally active cardiotropic B19V infection is clinically relevant and triggers adverse long-term mortality. During the study; we evaluated whether antiviral treatment with the nucleoside analogue telbivudine (LTD) is effective in suppressing transcriptional active B19V in endomyocardial biopsies (EMBs) of B19V positive patients and improving clinical outcomes. Seventeen B19V-positive patients (13 male; mean age 45.7 ± 13.9 years; mean left ventricular ejection fraction (LVEF) 37.7 ± 13.5%) with positive B19V DNA and transcriptional activity (B19V mRNA) in EMBs were treated with 600 mg/d LTD over a period of six months. Patients underwent EMBs before and after termination of the LTD treatment. B19V RNA copy numbers remained unchanged in 3/17 patients (non-responder) and declined or disappeared completely in the remaining 14/17 patients (responder) ($p \leq 0.0001$). Notably; LVEF improvement was more significant in patients who reduced or lost B19V RNA (responder; $p = 0.02$) in contrast to non-responders ($p = 0.7$). In parallel; responder patients displayed statistically significant improvement in quality of life (QoL) questionnaires ($p = 0.03$) and dyspnea on exertion ($p = 0.0006$), reflecting an improvement in New York Heart Association (NYHA) Classification ($p = 0.001$). Our findings demonstrated for the first time that suppression of B19V transcriptional activity by LTD treatment improved hemodynamic and clinical outcome significantly. Thus; the present study substantiates the clinical relevance of detecting B19V transcriptional activity of the myocardium.

Keywords: parvovirus B19; dilated inflammatory cardiomyopathy; telbivudine

Citation: Schultheiss, H.-P.; Bock, T.; Pietsch, H.; Aleshcheva, G.; Baumeier, C.; Fruhwald, F.; Escher, F. Nucleoside Analogue Reverse Transcriptase Inhibitors Improve Clinical Outcome in Transcriptional Active Human Parvovirus B19-Positive Patients. *J. Clin. Med.* **2021**, *10*, 1928. https://doi.org/10.3390/jcm10091928

Academic Editor: Stefan Peters

Received: 16 March 2021
Accepted: 25 April 2021
Published: 29 April 2021

1. Introduction

Virus-induced inflammatory cardiomyopathy (DCMi) represents a major cause of heart failure with potential for transition to the clinical picture of dilated cardiomyopathy (DCM). Human parvovirus B19 (B19V) is the predominant cardiotropic virus found in DCM hearts and chronic myocarditis [1–6]. Whereas latent B19V infection has presumably no effect on the course of DCMi [7,8], it was shown that transcriptionally active B19V leads to an altered cardiac gene expression in EMB. Furthermore, replicative B19V in DCMi is an unfavorable prognostic trigger of adverse mortality [9].

B19V is a member of the genus Erythroparvovirus of the family *Parvoviridae* harboring a linear, single-stranded DNA-genome of 5.6 kb that codes for the non-structural protein NS1 and two structural capsid proteins, VP1 and VP2. Viral gene and protein expression are controlled by a combination of alternative splicing and internal polyadenylation [10–13]. Based on its strong erythroid tropism and related acute disease association, it has been shown that B19V is infecting erythroid endothelial progenitor cells and causes endothelial dysfunction in myocardial tissue [14–16]. Moreover, the presence of B19V remains a single independent predictor for reduced cardiac capillary density in patients with cardiomyopathy. These results demonstrate the causality between B19V infection and reduced coronary blood flow leading to endothelial dysfunction and ischemia. This is an explanation for why acute endothelial cell B19V-infection in myocarditis is associated with a cardiac microvascular impairment mimicking myocardial infarction [17–19].

To date, therapeutic options against B19V infection have not yet been established. The first beneficial effects following telbivudine (LTD) treatment in B19V-associated DCMi were described in a case report of EMB analyses of our group, owing not only to its antiviral but presumably also to its immunomodulatory properties [20]. This drug is approved for the treatment of hepatitis B virus (HBV) infection [21]. LTD is a synthetic thymidine β-L-nucleoside analogue and impairs HBV DNA replication by incorporation into the HBV DNA intermediate by the HBV polymerase, competing with the natural substrate thymidine-50-triphosphate. This finally leads to chain termination by interruption of the HBV second strand synthesis [22,23]. Additionally, LTD shows a broad range of immune modulatory effects altering the expression of cytokines, such as tumor necrosis factor -(TNF-) α and interferon- (IFN)-γ, influences NF-κB level restoring cellular immune response, and reveals a direct effect on apoptosis [24–27].

In this observation, we retrospectively analyzed whether treatment with telbivudine is effective in suppressing B19V replicative activity in the myocardium and improving clinical outcomes.

2. Materials and Methods

2.1. Patients

Patients with clinical evidence of symptomatic heart failure of unknown cause and suspected inflammatory/viral cardiomyopathy underwent EMB after invasive exclusion of coronary artery disease by left heart catheterization. Indication of EMB was based on the position statement of the *ESC Working Group on Myocardial and Pericardial Diseases* [28]. Other clinical exclusion criteria were valvular disease, obstructive or restrictive cardiomyopathy, stroke, significant hepatic, renal, pulmonary, or endocrine disease, pregnancy or lactation, antiviral, immunomodulatory, or immunosuppressive therapy within six months prior to enrolment.

Patients complained of cardiac discomfort (e.g., angina pectoris at rest), atypical fatigue, and symptomatic heart failure (reduced physical capacity, dyspnea on exertion) for more than 3 months before first presentation in the clinics.

EMBs were analyzed using histology, immunohistology, and molecular virology. The inclusion criterion for this study was B19V positivity with transcriptional virus activity (viral mRNA) in EMBs. Exclusion criteria were active myocarditis in accordance with the Dallas classification [29], inflammatory cardiomyopathy without viral genomes, or other cardiotropic virus infections in EMB (Figure 1).

Seventeen patients (13 male; mean age 45.7 ± 13.9 years) with different baseline left ventricular ejection fraction (LVEF) (mean LVEF 37.7 ± 13.5; range [26.5–51.0]%), fitting the criteria of this study with positive B19V DNA and replicative intermediates (positive B19V mRNA) in EMBs, were included (Figure 1). The present study retrospectively investigates data from a prospective observational cohort from 1 single center, which neither includes randomization or matching of patients nor does it comprise a control group.

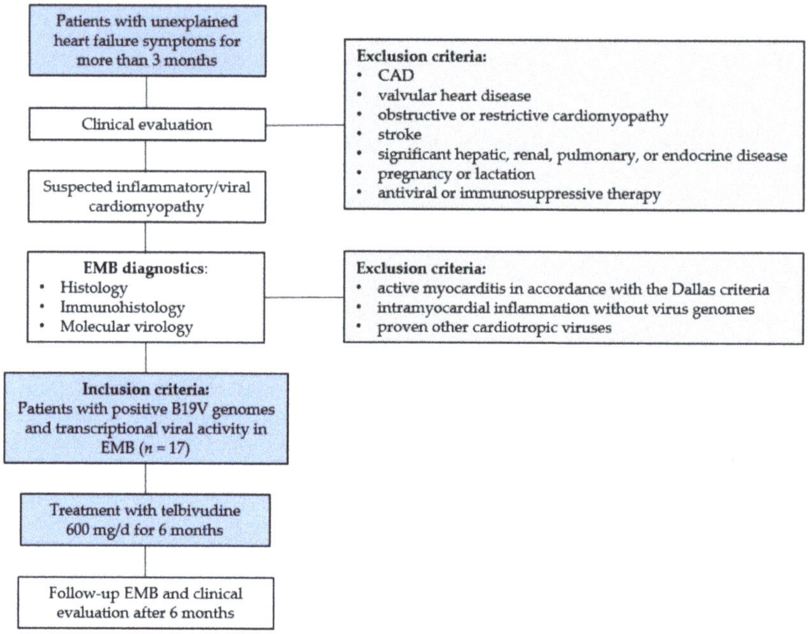

Figure 1. Study treatment scheme of patients with B19V transcriptional activity in EMB. B19V = parvovirus B19; CAD = coronary artery disease; EMB = endomyocardial biopsy.

Patients were treated with 600 mg/d LTD over a period of six months. Patients underwent EMBs before (pre/baseline) and immediately after termination (post/follow-up) of the LTD treatment. The clinical status of each patient was re-evaluated at follow-up after six months. A determination of LVEF was performed by echocardiography. Patients were examined with 2-dimensional echocardiography using the Philips iE33 ultrasound system (Philips Healthcare, Germany). LVEF measurements were performed with the Simpson method.

Initially, health insurance companies were informed from the clinicians and gave consent in "off-label" use reimbursement.

The analysis was performed within the CRC Transregio 19 (NCT02970227), which was approved by the local ethics committees of the participating clinical centers as well as by the committees of the respective federal states. Informed written consent was obtained from all patients.

2.2. Analysis of EMB

2.2.1. Genomic DNA Isolation from EMBs

EMBs were analyzed in the CAP-accredited laboratory Institute for Cardiac Diagnostic and Therapy Berlin, Germany (IKDT) by molecular workup: Genomic DNA from RNAlater (Thermo Fisher Scientific, Waltham, MA, USA) fixed EMBs were extracted by Gentra Puregene Mousetail Kit (Qiagen, Hilden, Germany). After isolation, the amount of DNA was quantified by Quantifiler™ Human DNA TaqMan assay (Thermo Fisher Scientific, Waltham, MA, USA), in order to calculate and standardize viral load in small EMBs (viral genomes per µg of isolated human genomic DNA) [30].

2.2.2. Detection of Viral Genomes in EMBs by Nested-PCR and Sequencing

Nested polymerase chain reaction (nested-PCR) and reverse transcriptase (RT)-PCR for qualitative detection of B19V, enteroviruses (including coxsackieviruses and echoviruses), adenoviruses, Epstein–Barr virus, and human herpesvirus 6 genome sequences in nucleic acids were extracted from EMB, performed as described previously [30].

The specificity of PCR products was confirmed by DNA sequencing and sequences were matched to the NCBI GenBank. DNA sequence analysis for quality control and genotype/species determination of generated nested-PCR amplicons was performed by PCR using corresponding primer pairs matching the amplified virus fragment.

2.2.3. Measurement of Viral DNA Load by Quantitative Real-Time PCR (TaqMan qPCR)

Subsequently, calculation of viral DNA load was performed by the ratio of viral genome copy number in TaqMan assay to the amount of isolated total human DNA measured by Quantifiler™ Human DNA TaqMan assay (Thermo Fisher Scientific, Waltham, MA, USA) [9].

2.2.4. RNA Isolation, Reverse Transcription (RT), and TaqMan qPCR for Measurement of Viral Transcripts

Total RNA was isolated from endomyocardial biopsies using TRIzol reagent (Thermo Fisher Scientific, Waltham, MA, USA), treated with DNAse (PeqLab, Erlangen, Germany) to remove any traces of DNA and reverse-transcribed to cDNA with the High-Capacity cDNA Reverse Transcription Kit (Applied Biosystems, Darmstadt, Germany) using random hexamers.

The amount of viral transcripts in cDNA was determined by real-time PCR using TaqMan Universal PCR master mix (Thermo Fisher Scientific, Waltham, MA, USA) in relation to housekeeping-gene HPRT (viral transcripts per μg of isolated human genomic RNA) (Applied Biosystems, Darmstadt, Germany) as described previously [31].

2.2.5. Histological and Immunohistochemical Staining for Assessment of Inflammation

Histology was developed by hematoxylin eosin staining in light microscopy. Myocardial inflammation was diagnosed by $CD3^+$ T-lymphocytes/mm^2 (Dako, Glostrup, Denmark), $CD11a^+$/$LFA\text{-}1^+$ lymphocytes/mm^2 (Immuno Tools, Friesoythe, Germany), $CD11b^+$/$Mac\text{-}1^+$ macrophages/mm^2 (ImmunoTools, Friesoythe, Germany), and $CD45R0^+$ T memory cells/mm^2 (Dako, Glostrup, Denmark). Stainings were quantified by digital image analysis as described previously [32]. Intramyocardial inflammation was assigned by >14 leucocytes [28]. Furthermore, we analyzed macrophages (threshold > 40.0 $CD11b^+$/$Mac\text{-}1^+$ macrophages/mm^2) and $CD45R0^+$ T Memory cells (threshold > 40 cells/mm^2).

2.3. *Statistics*

Qualitative data were compared using the Fisher's exact or $\chi 2$ test. Shapiro–Wilk normality tests were used to test for normal distribution of data. When data showed normal distribution, a two-tailed parametric paired *t*-test was used to analyze continuous variables; otherwise, Wilcoxon matched-pairs signed rank test was applied. Results for quantitative features are given as mean ± SD or median values. *p*-values below 0.05 were considered to indicate statistical significance. All statistical analyses were performed using the SPSS software version 23.0 (IBM Corp., Armonk, NY, USA) and GraphPad Prism 7.04 software (GraphPad Software Inc., La Jolla, CA, USA).

3. Results

Patients included in this analysis were in clinically stable condition with an impaired systolic mean LVEF of 37.7 ± 13.5 [range 26.5–51.0]% (Table 1). There was a history of infection preceding onset of symptoms < 12 weeks in 70.1% of patients (Table 1). Complaints included mostly dyspnea on exertion (88.2%), reflected in New York Heart Association (NYHA) class II/III (Table 1). Clinical data of the total patient cohort at baseline are summarized in Table 1.

Table 1. Baseline characteristics of patients.

Patient Characteristics	
Men, n (%)	13 (65)
Age, years, mean ± SD	45.7 ± 13.9
History, weeks ± SD	18.9 ± 11.4
LVEF, % ± SD; [range 25–75]	37.7 ± 13.5 [26.5–51.0]
Systolic blood pressure, mmHg ± SD	102 ± 27
Diastolic blood pressure, mmHg ± SD	69 ± 8
Infection preceding onset of symptoms < 12 weeks, %	70.7
Complaints at Baseline Biopsy	
MLHFQ total score, mean ± SD	68.1 ± 17.7
6MWD, m, mean ± SD	468.8 ± 73.3
Dyspnea on exertion, n (%)	15 (88.2)
NYHA class I/II/III/IV, %	0/47.0/47.0/5.9
Heart Failure Medication	
ACE inhibitors/Angiotensin receptor blockers, n (%)	17 (100)
Beta-blockers, n (%)	15 (88.2)
Aldosterone-antagonists, n (%)	13 (76.4)
Diuretics, n (%)	16 (94.1)

LVEF = left ventricular ejection fraction; MLHFQ = Minnesota Living with Heart Failure Questionnaire. The total score ranges from 0 to 105, with higher scores indicating worse health status; 6MWD = Six-Minute Walk Distance; NYHA class = New York Heart Association class. The data are presented as mean values ± standard deviation, as %, as range [25–75 percentile], or as number of subjects.

Patients with active myocarditis in accordance with the Dallas criteria or viral co-infections in EMB were excluded.

LTD treatment was started immediately after evaluation of baseline EMB. Interruptions in study medication were not reported.

3.1. EMB Analyses at Baseline and Follow-Up

At baseline, EMBs of all patients tested positive for presence of B19V DNA and viral replicative intermediates (B19V mRNA).

B19V RNA transcript numbers remained unchanged or increased in 3/17 patients (17.6% non-responder) and declined or disappeared completely in the remaining 14/17 patients (82.4%, responder) (mean viral RNA transcript numbers declined after treatment at follow-up in the responder group from 1168 ± 2142 to 3.0 ± 11.2 transcripts/μgRNA, $p \leq 0.0001$ (Figure 2)). In addition, a significant reduction of viral DNA load was observed for the responders (from 1514 ± 2383 to 539 ± 1033 copies/μg DNA; $p = 0.035$) in contrast to non-responders (from 561 ± 499 to 1768 ± 2878 copies/μg DNA; $p = 0.478$) pre- and post-treatment.

LVEF improvement was statistically significant in patients who reduced or resolved the replicative viral intermediates (LVEF from 39.6 ± 12.4 [range 27.7–52.5] %, to 52.9 ± 15.7 [range 38.7–65.0] %, (responder, $p = 0.02$)) (Figure 3). No significant improvement of LVEF was observed in the non-responder group from 29 ± 18.2 [range 19.0–48.0] % to 35 ± 21.2% [range 23.0–50.0] %, ($p = 0.7$) (Figure 3).

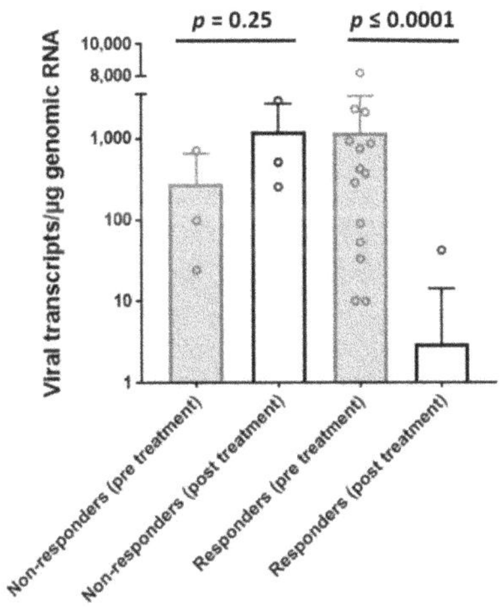

Figure 2. Number of viral RNA transcripts of non-responders and responders pre- and post-treatment. Bar height indicates the mean value ± SD expression rate of viral transcripts/µg RNA in non-responders' (n = 3) and responders' group (n = 14) pre (baseline) and post (follow-up) LTD-treatment. Dots indicate individual values. Whereas responders significantly reduce viral replication intermediates upon treatment, non-responders show a non-significant increase of viral RNA. Viral transcripts are given as mean value and error bars represent SD.

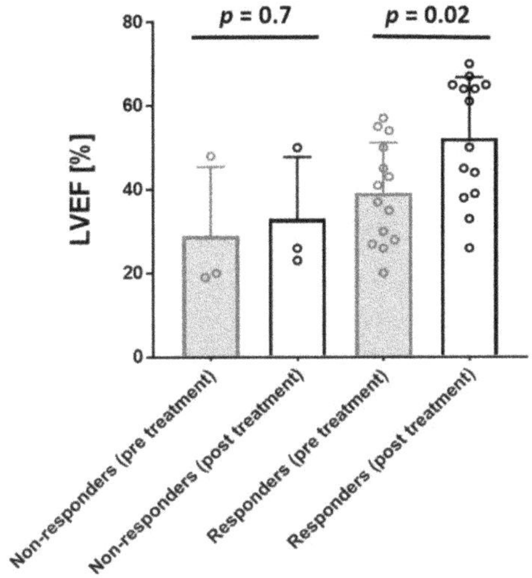

Figure 3. LVEF of non-responders and responders pre- and post-treatment. Bar height indicates LVEF (%) in non-responders' (n = 3) and responders' (n = 14) group pre (baseline) and post (follow-up) LTD-treatment. Dots indicate individual values. LVEF improvement was significantly improved in patients who reduced or lost the replicative viral intermediates (positive B19V RNA). LVEF is given as mean value and error bars represent SD.

Six-Minute Walk Distance (6MWD) results and quality of live (QOL) score by the Minnesota Living with Heart Failure Questionnaire (MLHFQ) before and after the treatment were assessed. Patients showed a statistically significant improvement in maximal 6MWD in responders (465.9 ± 82.8 vs. 559.8 ± 71.7 m, p = 0.04) and QOL total score (66.6 ± 17.7 vs. 43.2 ± 23.9; p = 0.03) after treatment (Table 2). In addition, a significant reduction of dyspnea on exertion (p = 0.0006), reflecting an improvement and New York

Heart Association (NYHA) Classification ($p = 0.001$), was noticed (Table 2). No significant improvements in clinical symptoms were observed in non-responders (Table 2).

Table 2. Course of clinical symptoms at baseline and at follow-up upon treatment in responders.

	Baseline	Follow-Up	*p*-Value
LVEF, % ± SD, [range 25–75]	39.6 ± 12.4 [27.7–52.5]	52.9 ± 15.7 [38.7–65.0]	$p = 0.02$
MLHFQ total score, mean ± SD	66.6 ± 16.4	43.2 ± 23.9	$p = 0.03$
6MWD, m, mean ± SD	465.9 ± 82.8	559.8 ± 71.7	$p = 0.04$
Dyspnea on exertion, n (%)	12 (85.7)	4 (28.5)	$p = 0.0006$
NYHA class I/II/III/IV, %	0/57.1/35.7/7.1	35.7/64.2/0/0	$p = 0.001$

LVEF = left ventricular ejection fraction; MLHFQ = Minnesota Living with Heart Failure Questionnaire. The total score ranges from 0–105, with higher scores indicating worse health status; 6MWD = Six-Minute Walk Distance; NYHA class = New York Heart Association class. The data are presented as mean values ± standard deviation, as %, as range [25–75 percentile], or as number of subjects.

The number of inflammatory cells ($CD3^+$ T-lymphocytes, $CD11a^+$/LFA-1^+ lymphocytes, $CD11b^+$/Mac-1^+ macrophages, $CD45R0^+$ T memory cells) was low at baseline EMB and did not change significantly upon LTD treatment, with no difference between responder and non-responder group (Table 3).

Table 3. Immunohistological biopsy findings at baseline and upon treatment at follow-up in responders.

	Baseline	Follow-Up	*p*-Value
$CD3^+$ cells/mm^2	8.7 ± 7.7	4.7 ± 4.0	0.1
LFA-1^+ cells/mm^2	15.9 ± 11.6	10.9 ± 8.3	0.09
$CD45R0^+$ cells/mm^2	23.5 ± 15.0	20.5 ± 17.5	0.4
MAC-1^+ cells/mm^2	42.9 ± 41.5	28.7 ± 17.9	0.3

CD3 = T cells; CD45R0 = T memory cells; LFA-1 = Lymphocyte function-associated antigen 1; MAC-1 = Macrophage-1 antigen. The data are presented as mean values ± SD.

3.2. LTD Side Effects

LTD antiviral treatment was well tolerated, and the majority of patients reported no drug-associated side effects. One male patient experienced an asymptomatic sudden increase of creatine kinase from <150 U/L to 3449 U/L at the time of the follow-up. This elevated creatine kinase level normalized within 5 days after immediate cessation of the treatment and remained at a normal level throughout the following 12 months.

4. Discussion

In this analysis, we demonstrated the beneficial effects from treatment with the antiviral drug LTD on hemodynamic and clinical outcomes in patients with transcriptionally active cardiotropic B19V in EMB.

B19V infection of the heart muscle and its association with DCMi is still a matter of discussion. Previous reports have shown that B19V is the predominant virus detected in EMBs of patients with suspected myocarditis and DCMi [28,33–35]. There is broad approval that latent B19V infection has no effect on the course of DCMi [7,8]. However, we could show previously that patients characterized by transcriptionally active cardiotropic B19V with detectable replication intermediates (viral mRNA) demonstrated an altered cardiac gene expression pattern. Furthermore, transcriptionally active B19V in DCMi is an unfavorable prognostic trigger of adverse mortality [9,36].

Recently, we demonstrated that endothelial dysfunction and clinical symptoms improved during antiviral treatment with interferon-β (IFN-β), whereas B19V viral DNA load was barely affected [37,38]. The underlying mechanisms of how IFN-β exerts such beneficial clinical effects without substantially clearing the virus are unknown. However, cell culture analyses using infected immortalized human microvascular endothelial cells (EC) have shown that IFN-β inhibits B19V reactivation and improves endothelial cell viability [38].

The first experimental data have provided evidence that antiviral nucleoside analogue reverse transcriptase inhibitors, such as LTD, may improve the viability of B19V infected endothelial cells in addition to their effectiveness in retroviral and para-retroviral (hepatitis B viruses) infections [39–41] and reduce apoptosis [20]. An advantage of the thymidine β-L-nucleoside analogue LTD is a significantly lower frequency of drug-specific side effects in comparison to IFN-β. The antiviral efficacy of LTD on non-hepatic infection is, however, less well documented [42–44].

Although this antiviral nucleoside analogue reverse transcriptase inhibitor is especially effective against retroviral and para-retroviral infections, it has some pleiotropic immunomodulatory/anti-inflammatory and interesting antiviral properties that might interfere with the unique replication mode of B19V. Since LTD modulates the innate and adaptive immune system through IFN-like functions in addition to its antiviral potential [45–47], we analyzed whether this drug may have an impact on the clinical outcome of patients with active B19V infection and persisting symptomatic heart failure during this present study, independently of baseline LVEF (Figure 1).

We could show that LTD treatment resulted in a significant amelioration of LVEF. B19V RNA transcript numbers remained unchanged in 3 of 17 patients (non-responder) and declined or disappeared completely in the remaining 14 of 17 patients (responder) (Figure 2). LVEF improvement was statistically significant in patients who reduced or lost B19V RNA (responder, $p = 0.02$) in contrast to non-responders (Figure 3). Although B19V DNA genomes in the myocardium alone are not of significant clinical relevance [7,8,34], we also observed a significant reduction of viral DNA in the responders group in contrast to non-responders.

In parallel, LTD treatment resulted in a significant amelioration of LVEF and a significant reduction of dyspnea on exertion, reflected in an improvement of NYHA class (Table 2).

The mode of action of the antiviral treatment of B19V with LTD is speculative. Clinical improvement may be associated with consecutive improvements of myocardial function or as a result of regeneration of B19V-associated endothelial dysfunction [38]. In addition, LTD shows pleiotropic immunomodulatory/anti-inflammatory and anti-viral properties that are hypothesized to interfere with the unique replication mode of B19V [48]. Since the number of inflammatory cells was low at baseline EMB, we were not able to investigate any anti-inflammatory effects upon evaluation of follow-up EMB. B19V uses the cellular DNA replication machinery for viral DNA replication by a rolling circle mechanism and induces DNA damage response and cell cycle arrest at late S phase, which facilitates viral DNA replication. DNA replication polymerase δ and polymerase α are responsible for B19V DNA replication [49]. Here, a nucleoside analogue can hypothetically interfere with the production of the obligatory dimer duplex replicative intermediate of B19V resembling second-strand synthesis of HBV DNA intermediates [50]; however, this hypothesis has to be proven in future experiments.

In a previous study by Hazebroek et al., intravenous immunoglobulin therapy does not significantly improve LVEF or functional capacity in patients with cardiac B19V persistence. However, inclusion criteria were solely based on B19 viral DNA load [51]. These results underline the importance of diagnostic differentiation of endomyocardial B19V infections (including viral replication) as a key approach for a more meaningful selection of candidates for future innovative anti-viral immunomodulatory treatment strategies.

5. Conclusions

In conclusion, the present study demonstrates the benefit of nucleoside-analogue treatment with respect to control of B19V replication and virus transcript reduction as well as the rapid improvement of symptoms of patients with active B19V infection. To further explore the direct and important clinical impact of our findings, a large randomized, placebo-controlled clinical study should evaluate the results and will be able to gain more insights into effective B19V treatment conditions.

6. Study Limitations

There are several limitations which have to be considered when interpreting the obtained results. The cohort was only adjusted to consecutive B19V-positive symptomatic patients with detectable replicative intermediates of B19V confirmed by measurement of B19V RNA transcripts. Findings do not include randomization or matching of patients nor evaluation of a placebo control. This is a retrospective analysis of data from a prospective observational cohort and, as such, a possible effect of selection bias cannot be denied.

Author Contributions: Conceptualization, H.-P.S.; methodology, H.-P.S., G.A., H.P., F.F. and F.E.; investigation, H.-P.S.; data curation, H.P., G.A. and F.E.; writing—original draft preparation, F.E., T.B., G.A., H.P. and C.B.; writing—review and editing, H.-P.S., T.B., G.A., H.P., C.B., F.F. and F.E.; visualization, H.P. and F.E.; supervision, H.-P.S., T.B. and F.E.; project administration, H.-P.S.; funding acquisition, H.-P.S. All authors have read and agreed to the published version of the manuscript.

Funding: This study was supported by the Deutsche Forschungsgesellschaft (DFG; CRC TR-19).

Institutional Review Board Statement: The study was conducted according to the guidelines of the Declaration of Helsinki, and performed within the CRC Transregio 19 (NCT02970227), which was approved by the local ethics committees of the participating clinical centers as well as by the committees of the respective federal states.

Informed Consent Statement: Informed consent was obtained from all subjects involved in the study.

Data Availability Statement: The data presented in this study are available on request from the corresponding author.

Acknowledgments: For their excellent technical assistance, we thank K. Winter, S. Ochmann, J. Klostermann, C. Liebig, and K. Errami, IKDT Berlin, Germany.

Conflicts of Interest: The authors declare no conflict of interest.

Abbreviations

B19V = parvovirus B19; CAD—coronary artery disease; DCM = dilated cardiomyopathy; CD3 = T cells; CD45R0 = T memory cells; DCMi = inflammatory dilated cardiomyopathy; DNA = deoxyribonucleic acid; EMB = endomyocardial biopsy; GE = genome equivalents; HBV = hepatitis B virus; HPRT = hypoxanthine phosphoribosyltransferase 1; IFN = interferon; LFA-1 = Lymphocyte function-associated antigen 1; LTD = telbivudine; MAC-1 = Macrophage-1 antigen; NYHA classification = New York Heart Association classification; QoL = quality of life; PCR = polymerase chain reaction; RT-PCR = reverse transcription PCR; TNF-α = Tumor necrosis factor-α.

References

1. Bock, C.-T.; Klingel, K.; Aberle, S.; Duechting, A.; Lupescu, A.; Lang, F.; Kandolf, R.; Bock, T. Human Parvovirus B19: A New Emerging Pathogen of Inflammatory Cardiomyopathy. *J. Veter-Med. Ser. B* **2005**, *52*, 340–343. [CrossRef] [PubMed]
2. Kühl, U.; Pauschinger, M.; Noutsias, M.; Seeberg, B.; Bock, T.; Lassner, D.; Poller, W.; Kandolf, R.; Schultheiss, H.-P. High Prevalence of Viral Genomes and Multiple Viral Infections in the Myocardium of Adults with "Idiopathic" Left Ventricular Dysfunction. *Circulation* **2005**, *111*, 887–893. [CrossRef] [PubMed]
3. Adamson-Small, L.A.; Ignatovich, I.V.; Laemmerhirt, M.G.; Hobbs, J.A. Persistent parvovirus B19 infection in non-erythroid tissues: Possible role in the inflammatory and disease process. *Virus Res.* **2014**, *190*, 8–16. [CrossRef] [PubMed]
4. Verdonschot, J.; Hazebroek, M.; Merken, J.; Debing, Y.; Dennert, R.; Rocca, H.-P.B.-L.; Heymans, S. Relevance of cardiac parvovirus B19 in myocarditis and dilated cardiomyopathy: Review of the literature. *Eur. J. Heart Fail.* **2016**, *18*, 1430–1441. [CrossRef]
5. Schultheiss, H.-P.; Fairweather, D.; Caforio, A.L.P.; Escher, F.; Hershberger, R.E.; Lipshultz, S.E.; Liu, P.P.; Matsumori, A.; Mazzanti, A.; McMurray, J.; et al. Dilated cardiomyopathy. *Nat. Rev. Dis. Prim.* **2019**, *5*, 32. [CrossRef]
6. Schultheiss, H.-P.; Kühl, U.; Cooper, L.T. The management of myocarditis. *Eur. Heart J.* **2011**, *32*, 2616–2625. [CrossRef] [PubMed]
7. Hjalmarsson, C.; Liljeqvist, J.-Å.; Lindh, M.; Karason, K.; Bollano, E.; Oldfors, A.; Andersson, B. Parvovirus B19 in Endomyocardial Biopsy of Patients With Idiopathic Dilated Cardiomyopathy: Foe or Bystander? *J. Card. Fail.* **2019**, *25*, 60–63. [CrossRef]
8. Verdonschot, J.A.; Cooper, L.T.; Heymans, S.R. Parvovirus B19 in Dilated Cardiomyopathy: There Is More Than Meets the Eye. *J. Card. Fail.* **2019**, *25*, 64–66. [CrossRef]

9. Kuhl, U.; Lassner, D.; Dorner, A.; Rohde, M.; Escher, F.; Seeberg, B.; Hertel, E.; Tschope, C.; Skurk, C.; Gross, U.M.; et al. A distinct subgroup of cardiomyopathy patients characterized by transcriptionally active cardiotropic erythrovirus and altered cardiac gene expression. *Basic Res. Cardiol.* **2013**, *108*, 1–10. [CrossRef]
10. Wan, Z.; Zhi, N.; Wong, S.; Keyvanfar, K.; Liu, D.; Raghavachari, N.; Munson, P.J.; Su, S.; Malide, D.; Kajigaya, S.; et al. Human parvovirus B19 causes cell cycle arrest of human erythroid progenitors via deregulation of the E2F family of transcription factors. *J. Clin. Investig.* **2010**, *120*, 3530–3544. [CrossRef]
11. Heegaard, E.D.; Brown, K.E.; Ablashi, D.V.; Chatlynne, L.G.; Whitman, J.J.E.; Cesarman, E. Human Parvovirus B19. *Clin. Microbiol. Rev.* **2002**, *15*, 439–464. [CrossRef]
12. Xu, P.; Zhou, Z.; Xiong, M.; Zou, W.; Deng, X.; Ganaie, S.S.; Kleiboeker, S.; Peng, J.; Liu, K.; Wang, S.; et al. Parvovirus B19 NS1 protein induces cell cycle arrest at G2-phase by activating the ATR-CDC25C-CDK1 pathway. *PLoS Pathog.* **2017**, *13*, e1006266. [CrossRef]
13. Rogo, L.D.; Mokhtari-Azad, T.; Kabir, M.H.; Rezaei, F. Human parvovirus B19: A review. *Acta Virol.* **2014**, *58*, 199–213. [CrossRef]
14. Schmidt-Lucke, C.; Zobel, T.; Escher, F.; Tschöpe, C.; Lassner, D.; Kühl, U.; Gubbe, K.; Volk, H.-D.; Schultheiss, H.-P. Human Parvovirus B19 (B19V) Up-regulates CXCR4 Surface Expression of Circulating Angiogenic Cells: Implications for Cardiac Ischemia in B19V Cardiomyopathy. *J. Infect. Dis.* **2017**, *217*, 456–465. [CrossRef]
15. Schmidt-Lucke, C.; Zobel, T.; Schrepfer, S.; Kuhl, U.; Wang, D.; Klingel, K.; Becher, P.M.; Fechner, H.; Pozzuto, T.; Van Linthout, S.; et al. Impaired Endothelial Regeneration Through Human Parvovirus B19–Infected Circulating Angiogenic Cells in Patients With Cardiomyopathy. *J. Infect. Dis.* **2015**, *212*, 1070–1081. [CrossRef] [PubMed]
16. Brown, K.; Anderson, S.M.; Young, N.S. Erythrocyte P antigen: Cellular receptor for B19 parvovirus. *Science* **1993**, *262*, 114–117. [CrossRef] [PubMed]
17. Bültmann, B.D.; Sotlar, K.; Klingel, K. Parvovirus B19. *N. Engl. J. Med.* **2004**, *350*, 2006–2007. [CrossRef]
18. Kühl, U.; Pauschinger, M.; Bock, T.; Klingel, K.; Schwimmbeck, C.P.L.; Seeberg, B.; Krautwurm, L.; Poller, W.; Schultheiss, H.-P.; Kandolf, R. Parvovirus B19 Infection Mimicking Acute Myocardial Infarction. *Circulation* **2003**, *108*, 945–950. [CrossRef] [PubMed]
19. Bültmann, B.D.; Klingel, K.; Sotlar, K.; Bock, C.; Baba, H.A.; Sauter, M.; Kandolf, R. Fatal parvovirus B19–associated myocarditis clinically mimicking ischemic heart disease: An endothelial cell–mediated disease. *Hum. Pathol.* **2003**, *34*, 92–95. [CrossRef] [PubMed]
20. Van Linthout, S.; Elsanhoury, A.; Klein, O.; Sosnowski, M.; Miteva, K.; Lassner, D.; Abou-El-Enein, M.; Pieske, B.; Kühl, U.; Tschöpe, C. Telbivudine in chronic lymphocytic myocarditis and human parvovirus B19 transcriptional activity. *ESC Heart Fail.* **2018**, *5*, 818–829. [CrossRef]
21. Lai, C.-L.; Gane, E.; Liaw, Y.-F.; Hsu, C.-W.; Thongsawat, S.; Wang, Y.; Chen, Y.; Heathcote, E.J.; Rasenack, J.; Bzowej, N.; et al. Telbivudine versus Lamivudine in Patients with Chronic Hepatitis B. *N. Engl. J. Med.* **2007**, *357*, 2576–2588. [CrossRef] [PubMed]
22. Keam, S.J. Telbivudine. *Drugs* **2007**, *67*, 1917–1929. [CrossRef] [PubMed]
23. Han, S.-H.B. Telbivudine: A new nucleoside analogue for the treatment of chronic hepatitis B. *Expert Opin. Investig. Drugs* **2005**, *14*, 511–519. [CrossRef]
24. Chen, Y.; Li, X.; Ye, B.; Yang, X.; Wu, W.; Chen, B.; Pan, X.; Cao, H.; Li, L. Effect of telbivudine therapy on the cellular immune response in chronic hepatitis B. *Antivir. Res.* **2011**, *91*, 23–31. [CrossRef] [PubMed]
25. Li, J.; Jia, M.; Liu, Y.; She, W.; Li, L.; Wang, J.; Jiang, W. Telbivudine therapy may shape CD4+ T-cell response to prevent liver fibrosis in patients with chronic hepatitis B. *Liver Int.* **2015**, *35*, 834–845. [CrossRef] [PubMed]
26. Wu, Q.; Huang, H.; Sun, X.; Pan, M.; He, Y.; Tan, S.; Zeng, Y.; Li, L.; Deng, G.; Yan, Z.; et al. Telbivudine Prevents Vertical Transmission of Hepatitis B Virus From Women With High Viral Loads: A Prospective Long-Term Study. *Clin. Gastroenterol. Hepatol.* **2015**, *13*, 1170–1176. [CrossRef]
27. Zobel, T.; Bock, C.-T.; Kühl, U.; Rohde, M.; Lassner, D.; Schultheiss, H.-P.; Schmidt-Lucke, C. Telbivudine Reduces Parvovirus B19-Induced Apoptosis in Circulating Angiogenic Cells. *Viruses* **2019**, *11*, 227. [CrossRef]
28. Aretz, H.T. Myocarditis: The Dallas criteria. *Hum. Pathol.* **1987**, *18*, 619–624. [CrossRef]
29. Kühl, U.; Lassner, D.; Pauschinger, M.; Gross, U.; Seeberg, B.; Noutsias, M.; Poller, W.; Schultheiss, H.-P. Prevalence of erythrovirus genotypes in the myocardium of patients with dilated cardiomyopathy. *J. Med. Virol.* **2008**, *80*, 1243–1251. [CrossRef]
30. Pietsch, H.; Escher, F.; Aleshcheva, G.; Lassner, D.; Bock, C.-T.; Schultheiss, H.-P. Detection of parvovirus mRNAs as markers for viral activity in endomyocardial biopsy-based diagnosis of patients with unexplained heart failure. *Sci. Rep.* **2020**, *10*, 1–9. [CrossRef]
31. Escher, F.; Kühl, U.; Lassner, D.; Poller, W.; Westermann, D.; Pieske, B.; Tschöpe, C.; Schultheiss, H.-P. Long-term outcome of patients with virus-negative chronic myocarditis or inflammatory cardiomyopathy after immunosuppressive therapy. *Clin. Res. Cardiol.* **2016**, *105*, 1011–1020. [CrossRef]
32. Caforio, A.L.P.; Pankuweit, S.; Arbustini, E.; Basso, C.; Gimeno-Blanes, J.; Felix, S.B.; Fu, M.; Heliö, T.; Heymans, S.; Jahns, R.; et al. Current state of knowledge on aetiology, diagnosis, management, and therapy of myocarditis: A position statement of the European Society of Cardiology Working Group on Myocardial and Pericardial Diseases. *Eur. Heart J.* **2013**, *34*, 2636–2648. [CrossRef]
33. Bock, C.-T. Parvovirus B19: A New Emerging Pathogenic Agent of Inflammatory Cardiomyopathy. *Chronic Viral Inflamm. Cardiomyopathy* **2006**, 83–97. [CrossRef]

34. Bock, C.-T.; Klingel, K.; Kandolf, R. Human Parvovirus B19–Associated Myocarditis. *N. Engl. J. Med.* **2010**, *362*, 1248–1249. [CrossRef] [PubMed]
35. Mahrholdt, H.; Wagner, A.; Deluigi, C.C.; Kispert, E.; Hager, S.; Meinhardt, G.; Vogelsberg, H.; Fritz, P.; Dippon, J.; Bock, C.-T.; et al. Presentation, Patterns of Myocardial Damage, and Clinical Course of Viral Myocarditis. *Circulation* **2006**, *114*, 1581–1590. [CrossRef] [PubMed]
36. Kühl, U.; Rohde, M.; Lassner, D.; Gross, U.; Escher, F.; Schultheiss, H.-P. miRNA as activity markers in Parvo B19 associated heart disease. *Herz* **2012**, *37*, 637–643. [CrossRef] [PubMed]
37. Schultheiss, H.-P.; Piper, C.; Sowade, O.; Waagstein, F.; Kapp, J.-F.; Wegscheider, K.; Groetzbach, G.; Pauschinger, M.; Escher, F.; Arbustini, E.; et al. Betaferon in chronic viral cardiomyopathy (BICC) trial: Effects of interferon-β treatment in patients with chronic viral cardiomyopathy. *Clin. Res. Cardiol.* **2016**, *105*, 763–773. [CrossRef] [PubMed]
38. Schmidt-Lucke, C.; Spillmann, F.; Bock, T.; Kühl, U.; Van Linthout, S.; Schultheiss, H.; Tschöpe, C. Interferon Beta Modulates Endothelial Damage in Patients with Cardiac Persistence of Human Parvovirus B19 Infection. *J. Infect. Dis.* **2010**, *201*, 936–945. [CrossRef]
39. Bonvicini, F.; Bua, G.; Manaresi, E.; Gallinella, G. Enhanced inhibition of parvovirus B19 replication by cidofovir in extendedly exposed erythroid progenitor cells. *Virus Res.* **2016**, *220*, 47–51. [CrossRef]
40. Ganaie, S.S.; Qiu, J. Recent Advances in Replication and Infection of Human Parvovirus B19. *Front. Cell. Infect. Microbiol.* **2018**, *8*, 166. [CrossRef]
41. Luo, Y.; Qiu, J. Human parvovirus B19: A mechanistic overview of infection and DNA replication. *Futur. Virol.* **2015**, *10*, 155–167. [CrossRef] [PubMed]
42. Gish, R.G. Improving outcomes for patients with chronic hepatitis B. *Hepatol. Res.* **2007**, *37*, S67–S78. [CrossRef] [PubMed]
43. Wang, Y.; Thongsawat, S.; Gane, E.J.; Liaw, Y.; Jia, J.; Hou, J.; Chan, H.L.Y.; Papatheodoridis, G.; Wan, M.; Niu, J.; et al. Efficacy and safety of continuous 4-year telbivudine treatment in patients with chronic hepatitis B. *J. Viral Hepat.* **2012**, *20*, e37–e46. [CrossRef] [PubMed]
44. Gao, Y.Q. Role of natural killer cells (NK) and toll-like receptor 9 (TLR9) in early responder to telbuvidine for chronic hepatitis B patients. *Hepatol. Int.* **2012**, *6*, 61.
45. Ma, L.; Cai, Y.-J.; Yu, L.; Feng, J.-Y.; Wang, J.; Li, C.; Niu, J.-Q.; Jiang, Y.-F. Treatment with Telbivudine Positively Regulates Antiviral Immune Profiles in Chinese Patients with Chronic Hepatitis B. *Antimicrob. Agents Chemother.* **2013**, *57*, 1304–1311. [CrossRef]
46. Pan, X.; Yao, W.; Fu, J.; Liu, M.; Li, L.; Gao, X. Telbivudine improves the function of myeloid dendritic cells in patients with chronic hepatitis B. *Acta Virol.* **2012**, *56*, 31–38. [CrossRef]
47. Tzang, B.-S.; Chiu, C.-C.; Tsai, C.-C.; Lee, Y.-J.; Lu, I.-J.; Shi, J.-Y.; Hsu, T.-C. Effects of human parvovirus B19 VP1 unique region protein on macrophage responses. *J. Biomed. Sci.* **2009**, *16*, 13. [CrossRef]
48. Meng, N.; Gao, X.; Yan, W.; Wang, M.; Liu, P.; Lu, X.-D.; Zhang, S.-J.; Lu, Y.-Q.; Tang, W.-X. Efficacy of telbivudine in the treatment of chronic hepatitis b and liver cirrhosis and its effect on immunological responses. *Acta Acad. Med.* **2015**, *35*, 230–234. [CrossRef]
49. Zou, W.; Wang, Z.; Xiong, M.; Chen, A.Y.; Xu, P.; Ganaie, S.S.; Badawi, Y.; Kleiboeker, S.; Nishimune, H.; Ye, S.Q.; et al. Human Parvovirus B19 Utilizes Cellular DNA Replication Machinery for Viral DNA Replication. *J. Virol.* **2017**, *92*. [CrossRef]
50. Cotmore, S.F.; Tattersall, P. Parvovirus DNA Replication. *Cold Spring Harb. Monogr. Arch.* **1996**, 799–813.
51. Hazebroek, M.R.; Henkens, M.T.; Raafs, A.G.; Verdonschot, J.A.; Merken, J.J.; Dennert, R.M.; Eurlings, C.; Hamid, M.A.A.; Wolffs, P.F.; Winkens, B.; et al. Intravenous immunoglobulin therapy in adult patients with idiopathic chronic cardiomyopathy and cardiac parvovirus B19 persistence: A prospective, double-blind, randomized, placebo-controlled clinical trial. *Eur. J. Heart Fail.* **2021**, *23*, 302–309. [CrossRef] [PubMed]

Journal of
Clinical Medicine

MDPI

Review

Noncompaction Cardiomyopathy—History and Current Knowledge for Clinical Practice

Birgit J. Gerecke [1,2,*] and Rolf Engberding [3]

1 Department of Cardiology and Pneumology, University Medical Center Göttingen, 37075 Göttingen, Germany
2 Department of Thoracic and Cardiovascular Surgery, University Medical Center Göttingen, 37075 Göttingen, Germany
3 Internal Medicine & Cardiology, amO MVZ, Academic Hospital Wolfsburg, 38440 Wolfsburg, Germany; rolf.engberding@gmx.de
* Correspondence: birgit.gerecke@med.uni-goettingen.de

Abstract: Noncompaction cardiomyopathy (NCCM) has gained increasing attention over the past twenty years, but in daily clinical practice NCCM is still rarely considered. So far, there are no generally accepted diagnostic criteria and some groups even refuse to acknowledge it as a distinct cardiomyopathy, and grade it as a variant of dilated cardiomyopathy or a morphological trait of different conditions. A wide range of morphological variants have been observed even in healthy persons, suggesting that pathologic remodeling and physiologic adaptation have to be differentiated in cases where this spongy myocardial pattern is encountered. Recent studies have uncovered numerous new pathogenetic and pathophysiologic aspects of this elusive cardiomyopathy, but a current summary and evaluation of clinical patient management are still lacking, especially to avoid mis- and overdiagnosis. Addressing this issue, this article provides an up to date overview of the current knowledge in classification, pathogenesis, pathophysiology, epidemiology, clinical manifestations and diagnostic evaluation, including genetic testing, treatment and prognosis of NCCM.

Keywords: noncompaction cardiomyopathy; NCCM-diagnostic-therapy-prognosis; cardiomyopathy classification; LVNC; LVHT; phenotype; congenital heart disease

Citation: Gerecke, B.J.; Engberding, R. Noncompaction Cardiomyopathy—History and Current Knowledge for Clinical Practice. *J. Clin. Med.* **2021**, *10*, 2457. https://doi.org/10.3390/jcm10112457

Academic Editors: Stefan Peters and Luisa Mestroni

Received: 4 May 2021
Accepted: 27 May 2021
Published: 1 June 2021

1. Introduction

When the World Health Organization (WHO) published the first definition of cardiomyopathy in 1980, noncompaction cardiomyopathy (NCCM) was not yet known [1]. Historically, cases with an embryonic spongy pattern of the left ventricle (LV) were described in newborns and infants with complex congenital heart disease, especially with aortic and pulmonary valve atresia [2–6]. In the early cases, diagnosis had to rely on autopsy data, whereas later, newer imaging techniques such as angiography have been used.

A real breakthrough in diagnosis of this myocardial anomaly in vivo could be achieved through 2D echocardiography as was described in 1984 and is presented in Figure 1. The echocardiographic and angiographic images of a 33-year-old female patient showed an embryonic spongy pattern of the LV myocardium in absence of congenital or other structural heart disease [7]. Retrospectively, this was the first published case of NCCM without other structural defects of the heart. In this publication, the myocardial anomaly was referred to as "persistence of isolated myocardial sinusoids", assuming the anomalous LV morphology was due to a developmental defect in regression of the embryonal sinusoids. This term was used in the following years by other authors for similar cases [8].

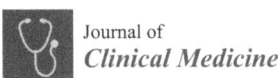

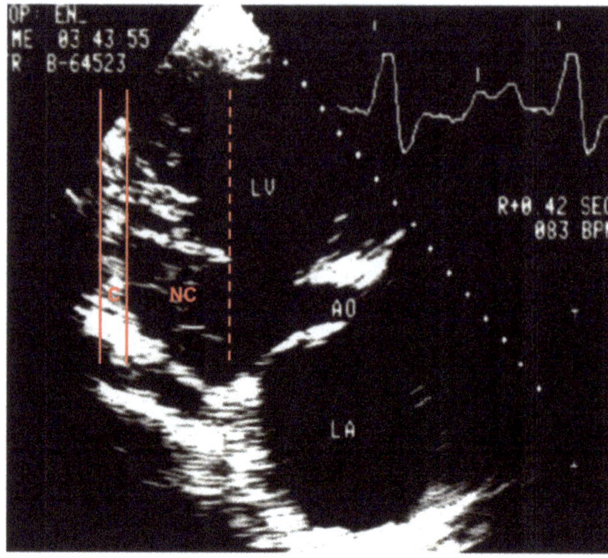

Figure 1. Echocardiography of the first published patient with NCCM without congenital heart disease. LV—left ventricle; LA—left atrium; Ao—aorta; C—compacted layer; NC—noncompacted layer of the left ventricular wall with deep recesses.

In 1990, Chin et al. suggested the term "isolated noncompaction of the left ventricular myocardium (INVM)", assuming that the myocardial anomaly occurred as a result of an arrest of the normal compaction process during embryonal endomyocardial morphogenesis [9].

Eventually, recent observations suggest, that LV noncompaction (LVNC) may not be the result of an arrest in the compaction process, but instead results from the compacted myocardium of the ventricular wall, growing into the ventricular lumen in a trabecular fashion [10].

Initially, the term isolated NCCM was used for cases without congenital or other structural heart defects. Today, some groups use the term for cases with areas of LVNC and normal LV function [11]. Table 1 shows a selection of terms and abbreviations used for noncompaction cardiomyopathy and the noncompacted morphology in the last nearly 100 years.

Table 1. A selection of terms and abbreviations for noncompacted cardiomyopathy and the noncompacted phenotype.

Term	Abbreviation
Spongy myocardium	
Fetal myocardium	
Honeycomb myocardium	
Persistent sinusoids	
Isolated noncompaction of the left ventricular myocardium	INVM
Left ventricular noncompaction	LVNC
Noncompaction cardiomyopathy	NCCM
Left ventricular hypertrabeculation	LVHT
Hypertrabeculation syndrome	
Left ventricular myocardial noncompaction cardiomyopathy	
Non-compaction of the left ventricular myocardium	

During the years, a wide range of morphological variants could be observed. Some authors, therefore, propose to consider a differentiation in several subtypes, especially in the pediatric population [12].

In the last five years, a number of studies described the usefulness of contemporary diagnostic tools, including echocardiographic imaging techniques, magnetic resonance (CMR), computed tomographic (CT) imaging and genetic testing, and revealed that some cases seemed to occur in patients with neuromuscular disease [13–17]. Towbin and Jefferies discussed NCCM in association with metabolic abnormalities [18].

Of major interest are results from CMR imaging studies, which detected the phenotype of LVNC in healthy athletes and pregnant women, suggesting a physiologic adaptation [19,20]. The same can be found in normal healthy persons, in parts depending on the ethnic group [11]. In this context, future research needs to unravel when the phenotype of LVNC represents pathologic remodeling and when it is a morphologic variant in a healthy person.

2. Noncompaction Cardiomyopathy in the Cardiomyopathy Classifications

The classification and definition of cardiomyopathies have been developed in the last six decades with more precise and elaborated recommendations due to increasing abilities in diagnostic and therapeutic modalities.

In 1957, the term cardiomyopathy was proposed for uncommon, noncoronary heart muscle diseases [21]. In 1972, Goodwin and Oakley described cardiomyopathies as myocardial diseases of unknown origin and suggested a first classification [22]. When the first definition and classification of cardiomyopathies by the WHO/ISFC Task Force was reported in 1980, a cardiomyopathy was defined as a heart muscle disease of unknown cause and classified as a dilated, hypertrophic and restrictive cardiomyopathy. "Unclassified cardiomyopathy covered a few cases, which do not fit readily into any group" [1].

The WHO/ISFC updated its classification in 1995 as diseases of the myocardium associated with myocardial dysfunction and now included arrhythmogenic right ventricular cardiomyopathy. The cardiomyopathies were classified by "the dominant pathophysiology or, if possible, by etiological/pathogenetic factors" [23]. Once more the unclassified cardiomyopathies included a few cases that "do not fit readily into any group" (e.g., fibroelastosis, noncompacted myocardium, systolic dysfunction with minimal dilatation, mitochondrial involvement) [23].

In 2006, the AHA defined cardiomyopathies as diseases of the myocardium associated with mechanical and/or electrical dysfunction, which usually exhibit inappropriate ventricular hypertrophy or dilation due to a variety of causes that frequently are genetic, classified as primary or secondary. This classification presented the first attempt to classify primary cardiomyopathy by origin (genetic, acquired, or mixed) and NCCM was assigned a genetic cardiomyopathy [24]. The 2008 ESC proposal defined a cardiomyopathy as a myocardial disorder in which the heart muscle is structurally and functionally abnormal in the absence of coronary artery disease, hypertension, valvular disease and congenital heart disease sufficient to cause the observed myocardial abnormality. The familial diseases included unclassified forms such as NCCM, Barth syndrome, Lamin A/C, ZASP and a-dystrobrevin [25].

Today, NCCM is classified as a genetic cardiomyopathy by the AHA, while the ESC working group for myocardial and pericardial disease and the WHO classified it a familial/genetic unclassified cardiomyopathy [23–25].

In 2013 a nosology for cardiomyopathies was proposed with a descriptive genotype–phenotype system, the MOGE(S) nosology [26]. This classification system embodies the morphofunctional phenotype (M), organ involvement (O), genetic inheritance pattern (G), etiological annotation (E), including the genetic defect or underlying disease/substrate, and the functional status (S) of the disease using the American College of Cardiology (ACC)/American Heart Association (AHA) stage and New York Heart Association (NYHA) functional class. The morphofunctional (M) notation provides a descriptive diagnosis of the phenotype (M_D: dilated cardiomyopathy; M_H: hypertrophic cardiomyopathy; M_A: arrhythmogenic right ventricular (RV) cardiomyopathy; M_R: restrictive cardiomyopathy; M_{LVNC}: Noncompaction Cardiomyopathy) [26]. In the MOGE(s) nosology, LVNC is characterized by excessive trabeculation of the LV in echocardiography and cardiac magnetic resonance imaging. The noncompacted ventricular muscle layer is "substantially thicker than the compact layer"; an exact ratio of the layers is not documented. LVNC can occur as an isolated morphological phenotype in association with LV systolic dysfunction or with LV hypertrophy and with mutations in genes typically causing DCM and HCM. The MOGE(S) system distinguishes LVNC with LV dilation and dysfunction ($M_{LVNC \cdot D}$) or with LV hypertrophy ($M_{LVNC \cdot H}$) from pure LVNC (M_{LVNC}) [26].

3. Subtypes of Noncompaction Cardiomyopathy

LVNC remains a heterogeneous morphological anomaly of the heart with multiple possible concomitant phenotypes. Initially, isolated NCCM was characterized by the absence of an additional structural heart disease, especially congenital heart disease; later this definition was changed to those with normal systolic LV dimensions.

In 2015, LVNC was considered to consist of nine distinct subtypes in the pediatric population, whereas another classification was suggested in 2016 [12,27]. These subtypes are listed in Table 2a,b.

Table 2. Subtypes of noncompaction cardiomyopathies.

(a) Subtypes of NCCM in the Pediatric Population, modified after [12]
1. The isolated or benign form of LVNC, (M_{LVNC});
2. The arrhythmogenic form of LVNC;
3. The dilated form of LVNC, ($M_{LVNC + D}$);
4. The hypertrophic form of LVNC, ($M_{LVNC + H}$);
5. The "mixed" form of LVNC;
6. The restrictive form of LVNC, ($M_{LVNC + R}$);
7. The biventricular form of LVNC;
8. The right ventricular hypertrabeculation with normal LV form;
9. The congenital heart disease form of LVNC.
(b) Subtypes of NCCM, modified after [27]
1. iLVNC. NC morphology in left ventricles with normal systolic and diastolic function, size, and wall thickness;
2. LVNC with LV dilation and dysfunction at onset, such as in the paradigmatic infantile CMP of Barth syndrome;
3. LVNC in hearts fulfilling the diagnostic criteria for DCM, HCM, RCM, or ARVC;
4. LVNC associated with congenital heart disease;
5. Syndromes with LVNC, either sporadic or familial, in which the noncompaction morphology is one of the cardiac traits associated with both monogenic defects and chromosomal anomalies, i.e., complex syndromes with several multiorgan defects;
6. Acquired and potentially reversible LVNC, which has been reported in athletes; it has also been reported in sickle cell anemia, pregnancy, myopathies, and chronic renal failure;
7. Right ventricular noncompaction, concomitant with that of the left ventricle, or present as a unique anatomic area of NC.

In the literature, the most cohorts were analyzed as a whole, and only a few were divided into subgroups for analysis; for example, the isolated NCCM form that met the echocardiographic criteria, but did not have LV dilatation or hypertrophy, or the subtypes with concomitant dilatation or hypertrophy of the LV. Van Waning et al. described four subtypes in their cohort of 349 patients: Isolated NCCM $n = 95$ (27%); NCCM/HCM $n = 47$ (13%); NCCM/DCM $n = 195$ (56%) and NCCM/HCM/DCM $n = 12$ (3%) [28].

Right ventricular noncompaction cardiomyopathy is a challenging diagnosis due to an increased physiological trabeculation of the right ventricle. Nevertheless, there are some cases reported in the literature [29,30].

4. Epidemiology

NCCM in the pediatric and adult population probably has a different background. The National Australian Childhood Cardiomyopathy study documented 9.2% of the primary cardiomyopathies in children younger than 10 years of age as NCCM [31,32]. Jefferies et al. observed in the pediatric cardiomyopathy registry of the National Heart, Lung, and Blood Institute 4.8% of children with NCCM [32]. Therefore, NCCM was the third most common type of cardiomyopathy after DCM and HCM [31–33].

The percentage in adults seems lower: 4.1% in the EORP Cardiomyopathy registry and 5% in the German Torch registry [34,35].

In men, NCCM is twice to three times more common than in women. The diagnosis can be achieved in adults, adolescents, children, newborns and even prenatal [36,37]. The prenatal identification of isolated NCCM is feasible with current ultrasonographic technology in the hands of an experienced examiner who is familiar with the features of this rare anomaly. Fetal IVNC can involve the LV, the RV, or both ventricles [38]. Sato described a patient with NCCM in the 10th decade of life presenting with a transient cerebral ischemia [39].

Left ventricular noncompaction is estimated to affect 8 to 12 per one million individuals per year, but the condition is likely more common because asymptomatic individuals are not diagnosed. Increased awareness of this condition and improvements in noninvasive cardiac imaging have led to a higher detection rate.

Familial occurrence is seen in up to 40% of the cases. The clinical phenotype is very variable, even in a single family. In a systematic family screening, a quarter of the examined relatives showed echocardiographic abnormalities, including LV dysfunction with and without noncompaction [40].

In experienced echocardiography departments NCCM has a prevalence of 0.014% to 0.26% [17,41–43]. With more sensitive imaging techniques the numbers increased. The prevalence with echocardiographic imaging in cardiac patient cohorts rose to about 0.9%, in healthy controls 1.05%, in athletic cohorts 3.16% and in pregnant cohorts up to 18.6% [44]. With MR imaging the numbers were significantly higher, with 9.6% in cardiac patients and up to 36.2% in subgroups [44]. Cardiac MR imaging in asymptomatic, healthy volunteers met varying noncompaction criteria in 1.3 to 14.8% [45], in other adult populations the numbers differed with the diagnostic criteria applied between 3% and 39% [15]. Thus, the real number seems to be unclear due to selection bias in different cohorts. The significance of the findings in asymptomatic peoples remains unclear.

5. Clinical Features

There is a broad spectrum of clinical presentations with primarily heart failure symptoms, different forms of arrhythmias and thromboembolic events. Between the onset of symptoms and the diagnosis there can be a delay of up to 3 to 4 years [43].

Heart failure symptoms can be mild, but severe symptoms with need for heart transplantation or LV assist device implantation can arise. In the German NCCM registry, 61% of patients showed heart failure symptoms at the time of initial diagnosis of NCCM and 15% developed heart failure symptoms during the follow-up of 27 months or deteriorated [46].

Arrhythmias are frequent in NCCM, ventricular as well as supraventricular arrhythmias. In the German NCCM registry 26% of the patients presented with arrhythmias and were subsequently diagnosed with cardiomyopathy. In 17%, atrial fibrillation was found. Atrial fibrillation was more often observed in patients with reduced LV function. Bradycardia requiring pacemaker implantation was seen in 5% of the cohort. Supraventricular arrhythmias occurred in 4%, WPW syndrome was observed in 1.5%, AV nodal reentry tachycardia in 1% and typical atrial flutter in 1.5%. Sustained ventricular tachycardia and ventricular fibrillation were observed in patients with severely reduced LV function. In patients with an LV ejection fraction above 35%, sudden cardiac deaths were found only rarely [47,48]. In children, up to 20% presented with WPW syndrome and with sinus bradycardia; WPW syndrome can be associated with cardiac dysfunction [49]. Table 3 summarizes observed arrhythmias in the German NCCM registry.

Table 3. Observed arrhythmias in patients with NCCM.

Type of Arrhythmia	Subtype	Prevalence
Bradyarrhythmias	Sinus bradycardia First-degree AV block Second-degree AV block Mobitz II Third-degree AV block indication for pacemaker implantation	5%
Supraventricular	Atrial fibrillation	18%
Tachycardias	Atrial flutter	1.5%
	Atrial tachycardia	
	AV nodal reentrant tachycardia	1.0%
	AV reentrant tachycardia	1.5%
Ventricular arrhythmias	Premature ventricular contractions	
	Monomorphic ventricular tachycardia Bidirectional ventricular tachycardia Polymorphic ventricular tachycardia Ventricular fibrillation	6%

AV—atrioventricular. Data from the German NCCM registry [47,48].

Thromboembolic events mainly occur in patients with NCCM and atrial fibrillation. Stasis of blood flow can appear in the deep intertrabecular recesses notably in reduced LV function. Neurologic departments occasionally diagnose NCCM in patients with otherwise not explained stroke. In cohorts with NCCM, a percentage of about 10–15% suffer from stroke [50].

There are several case reports of patients with NCCM and specific neuromuscular disorders or hereditary neuropathy such as Charcot–Marie–Tooth, Becker muscular dystrophy, Emery–Dreifuss muscular dystrophy, myotonic dystrophy, Leber's hereditary optic neuropathy, and Barth syndrome, and also with neuromuscular problems not specified in more detail [17,51]. These findings support the necessity of systematic neurological examination in patients with NCCM [52].

Several congenital heart defects were described with NCCM [53,54]. A patient with pulmonic valve atresia was described in 1964 and patients with Ebstein anomaly in 2005 [5,55]. Friedberg described a patient with atrial isomerism [56]. Shunt defects such as ventricular septal defect, atrial septal defect and patent ductus arteriosus Botalli were described as well [57]. Stähli described noncompaction in patients with congenital heart disease, in Epstein anomaly, subaortic VSD, bicuspid aortic valve and tetralogy of Fallot [54]. This in fact strengthens the need for a comprehensive echocardiographic evaluation of any patient with newly diagnosed NCCM to rule out congenital heart disease. In about 50% of children with concomitant face dysmorphisms or a neutropenia (Barth syndrome), cardiomyopathy with and without noncompaction was described [58].

Coronary heart disease is uncommon in NCCM, but severe coronary heart disease that needs revascularization therapy has been found in some patients with NCCM [7,59–61].

6. Diagnostic Criteria

Up to now, the diagnostic criteria of LVNC are far from being perfect [62]. The differential diagnosis between NCCM and normal phenotypic variants cannot be established properly in a lot of cases. Even using multimodality imaging, including echocardiography and cardio MR, the criteria are not specific enough to properly avoid under- or overdiagnosis with important implications on treatment strategies or prognostic estimations. The current available diagnostic imaging criteria show a propensity towards overdiagnosing NCCM [63].

6.1. Diagnostic Criteria for Echocardiography

Echocardiography with its widespread availability, low costs and nearly zero complications is the first-choice procedure in diagnosis of LVNC. Echocardiography can detect the pathognomonic features of a thick, bilayered myocardium with prominent trabeculations and intertrabecular recesses communicating with the LV cavity (Figure 2). If conventional echocardiography is not diagnostic, additional contrast echocardiography is suggested in the EACVI recommendations [64]. Transesophageal echocardiography or real time 3D echocardiography—if applicable, combined—have also been shown to be helpful diagnostic procedures in cases with LVNC [65,66].

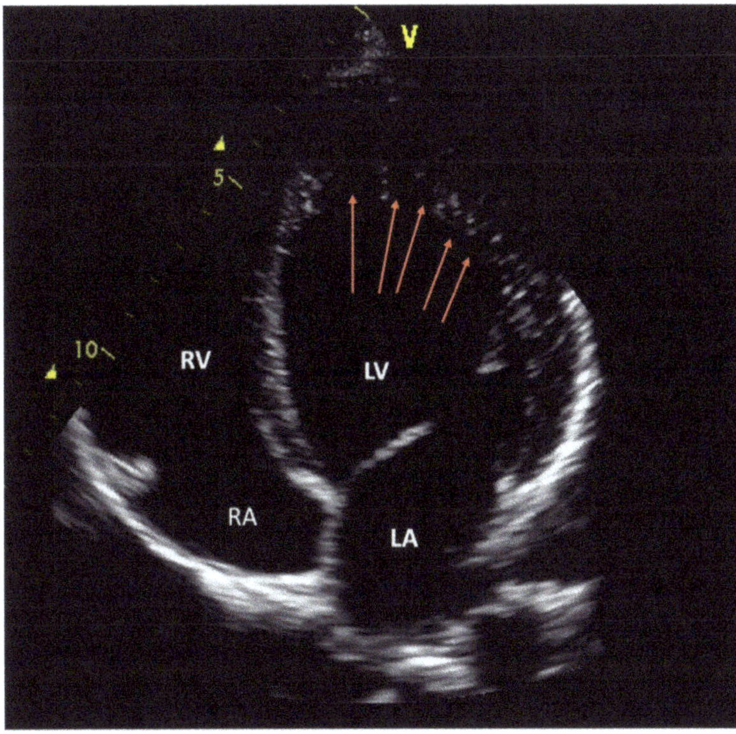

Figure 2. An echocardiographical apical 4-chamber view in a patient with NCCM. LV shows mild dilatation. The arrows mark the deep recesses in the noncompacted layer of the apical and lateral LV wall. LV—left ventricle; LA—left atrium; RV—right ventricle; RA—right atrium.

LVNC can be mainly observed at the cardiac apex and in the mid-inferior, mid-anterior, and mid-lateral areas of the LV wall [67]. A low-Nyquist limit color mapping is recommended to show blood flow into the recesses.

Although the first echocardiographic diagnosis of NCCM was published more than 37 years ago and the term noncompaction was introduced more than 30 years ago, there are no globally accepted diagnostic criteria [7,9,68]. Chin et al. were the first who introduced the term noncompaction and suggested diagnostic criteria for their cohort of children and young adults (California criteria). Jenni et al. described the criteria in a group of adults (Zurich criteria), both using the ratio between the compacted and the noncompacted layer, but with different measurements and timing in the cardiac cycle [8,9]. Stöllberger in contrast focused on the number of trabeculations and only later used the ratio as an additional diagnostic attribute (Vienna criteria) [17]. The German noncompaction registry used the combination of Jenni and Stöllberger criteria (Table 4.) [62,69]. Each group excluded patients with additional heart disease. In 2012, Paterick altered the measurement interval of the Jenni criteria; thus, creating the Milwaukee criteria [70].

Table 4. Echocardiographic criteria for the diagnosis of NCCM in the German NCCM registry [62].

1. At least four prominent trabeculations and deep intertrabecular recesses;
2. Blood flow between the cavity of the left ventricle and the recesses demonstrable by color Doppler echocardiography or by the use of ultrasonographic contrast medium;
3. The left ventricular wall segments show a typical bilaminar structure, and the noncompact subendocardial layer is at least twice as thick as the compact subepicardial layer in systole;
4. No other cardiac abnormalities present.

Frischknecht recommended the combination of criteria as specific, and Belanger in 2008 proposed different criteria with an additional classification of the severity derived from the noncompaction/compaction ratio and the affected planimetered area in cm^2 on an apical 4-chamber view, with three categories: mild, moderate and severe [71,72].

In the last decade of the last century and the first decade of this century, the diagnosis of NCCM was confirmed mainly in heart failure patients, and underdiagnosis of the disease was of major concern. Since more common recognition of the disease and introduction of newer imaging techniques occurred, the problem of overdiagnosis arose. To overcome these problems, additional criteria were introduced by the Swiss group in 2012: the compacta thickness; a compacta thickness of below 8 mm being a discriminator between the groups [73]. Sabatino tried to discriminate between NCCM and LVHT in a pediatric cohort using the noncompacted to compacted end diastolic myocardial ratio: the noncompaction cardiomyopathy with >2.3, the LVHT with <2.3 and >1.7 [74].

The Rotterdam group was the first to show that the absence of twist in speckle tracking tissue Doppler echocardiography can be a marker for NCCM. They demonstrated the loss of LV twist in 83% of 34 adults with NCCM [75]. The radial wall motion and the longitudinal LV wall velocity is impaired in NCCM, but the findings do not correlate with the extent or severity of noncompaction [76]. Further studies also showed impaired LV twist and the presence of rigid body rotation in NCCM but not in LVHT. A correlation between LV twist reduction in apical rotation and LV function was observed [77]. Table 5 shows an overview of different echocardiographic criteria.

Table 5. Different echocardiographic criteria for the diagnosis of NCCM.

Author Year; [ref.]	Appellation	Used Criteria						Cardiac Phase Used for Measurement	Recommended Views
		Trabeculations	Intertrabecular Recesses	Two-Layered Myocardial Structure	NC/C Ratio	Coexisting Cardiac Disease	Additional Criteria		
Chin 1990; [9]	California	Excessive prominent	Deep intertrabecular		X/Y ratio decrease i.e., C/NC+C; no exact cut-off value	Abnormalities excluded		End diastole	Apical view; subcostal view
Jenni 2001; [8,78]	Zurich	Excessive prominent trabeculations	Deep intertrabecular recesses	Compacted thin epicardial and much thicker non-compacted endocardial	NC/C > 2	Abnormalities absent	Perfused recesses in color Doppler	End systole	Short axis view
Stöllberger 2004; [17]	Vienna	>3 prominent trabeculations	Intertrabecular spaces	Trabeculations as part of non-compacted layer	No exact cut-off value		Perfusion of intertrabecular spaces by color Doppler	Trabeculations in end diastole; two-layered myocardium in end systole	Parasternal short axis and apical level; atypical apical 2-Ch view
Engberding 2007; [62]	Germany	At least 4 prominent trabeculations	Deep intertrabecular recesses	Bilaminar structure	NC/C ≥ 2	No other cardiac abnormalities	Blood flow in recesses in color Doppler or with echo contrast	Systole	
Belanger 2008; [72]	New York	Trabeculations	Recesses		NC/C	Absence of cardiomyopathy, congenital HD or coronary HD	Planimetered area of non-compacted myocardium	Systole	All standard views
Paterick 2012; [70]	Milwaukee	Trabeculations			NC/C > 2		Abnormal ventricular function	Total cardiac cycle; NC/C ratio end diastole	Multiple imaging windows
Van Dalen 2008; [75]	Rotterdam						Absence of LV twist		
Gebhard 2012; [73]	Additional						Compacta thickness < 8 mm		

Arunamata et al. investigated the speckle tracking strain results in a pediatric study group with NCCM, with and without congenital heart defects. Segmental radial, circumferential, and longitudinal strain decreased in NCCM compared with control subjects. Strain measurements were lowest in those with adverse compared with favorable outcomes. In NCCM, deformation was affected in all regions, including compacted myocardial segments [79].

Sabatino et al. assessed global and regional longitudinal strains in a pediatric population using apical 4-chamber, 3-chamber, and 2-chamber views; radial and circumferential strains were measured using LV short-axis views at different levels. LV twist was calculated as the difference between peak apical rotation and basal rotation at a time interval corresponding to the ejection phase of the systole. The measurements could discriminate between a normal counterclockwise pattern with reduced apical rotation peak values in LVHT and NCCM with rigid body rotation presenting with a sensitivity of 82% and a specificity of 92% [74]. In contrast, Huttin et al. showed that myocardial deformation was preserved in the apical region [80].

The World Heart Federation MOGE(S) classification graded LVNC as a morphological entity with an excessive trabeculation of the LV on echocardiography or cardiac magnetic resonance imaging. The noncompacted ventricular muscle layer was substantially thicker than the compact layer. No ratio was specified [26].

Even in experienced groups the interobserver agreement of the echocardiographic diagnosis was limited, with about 11% of questionable cases [81,82]. Measurements, according to existing diagnostic criteria for NCCM, vary due to the echocardiographic view and segment with different interobserver reliability and predictive validity. In a pediatric population, Joong et al. observed that the NC/C ratio showed the lowest reliability and predictive validity [83]. They found that the end diastolic measurements were more precise than the end systolic. A single echocardiographic diagnostic study may be too sensitive and may lead to overdiagnosis. Kohli et al. reported that 23.6% of patients presenting to their heart failure clinic met at least one of the three echocardiographic criteria for NCCM, including 8.3% of healthy control subjects, 50% of the control persons were black [84].

6.2. Diagnostic Criteria for Magnet Resonance Imaging

NCCM can be diagnosed using CMR (Figure 3.) There are several different methods that have been proposed to diagnose NCCM using CMR. Peterson et al. evaluated an end diastolic NC:C Ratio ≥ 2.3 measured in long axis cine views at the site with the most pronounced trabeculations, while Stacey defined an end systolic ratio > 2 in short axis views to diagnose NCCM [85,86]. Jacquier used short axis views to measure trabecular mass, where more than 20% of noncompacted mass were defined as NCCM [87]. Captur et al. described an end-diastolic loss of the base to apex fractal dimension gradient ≥ 1.3 for NCCM patients [88]. Grothoff redefined and extended the MR imaging criteria for diagnosing and discriminating NCCM from other cardiomyopathies using four basic criteria: the percentage of LV noncompacted myocardial mass (positive with >25%), the total amount of LV noncompacted myocardial mass (MM; positive >15 g/m^2), a noncompacted to compacted myocardium ratio of $\geq$3:1 in at least one of the segments 1–3 or 7–16 excluding the apical segment 17 and trabeculation in segments 4–6 $\geq$ 2:1 (noncompacted to compacted ratio) [89]. Dreisbach et al. used strain on MR imaging and Dodd et al. examined trabecular hyperenhancement on cardiac MR imaging [90,91]. The different MR criteria are listed in Table 6.

Table 6. Different CMR criteria for the diagnosis of NCCM.

Author Year; [ref.]	Used Criteria					Cardiac Phase Used for Measurement	Recommended Views
	Trabeculations	Recesses	Two-layered structure	NC/C ratio	Additional criteria		
Petersen 2005; [85]	Trabecular layering		Compacted epicardial and noncompacted endocardial layer	NC/C > 2.3	True apex excluded	End diastole	Long axis
Jacquier 2010; [87]	Trabeculated LV mass	Perfused, deep recesses	Jenni echo criteria		Trabeculated mass > 20%	End diastole	Short axis
Stacey 2012; [86]	Trabeculation	Flow in the recesses	Noncompacted and compacted layer	NC/C > 2.0	16–24 mm from the true apex	End systole	Short axis
Captur 2015; [83]	Abnormal trabecular pattern		Jenni echo criteria and #		Maximum apical fractal dimension > 1.3; global fractal dimension > 1.26	End diastole	Short axis
Grothoff 2012; [89]	Trabeculations	Recesses communicating with the left ventricular cavity	Noncompacted/compacted myocardium ratio	NC/C > 2 (segments 4–6) NC/C > 3 (segments 1–3, 7–16) *	Trabeculated mass > 25% of total LV mass; Trabeculated LV mass/BSA > 15 g/m^2	End diastole	Short axis
Choi 2016; [92]	Trabeculated mass		Most prominent noncompacted to compacted ratio	NC/C > 3.15 apical	Trabeculated mass > 35% of total LV volume	End diastole	Short axis

One of the following: family history, neuromuscular disorders, regional wall motion abnormality, arrhythmia, heart failure, thromboembolic event. * According to the 17-segments model of the left ventricle.

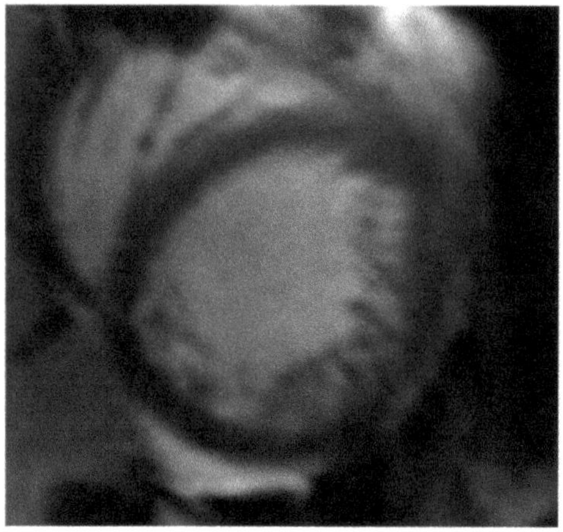

Figure 3. Magnetic resonance imaging: short axis of the left ventricle with excessive trabeculations. Notable, the septum shows no trabeculation.

7. Additional Diagnostic Armamentarium

7.1. The Multimodality Imaging Approach

A combination of different echocardiographic criteria and, if appropriate, a combination with an additional diagnostic technique should help to diagnose NCCM definitely or reject the diagnosis. However, there may be some borderline cases with a possible, but not definite, diagnosis of NCCM. In these cases, the imaging approach has to integrate clinical findings, family history and genetic data. However, at this time, a negative genetic test is not a marker, that diagnosis of NCCM is unlikely [28,93].

7.2. Left Ventricular Angiography

Diagnosis of NCCM can also be performed by LV angiography. Sometimes it is a diagnosis at a glance, but there are no definite criteria for the diagnosis of NCCM by LV angiography [7,62].

7.3. Computer Tomography

Cardiac CT is an imaging tool with increasing significance. In patients with dilated cardiomyopathy, cardiac CT is used to exclude coronary heart disease [94]. Conces et al. reported the first diagnosis of NCCM using cardiac CT [95]. For diagnosis of NCCM by cardiac CT, Melendez-Ramirez et al. proposed a ratio of noncompacted to compacted layer of 2.2 in one segment [96]. Fuchs et al. analyzed ECG-triggered low-dose cardiac CT and could discriminate patients with NCCM from normal individuals by using an NC:C ratio of >1.8 in diastole. Their results showed a good correlation of NC:C ratio between transthoracic echocardiography (TTE) and cardiac CT with the threshold of 1.8 [97].

7.4. Electrocardiography

An ECG does not show specific alterations in cases with NCCM. Alterations in the ST segments and T waves are common, as also are different types of bundle branch blocks. Some publications reported that nearly 90% of the patients presented with ECG alterations [98]. Conduction delay, P-wave abnormalities, QRS-axis deviation, interventricular conduction defects and various forms of bradyarrhythmias and tachyarrhythmias have been observed in affected patients. Alterations induced by a Wolff–Parkinson–White (WPW) syndrome may especially occur in children [49]. Atrial fibrillation is frequently observed [47,48].

7.5. Biomarkers

NTproBNP is a marker for heart failure. High NTproBNP levels were investigated for being an indicator for death and heart transplantation in patients with NCCM [99]. An elevated troponin level can refer to myocarditis but may also be present in patients with NCCM [100].

7.6. Endomyocardial Biopsy

Endomyocardial biopsy continues to be the gold standard in the detection of myocardial inflammation. Myocarditis is a potential differential diagnosis in cases with NCCM. Biopsy findings can offer clear therapeutic recommendations, especially in cases with giant cell myocarditis or sarcoidosis.

8. Differential Diagnosis

Prominent LV trabeculation can be found in healthy hearts, as well as in hypertrophic cardiomyopathy (HCM) and in LV hypertrophy secondary to dilated, valvular, or hypertensive cardiomyopathy. Thus, the differentiation between variants and LVNC may often be challenging [101]. Differential diagnosis of NCCM includes apical and other located LV thrombus, false tendons, aberrant chords, cardiac fibromas, eosinophilic heart disease, endomyocardial fibrosis and cardiac metastasis [102]. Other cardiomyopathies or localized LV hypertrophy have to be discriminated. Myocarditis may imitate NCCM.

In 25% of normal pregnancies, an increase in LV trabeculations can be assessed [20,103]. A LVNC pattern in pregnancy was reported in several studies [20,104,105]. Diagnosis of NCCM, therefore, is more difficult in pregnant women. A peripartum cardiomyopathy and a preexisting NCCM are important differential diagnoses in pregnant women or women after delivery with heart failure symptoms, requiring different treatment options. Noncompaction of the LV myocardium may be the morphological trait of a physiological remodeling in these cases.

Some persons affected with noncompacted areas do not have any symptoms and are diagnosed by chance. A major number of these persons are athletes, and noncompaction perhaps may be a physiological remodeling process in these persons [19]. Luijkx et al. even found ethnic differences in athletes with a greater degree of LV trabeculation in healthy African athletes, combined with biventricular EF reduction at rest [106]. De la Chica et al. found hypertrabeculation in persons with vigorous physical activity [107]. To exclude NCCM in athletes, a pre-participation screening with clinical and family history, ECG and echocardiography, and, in suspicious findings in these examinations, a CMR was recommended [19].

A noncompaction pattern can be a myocardial response to acquired triggers, Loria et al. discussed chemotherapy with drug toxicity as a possible trigger [108]. A report of 2009 described diagnosis of LVNC in a group of family members, including a pair of identical twins; each of them suffered from thalassemia major requiring multiple transfusions, and suggested a possible association with cardiac siderosis [109]. Chronic renal failure and polycystic kidney disease were reported likewise [27]. Figure 4 proposes a pathway for differential diagnostic considerations.

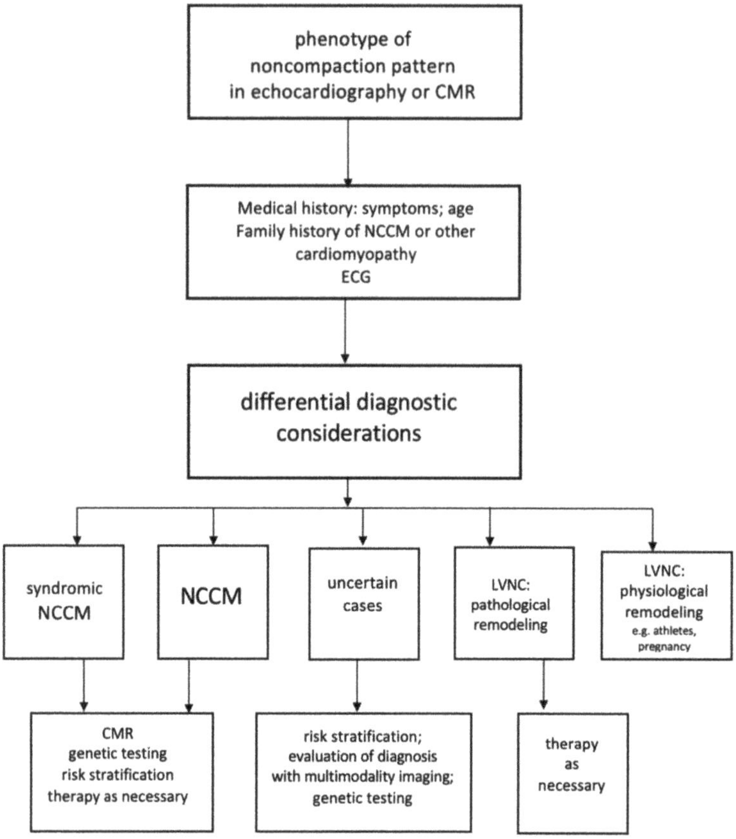

Figure 4. A pathway for differential diagnosis and risk stratification in patients with noncompacted myocardium (LVNC).

9. Pathogenesis—Embryogenesis and the Pathophysiological Concept

In the first series of patients with NCCM, the disease was familial to a large extent. Noncompaction areas resembled the fetal heart and the hypothesis of an arrest in the normal compaction process of the heart seemed adequate.

The development of the heart is a complex, precisely regulated molecular and embryogenetic process. The different steps of the development are triggered by specific signaling molecules and mediated by tissue-specific transcription factors [110,111]. Trabeculations appear at the end of the fourth gestational week in humans, when the heart tube consists of an external myocardial layer and an internal endocardial epithelium. The first trabeculations appear in the cardiac jelly between endocardial–myocardial contact points and extend radially into the ventricular lumen [112]. During myocardial development, two different myocardial layers are formed within the ventricular wall, a trabecular layer and a compact subepicardial layer [113–115]. In gestational week 12, development of trabeculations increases the surface to enhance the blood, respectively oxygen supply of the growing myocardium prior to the developing of the coronary arteries. The resulting intertrabecular recesses communicate with the LV cavity. The next step in the development is a compaction process from basal and septal to apical and lateral LV areas. This process underlies a complex genetic regulation as well. An arrest of the compaction process can occur if signal molecules are not expressed at the correct time [116].

The NOTCH pathway is required for proliferation, differentiation and tissue patterning in various tissues, including the heart [117]. The NOTCH pathway seems to independently regulate cardiomyocyte proliferation and differentiation, two balanced processes whose perturbation may result in congenital heart disease. Mutations in the NOTCH pathway regulator MIB1 cause NCCM by impaired growths of the trabecular instead of the compacted layer [118]. Other mutations in the NOTCH pathway lead to incorrect marker expression (e.g., EphrinB2, NRG1, BMP10, and MIB1) and decreased myocardial proliferation [112]. Neuregulin, ErbB2, ErbB4 and Nkx2.5 code other signaling proteins regulating organ proliferation and are described to control myocardial cell outgrowth that ultimately results in trabeculation [119–121]. The significance of the mutations in the NOTCH pathway was demonstrated by mutations in mice that lead to noncompacted myocardium [118].

In 2016, Jensen in contrary described the excessive trabeculations in noncompaction not to have the embryonic identity and drew the conclusion that noncompaction is probably not the result of failed compaction, but likely the result of abnormal growth of the compact wall [10]. This means that no compaction process may be present in the embryonic endomyocardial morphogenesis and that the term LVHT may be more appropriate than LVNC [68]. However, up to now, the concept of an arrest in the endomyocardial development is not completely understood [117].

10. Pathology

Pathoanatomical studies of NCCM revealed a marked trabecular meshwork with many intertrabecular recesses in the involved mural segments of the LV myocardium (Figure 5) [8,43,122]. The intertrabecular recesses are lined with endothelium [9], ending blindly in the external compact layer without a connection to the coronary circulation [9,122]. In autopsy studies, prominent trabeculations were found in the LV in up to 70% of a group of subjects without apparent clinical heart disease [123]. However, more than three trabeculations were found in only 4% of the patients. On basis of these data, Stöllberger et al. defined pathological LV trabeculations when more than three trabeculations apical to the papillary muscles were present on echocardiography [124].

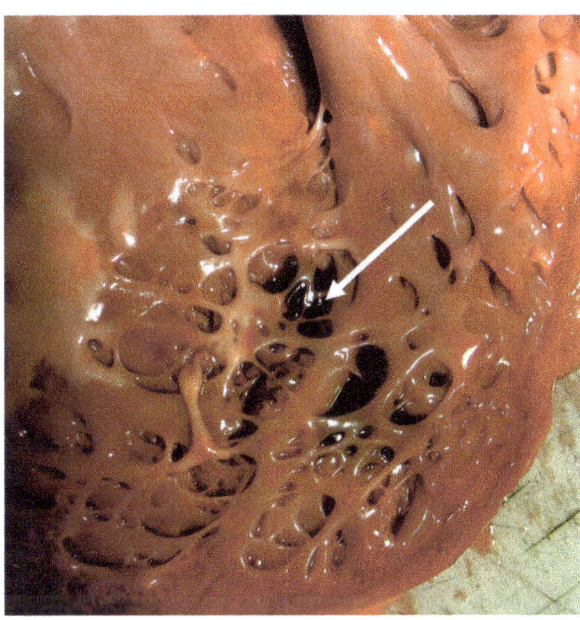

Figure 5. Autopsy specimen: left ventricle of a patient with NCCM and sudden cardiac death. A thin compacted layer and extensive trabeculation in the apical region. Small thrombi between the trabeculations (arrows).

Burke examined hearts in cases with NCCM by autopsies and found poorly formed papillary muscles in the LV, a distinct noncompacted zone in the LV and, often, in the right ventricle [125]. The patterns of the noncompacted area include anastomosing trabeculations and a polypoid endocardial surface. None of the pathological or histological findings was typical for either the isolated or nonisolated form of NCCM. Different cardiac abnormalities were seen in the nonisolated form, including epicardial coronary malformation, histiocytoid cardiomyopathy, ventricular septal defects, and conotruncal diseases [125]. Jenni reported scar tissue within the trabeculations and in the subendocardial area but not in the epicardial zone [78].

In histological examinations the trabeculations were covered with excessive fibrous tissue and elastin deposits, perhaps suggestive of some degree of subendocardial ischemia [115,125]. Oechslin et al. found an increased number of normally formed trabeculations in hypertrabeculation, while the histological appearance of NCCM was "far beyond being normal" [41]. Burke found no difference between the hearts of isolated and nonisolated noncompaction cardiomyopathy [125].

Ultrastructural investigations could give additional impact on the discussion of pathogenesis of noncompaction areas. Ultrastructural investigations of hearts with noncompaction/hypertrabeculation demonstrated alterations in the shape and number of mitochondria, sarcomeric alterations, and other morphological abnormalities such as lipid-like inclusions and enlarged interstitial spaces [126]. The findings were generally nonspecific. The reported abnormalities were most prominent in patients with neuromuscular disorders. The changes included elongated mitochondria, swollen mitochondria, and disruption of the usual parallel orientation between mitochondria and sarcomeres. Other myocardial diseases such as myocardial ischemia and hibernation have been reported to involve abnormalities in mitochondria equally [127].

11. Genetics in Noncompaction Cardiomyopathy

11.1. Basic Aspects

Familial cumulation of NCCM assumes a genetic background. Basic research showed that trabeculation is regulated by genes and that mutations in the NOTCH pathway regulator MIB1 cause noncompacted myocardium [118].

The genetic pathogenesis of NCCM is heterogeneous. In a majority of the adult patients with noncompaction cardiomyopathy, it is an autosomal dominant disorder. X-linked disorders, autosomal recessive, and mitochondrial (maternal) inheritance have also been described. The first genetic cause of isolated NCCM was initially described by Bleyl et al., when they identified mutations in the X-linked G4.5-Gen encoding for Tafazzin, the gene also responsible for Barth syndrome [128]. Affected children show cardiomyopathies, half of them with noncompaction, neutropenia and myopathy. Emery–Dreifuss muscular dystrophy is caused by a G4.5 mutation as well.

Gene mutations have been identified, that cause congenital heart disease with noncompaction; in patients with hypoplastic left heart syndrome and noncompaction a DTNA (α- dystrobrevin) mutation was identified. Dystrophin mutations are also involved in boys with Duchenne and Becker muscular dystrophies [129]. Whereas mutations in Nkx-2.5 mutations were reported in children with noncompaction, atrial septal defect and β-myosin heavy chain (MYH7) in patients with noncompaction and Ebstein anomaly [129]. Chromosomal abnormalities and syndromic patients have also been identified with noncompacted myocardium such as Coffin-Lowry syndrome, Sotos syndrome, Hunter–McAlpine syndrome, and Charcot–Marie–Tooth disease [130].

NCCM is often familial with an autosomal dominant inheritance but with variable penetrance and a high intrafamilial variability [131]. Studies in the 1980s and 1990s led to the discoveries that the sarcomere mutations cause cardiomyopathies. Mutations of genes, that are responsible for hypertrophic or dilated cardiomyopathy, were found in patients with NCCM as well [132]. Even primary restrictive cardiomyopathy shares the same sarcomeric genetic background [133]. Recent publications showed that nearly half of the affected genes in patients with NCCM were sarcomere genes relevant for the structure of contractile and non-contractile elements with single missense mutations [134]. MYH7 was involved in 48% of the sarcomere gene mutations. MYH7 and ACTC1 mutations had significant lower risk for MACE than MYBPC3 and TTN mutations [28]. Arrhythmic genes, non-sarcomere/non-arrhythmic genes, X-linked genes, genes associated with congenital heart disease, mitochondrial dysfunction genes and complex genotypes were found as well but in small numbers [28]. In some families with autosomal dominant NCCM associated with congenital heart disease (CHD), affected members may have very minor forms of CHD that may have normalized spontaneously, whereas other family members may have severe forms of CHD. In addition, mutations in the sodium channel gene SCN5A, were reported to cause noncompacted myocardium and rhythm disturbance [135]. Genetic testing in patients with NCCM appears to detect clinically significant variants in 35% to 40% of tested individuals. Table 7 shows a selection of affected genes.

Table 7. Genes involved in different forms of noncompaction cardiomyopathy.

Genes	Mutations in Gen:
Sarcomere genes (Contractile and non-contractile Structures)	MYH7; MYBPC3; ACTC1; TNT; TPM1; AN2; ACTN2; DES; LDB3; MYL2; NEBL; OBSCN; TNNC1; TNNI3
Arrhythmia genes	HCN4; RYR2; SCN5A; ABCC9; ANK2; CACNA2D1; CASQ2; KCNE3 KCNH2; KCNQ1
Non-sarcomere/non-arrhythmia Cardiomyopathy genes	MMPK; DSP; DTNA; FKTN; HFE; JUP; LMNA (Lamin A/C); PKP2; PLEC; PLN; PRDM16; RBM20; SGCD
X-linked genes	G4.5 (TAZ); DMD; FHL1; GLA; LAMP2: RPS6KA3
Genes associated with congenital heart disease	MIB1; MIB2; NKX2.5; NOTCH1; NSD1; PTPN11; TXB20; TBX5
Mitochondrial dysfunction genes	HADHB; HMGCL; MIPEP; MLYCD MT-ATP6; MT-CO3; MTFMT; MT-ND1; MT-ND2; SDHA; SDHD; TMEM70; VARS2
Complex genotypes	Multiple mutations in one patient. Complex MYBPC3 mutations with severe clinical phenotype, observed only in children

Adapted from [28,134].

Children more frequently had an X-linked or mitochondrial inherited defect or chromosomal anomalies. In multivariate analysis MYBPC3, TTN, arrhythmia—non-sarcomere non-arrhythmia cardiomyopathy—and X-linked genes were genetic predictors for MACE. The presence of pathogenic variants was an independent risk factor for adverse outcomes in other cohorts as well and may aid in risk stratification in patients. Biallelic mutations and double pathogenic variants were found to have a worse prognosis [136,137].

Current investigations in more than 800 patients showed a genetic overlap indicating that NCCM often represents a phenotypic variation of DCM or HCM, but also variants uniquely associated with NCCM [138].

11.2. Genetic Testing in Familial Noncompaction Cardiomyopathy

Up to 40% of NCCM cases may be familial, so family screening is recommended when the diagnosis of NCCM is assessed in a child [12]. NCCM is a heterogeneous condition, and genetic stratification plays a role in clinical management. Distinguishing genetic from nongenetic noncompaction should help to predict an outcome and to find adequate management and follow-up decisions tailored to genetic status [137]. When a definite diagnosis of NCCM is assessed, the diagnostic process should include genetic testing which will provide a relatively high probability to find sarcomeric mutations [28]. No pathogenetic variants were identified in patients with isolated LVNC in the absence of cardiac dysfunction or syndromic features. Consequently, the diagnostic yield of genetic testing in adult index patients with LVNC is low. Genetic testing is most beneficial in LVNC associated with other cardiac and syndromic features, in which it can facilitate the correct diagnosis, and is least useful in adults with isolated LVNC without a family history of noncompaction [139,140].

HRS/EHRA in 2011 recommended mutation specific testing of family members and appropriate relatives following the identification of a NCCM causative mutation in the index case (Class I). NCCM genetic testing can be useful (Class II a) for patients in whom a cardiologist has established a clinical diagnosis of NCCM, based on an examination of the patient's clinical history, family history, and electrocardiographic/echocardiographic phenotype [141]. The German position paper for "Gendiagnostik bei kardiovaskulären Erkrankungen" in 2015 conferred genetic testing in a patient with an established clinical diagnosis of NCCM a Class IIA recommendation. The recommendations include a mutation-specific test in family members after identification of the causative mutation in the index case (Class I) [142]. Sensitivity for a genetic test at that time was 20–30%. [142]. The AHA in 2020 recommends a family history for $\geq$3 generations and clinical screening for cardiomyopathy in asymptomatic first-degree relatives. Genetic testing should be considered for the most clearly affected person in a family to facilitate family screening and management. For NCCM the use of the gene panel for the cardiomyopathy identified in association with the NCCM phenotype is proposed, following the data of Hershberger [140,143].

In the pediatric population, genetic testing should be considered in individuals with cardiomyopathy co-occurring with NCCM. The actual database does not suggest an indication for cardiomyopathy gene panel testing in individuals with isolated noncompaction in the absence of a family history of cardiomyopathy phenotype with dilatation or hypertrophy [93].

12. Prognosis

With no underlying common diagnostic criteria, the comparison of different cohorts is difficult. The prognosis of the patient populations with NCCM is dependent on the occurrence of heart failure, death and on the need for heart transplantation. Systolic function is an important risk factor; heart failure with a reduced ejection fraction (HFrEF) with an LV ejection fraction below 35% has a worse prognosis. Several MR imaging studies demonstrated a good prognosis in preserved LV function [13,45,144,145].

Long term survival of patients with isolated apical noncompaction and preserved ejection fraction was shown to be comparable with the general population [16]. The end diastolic diameter of the LV assessed by echocardiography and heart failure symptoms have prognostic impact as well. No major cardiovascular events occurred in the non-symptom-based group, whereas 15/48 (31%) symptomatically diagnosed patients experienced cardiovascular death or heart transplantation. Independent predictors of cardiovascular death or heart transplantation were heart failure patient graded NYHA III-IV, sustained ventricular arrhythmias and left atrial size [146]. Left bundle branch block, atrial fibrillation and neuromuscular comorbidities have also been identified as risk factors [51,62,147]

Murphy et al. found that 62% of the patients developed heart failure symptoms. The death rate was found to be only 2% in a follow-up time of up to 15 years with regular visits [40]. In children, Pignatelli et al. described a mortality rate of 14% in 3 years, but transient recovery as well [148]. The Australian childhood cardiomyopathy registry has found the prognosis in children usually present with predominant noncompaction phenotype to be worse than the prognosis for matched children with DCM. In this registry, the freedom from death or heart transplantation at 10 years was 48% and at 15 years 45% [32]. The data of the RICARDA study in contrast show a better prognosis in those with hypertrabeculation, long term results are still lacking [149]. Whether the prognosis of

NCCM differs from the prognosis of DCM in adults is unclear. A multicenter study from the Netherlands showed no difference between the groups, while the Heidelberg group showed a better prognosis in DCM compared to NCCM [150,151]. Aung et al. reported that LVNC patients had a similar risk of cardiovascular mortality compared with a DCM control group. The incidence rates of all-cause mortality, stroke and systemic emboli, heart failure admission, cardiac transplantation, ventricular arrhythmias, and cardiac device implantation were 2.16, 1.54, 3.53, 1.24, 2.17, and 2.66, respectively per 100 person-years. Meta-regression and subgroup analyses of these data revealed that LV ejection fraction, and not the extent of LV trabeculation, showed an important influence on the variability of incidence rates [152]. CMR studies compared the outcome of adults with NCCM compared to DCM patients and found no difference in the prognosis [14,15,153].

Genetic testing also has an impact on the prognostic stratification (see genetics).

Romano et al. demonstrated global longitudinal strain (GLS) derived with CMR to be a prognostic factor even in NCCM [154]. The existence of late enhancement in MR imaging was found to be an additional risk factor [155,156]. Vaidya et al. examined a study group with isolated apical noncompaction versus a patient group of mid basal noncompaction localization and found a lower risk of all-cause mortality compared to the mid basal noncompaction localization even in groups with comparable cardiovascular risk factors. However, in general, patients with isolated apical NCCM showed a higher LV ejection fraction and were more frequently asymptomatic than those with mid basal noncompaction localization [16]. Additionally, a correlation of 5 years mortality to the number of affected segments was found [137]. Vaidya et al. compared patients with and without left atrial dilatation, defined as LAVI > 34 cm^2/m^2. Left atrial dilatation was present in half of the patients. Among the patients with left atrial dilatation 25% died, compared to 8% without left atrial dilatation. However, the patients with left atrial dilatation were significantly older, showing a greater frequency of hypertension, congestive heart failure, and atrial fibrillation [16]. Regression of noncompacted areas was associated with an improvement in LV systolic function and might be associated with a favorable prognosis in these patients [157].

13. Therapy

There is no specific therapy for NCCM today. Therapy has to address the clinical symptoms and to cover prognostic aspects. Heart failure therapy in patients with NCCM and reduced LV systolic function can be applied according to the heart failure guidelines [62]. Cardiac resynchronization therapy results in an improvement of LV function in patients with left bundle branch block [158]. The implantation of an LV assist device is documented in several case reports [159]. In a single heart transplantation center, NCCM was a rare cause for transplantation with 2% of the cohort [160].

Antiarrhythmic therapy depends on the clinical situation, the use of ablation therapy in supraventricular and ventricular tachycardia, pacemaker and ICD systems have been reported [48,161,162]. Ablation of an accessory pathway in WPW-syndrome in children could be successfully performed in 83% with improvement of a reduced LV function in three of four of those with reduced LV function [49]. Therapy of atrial fibrillation in patients with cardiomyopathies is challenging [163].

The 2008 ACC/AHA guidelines graded ICD implantation a Class II b indication in NCCM independent of the systolic LV function [164]. The current guidelines on the prevention of sudden cardiac death do not mention NCCM (AHA), or state that there are only few data that LV noncompaction by itself is an indication for an ICD implantation (ESC) [165,166].

Anticoagulation with VKA is recommended in cases with NCCM and reduced ejection fraction with LVEF < 40%, as proposed in the literature [40,41,62]. The patients with NCCM after thromboembolic events and those with atrial fibrillation should also receive anticoagulation therapy. In patients with atrial fibrillation NOAC can be used instead of VKA as well.

Recently, there were case reports on resection of the noncompacted myocardium that showed recovery of the cardiac function. Long term follow-up is recommended [167].

Regular physical activity, including systematic exercise, is an important component of prevention and therapy for most cardiovascular diseases and is associated with reduced mortality [168]. The 2020 ESC Guideline on sports cardiology regard NCCM patients and allow participation in high-intensity exercise and competitive sports only in asymptomatic individuals with an LVEF > 50% and the absence of arrhythmias, and in recreational exercise programs only in patients with an LVEF > 40%. Follow-up visits are recommended [168]. Figure 6 shows a proposal for a clinical algorithm for the management of noncompaction cardiomyopathy.

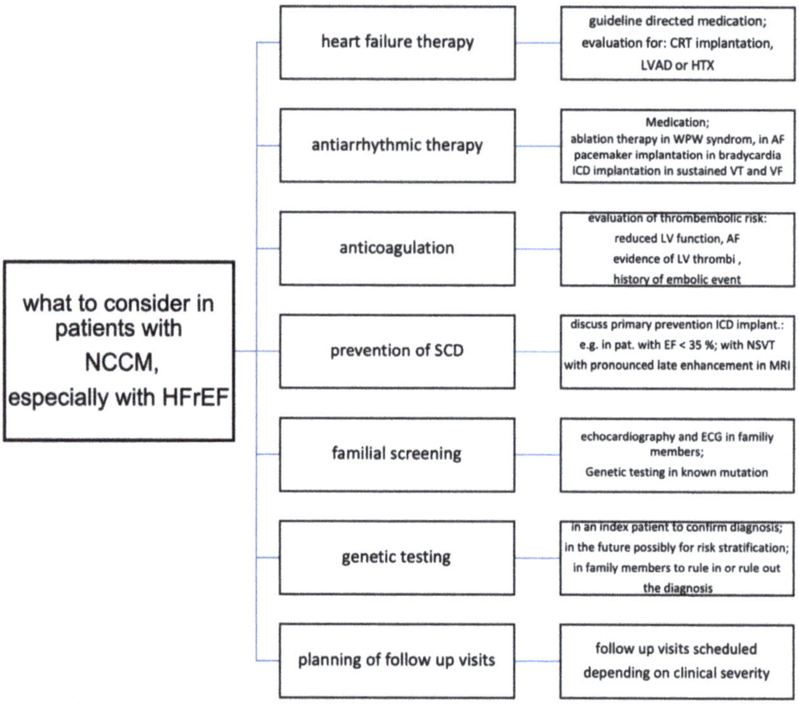

Figure 6. Treatment algorithm for patients with NCCM.

14. Future Work

Today, we know that the morphological noncompaction pattern is not restricted to the genetically determined NCCM. LVNC can occur in both, physiologic and pathologic remodeling. However, the same is true for other structural features such as dilatation of the LV or for LV hypertrophy, which can also be detected in a variety of clinical settings and require a differentiated approach.

Nevertheless, we need diagnostic consensus criteria to streamline future research efforts and be able to better compare patients' subgroups with statistical meaningful volume. A big international registry could be the basis for more evidence-based recommendations to avoid unnecessary diagnostic testing and to formulate specific treatment options for this elusive cardiomyopathy.

There are ample areas of need for future research to help unravel the mysteries of this rare disease, NCCM. Future basic research should investigate the role of genetics as well as the ultrastructural features of cardiomyocytes to help discover targeted treatments. Future clinical studies need to focus on improving diagnostic imaging and laboratory testing.

In the meantime, patients with NCCM should receive early diagnosis, counselling and optimal treatment, while avoiding overdiagnosis and overtreatment in those with only a physiologic remodeling.

Author Contributions: Writing—original draft preparation, B.J.G.; writing—review and editing, B.J.G. and R.E. All authors have read and agreed to the published version of the manuscript.

Funding: This research received no external funding.

Institutional Review Board Statement: Not applicable.

Acknowledgments: Acknowledgments to all friends and the countless colleagues who discussed this subject with us in the last decades.

Conflicts of Interest: The authors declare no conflict of interest.

References

1. Brandenburg, R.O. Report of the WHO/ISFC task force on the definition and classification of cardiomyopathies. *Br. Heart J.* **1980**, *44*, 672–673. [CrossRef]
2. Grant, R.T. An unusual anomaly of the coronary vessels in the malformed heart of a child. *Heart* **1926**, *1*, 273–283.
3. Bellet, S.; Gouley, B.A. Congenital heart disease with multiple cardiac anomalies: Report of case showing aortic atresia, fibrous scar in myocardium, and embryonal sinusoidal remains. *Am. J. Med. Sci.* **1932**, *183*, 458–465. [CrossRef]
4. Dusek, J.; Ostádal, B.; Duskova, M. Postnatal persistence of spongy myocardium with embryonic blood supply. *Arch. Pathol.* **1975**, *99*, 312–317.
5. Lauer, R.M.; Fink, H.P.; Petry, E.L.; Dunn, M.I.; Diehl, A.M. Angiographic Demonstration of Intramyocardial Sinusoids in Pulmonary-Valve Atresia with Intact Ventricular Septum and Hypoplastic Right Ventricle. *N. Engl. J. Med.* **1964**, *271*, 68–72. [CrossRef]
6. Feldt, R.H.; Rahimtoola, S.H.; Davis, G.D.; Swan, H.; Titus, J.L. Anomalous ventricular myocardial patterns in a child with complex congenital heart disease. *Am. J. Cardiol.* **1969**, *23*, 732–734. [CrossRef]
7. Engberding, R.; Bender, F. Identification of a rare congenital anomaly of the myocardium by two-dimensional echocardiography: Persistence of isolated myocardial sinusoids. *Am. J. Cardiol.* **1984**, *53*, 1733–1734. [CrossRef]
8. Jenni, R.; Goebel, N.; Tartini, R.; Schneider, J.; Arbenz, U.; Oelz, O. Persisting myocardial sinusoids of both ventricles as an isolated anomaly: Echocardiographic, angiographic, and pathologic anatomical findings. *Cardiovasc. Interv. Radiol.* **1986**, *9*, 127–131. [CrossRef]
9. Chin, T.K.; Perloff, J.K.; Williams, R.G.; Jue, K.; Mohrmann, R. Isolated noncompaction of left ventricular myocardium. A study of eight cases. *Circulation* **1990**, *82*, 507–513. [CrossRef]
10. Jensen, B.; van der Wal, A.C.; Moorman, A.F.M.; Christoffels, V.M. Excessive trabecularions in noncompaction do not have the embryonic identity. *Int. J. Cardiol.* **2017**, *227*, 325–330. [CrossRef]
11. Nel, S.; Khandheria, B.K.; Libhaber, E.; Peters, F.; dos Santos, C.F.; Matioda, H.; Grinter, S.; Maharaj, N.; Essop, M.R. Prevalence and significance of isolated left ventricular non-compaction phenotype in normal black Africans using echocardiography. *IJC Heart Vasc.* **2020**, *30*, 100585. [CrossRef]
12. Towbin, J.; Lorts, A.; Jefferies, J.L. Left ventricular non-compaction cardiomyopathy. *Lancet* **2015**, *386*, 813–825. [CrossRef]
13. Zemrak, F.; Ahlman, M.A.; Captur, G.; Mohiddin, S.; Kawel-Boehm, N.; Prince, M.R.; Moon, J.C.; Hundley, W.G.; Lima, J.A.; Bluemke, D.; et al. The Relationship of Left Ventricular Trabeculation to Ventricular Function and Structure Over a 9.5-Year Follow-Up. *J. Am. Coll. Cardiol.* **2014**, *64*, 1971–1980. [CrossRef] [PubMed]
14. Andreini, D.; Pontone, G.; Bogaert, J.; Roghi, A.; Barison, A.; Schwitter, J.; Mushtaq, S.; Vovas, G.; Sormani, P.; Aquaro, G.D.; et al. Long-Term Prognostic Value of Cardiac Magnetic Resonance in Left Ventricle Noncompaction. *J. Am. Coll. Cardiol.* **2016**, *68*, 2166–2181. [CrossRef]
15. Ivanov, A.; Dabiesingh, D.S.; Bhumireddy, G.P.; Mohamed, A.; Asfour, A.; Briggs, W.M.; Ho, J.; Khan, S.A.; Grossman, A.; Klem, I.; et al. Prevalence and Prognostic Significance of Left Ventricular Noncompaction in Patients Referred for Cardiac Magnetic Resonance Imaging. *Circ. Cardiovasc. Imaging* **2017**, *10*, e006174. [CrossRef] [PubMed]
16. Vaidya, V.R.; Lyle, M.; Miranda, W.R.; Farwati, M.; Isath, A.; Patlolla, S.H.; Hodge, D.O.; Asirvatham, S.J.; Kapa, S.; Deshmukh, A.J.; et al. Long-Term Survival of Patients with Left Ventricular Noncompaction. *J. Am. Heart Assoc.* **2021**, *10*, e015563. [CrossRef]
17. Stöllberger, C.; Finsterer, J.; Blazek, G. Isolated left ventricular abnormal trabeculation is a cardiac manifestation of neuromuscular disorders. *Cardiology* **2000**, *94*, 72–76. [CrossRef]
18. Towbin, J.A.; Jefferies, J.L. Cardiomyopathies Due to Left Ventricular Noncompaction, Mitochondrial and Storage Diseases, and Inborn Errors of Metabolism. *Circ. Res.* **2017**, *121*, 838–854. [CrossRef]
19. Caselli, S.; Jost, C.H.A.; Jenni, R.; Pelliccia, A. Left Ventricular Noncompaction Diagnosis and Management Relevant to Pre-participation Screening of Athletes. *Am. J. Cardiol.* **2015**, *116*, 801–808. [CrossRef]
20. Gati, S.; Papadakis, M.; Papamichael, N.D.; Zaidi, A.; Sheikh, N.; Reed, M.; Sharma, R.; Thilaganathan, B.; Sharma, S. Reversible De Novo Left Ventricular Trabeculations in Pregnant Women. *Circulation* **2014**, *130*, 475–483. [CrossRef]

21. Brigden, W. Uncommon myocardial diseases the non-coronary cardiomyopathies. *Lancet* **1957**, *270*, 1179–1184. [CrossRef]
22. Goodwin, J.F.; Oakley, C.M. The cardiomyopathies. *Br. Heart J.* **1972**, *34*, 545–552. [CrossRef]
23. Richardson, P.; McKenna, W.; Bristow, M.; Maisch, B.; Mautner, B.; O´Connell, J.; Olsen, E.; Thiene, G.; Goodwin, J.; Gyarfas, I.; et al. Report of the 1995 World Health Organization/International Society and Federation of Cardiology Task Force on the Definition and Classification of Cardiomyopathies. *Circulation* **1996**, *93*, 841–842. [PubMed]
24. Maron, B.J.; Towbin, J.A.; Thiene, G.; Antzelevitch, C.; Corrado, D.; Arnett, D.; Moss, A.J.; Seidman, C.E.; Young, J.B. Contemporary definitions and classifications of the cardiomyopathies: An American Heart Association Scientific Statement form the Council on Clinical Cardiology, Heart Failure and Transplantation Committee: Quality of Care and Outcomes Research and functional genomics and translational biology interdisciplinary working groups; and the Council on Epidemiology and Prevention. *Circulation* **2006**, *113*, 1807–1816. [CrossRef]
25. Elliott, P.; Andersson, B.; Arbustini, E.; Bilinska, Z.; Cecchi, F.; Charron, P.; Dubourg, O.; Kuhl, U.; Maisch, B.; McKenna, W.J.; et al. Classification of the cardiomyopathies: A position statement from the European Society of Cardiology Working Group on myocardial and pericardial diseases. *Eur. Heart J.* **2008**, *29*, 270–276. [CrossRef]
26. Arbustini, E.; Narula, N.; Dec, G.W.; Reddy, K.S.; Greenberg, B.; Kushwaha, S.; Marwick, T.; Pinney, S.; Bellazzi, R.; Favalli, V.; et al. The MOGE(S) Classification for a Phenotype–Genotype Nomenclature of Cardiomyopathy: Endorsed by the World Heart Federation. *Glob. Heart* **2013**, *8*, 355–382. [CrossRef] [PubMed]
27. Arbustini, E.; Favalli, V.; Narula, N.; Serio, A.; Grasso, M. Left ventricular noncompaction. A distinct genetic cardiomyopathy. *J. Am. Coll. Cardiol.* **2016**, *68*, 949–966. [CrossRef]
28. van Waning, J.I.; Moesker, J.; Heijsman, D.; Boersma, E.; Majoor-Krakauer, D. Systematic Review of Genotype-Phenotype Correlations in Noncompaction Cardiomyopathy. *J. Am. Heart Assoc.* **2019**, *8*, e012993. [CrossRef]
29. Maheshwari, M.; Gokroo, R.K.; Kaushik, S.K. Isolated non-compacted right ventricular myocardium. *J. Assoc. Physicians India* **2012**, *60*, 56–57.
30. Gomathi, S.B.; Makadia, N.; Ajit, S.M. An unusual case of isolated non-compacted right ventricular myocardium. *Eur. J. Echocardiogr.* **2008**, *9*, 424–425. [CrossRef]
31. Nugent, A.W.; Daubeney, P.E.; Chondros, P.; Carlin, J.B.; Cheung, M.; Wilkinson, L.C.; Davis, A.M.; Kahler, S.G.; Chow, C.; Wilkinson, J.L.; et al. The Epidemiology of Childhood Cardiomyopathy in Australia. *N. Engl. J. Med.* **2003**, *348*, 1639–1646. [CrossRef]
32. Shi, W.Y.; Moreno-Betancur, M.; Nugent, A.W.; Cheung, M.; Colan, S.; Turner, C.; Sholler, G.F.; Robertson, T.; Justo, R.; Bullock, A.; et al. Long-Term Outcomes of Childhood Left Ventricular Noncompaction Cardiomyopathy. *Circulation* **2018**, *138*, 367–376. [CrossRef]
33. Jefferies, J.L.; Wilkinson, J.D.; Sleeper, L.A.; Colan, S.D.; Lu, M.; Pahl, E.; Kantor, P.; Everitt, M.D.; Webber, S.A.; Kaufman, B.D.; et al. Cardiomyopathy Phenotypes and Outcomes for Children with Left Ventricular Myocardial Noncompaction: Results From the Pediatric Cardiomyopathy Registry. *J. Card. Fail.* **2015**, *21*, 877–884. [CrossRef]
34. Charron, P.; Elliott, P.M.; Gimeno, J.R.; Caforio, A.L.P.; Kaski, J.P.; Tavazzi, L.; Tendera, M.; Maupain, C.; Laroche, C.; Rubis, P.; et al. The Cardiomyopathy Registry of the EURObservational Research Programme of the European Society of Cardiology: Baseline data and contemporary management of adult patients with cardiomyopathies. *Eur. Heart J.* **2018**, *39*, 1784–1793. [CrossRef]
35. Seyler, C.; Meder, B.; Weis, T.; Schwaneberg, T.; Weitmann, K.; Hoffmann, W.; Katus, H.A.; Dösch, A. TranslatiOnal Registry for CardiomyopatHies (TORCH)—rationale and first results. *ESC Heart Fail.* **2017**, *4*, 209–215. [CrossRef]
36. Arunamata, A.; Punn, R.; Cuneo, B.; Bharati, S.; Silverman, N.H.; Silverman, N.H. Echocardiographic Diagnosis and Prognosis of Fetal Left Ventricular Noncompaction. *J. Am. Soc. Echocardiogr.* **2012**, *25*, 112–120. [CrossRef]
37. Vinograd, C.A.; Srivastava, S.; Panesar, L.E. Fetal Diagnosis of Left-Ventricular Noncompaction Cardiomyopathy in Identical Twins with Discordant Congenital Heart Disease. *Pediatr. Cardiol.* **2012**, *34*, 1503–1507. [CrossRef]
38. Tian, L.; Zhou, Q.; Zhou, J.; Zeng, S.; Cao, D.; Zhang, M. Ventricular non-compaction cardiomyopathy: Prenatal diagnosis and pathology. *Prenat. Diagn.* **2014**, *35*, 221–227. [CrossRef]
39. Sato, Y.; Matsumoto, N.; Matsuo, S.; Yoda, S.; Iida, K.; Kunimasa, T.; Kunimoto, S.; Saito, S. Isolated noncompaction of the ventricular myocardium in a 94-year-old patient: Depiction at echocardiography and magnetic resonance imaging. *Int. J. Cardiol.* **2007**, *119*, e32–e34. [CrossRef] [PubMed]
40. Murphy, R.T.; Thaman, R.; Blanes, J.G.; Ward, D.; Sevdalis, E.; Papra, E.; Kiotsekolglou, A.; Tome, M.T.; Pellerin, D.; McKenna, W.J.; et al. Natural history and familial characteristics of isolated left ventricular non-compaction. *Eur. Heart J.* **2004**, *26*, 187–192. [CrossRef]
41. Oechslin, E.N.; Jost, C.H.A.; Rojas, J.R.; Kaufmann, P.; Jenni, R. Long-term follow-up of 34 adults with isolated left ventricular noncompaction: A distinct cardiomyopathy with poor prognosis. *J. Am. Coll. Cardiol.* **2000**, *36*, 493–500. [CrossRef]
42. Sandhu, R.; Finkelhor, R.S.; Gunawardena, D.R.; Bahler, R.C. Prevalence and characteristics of left ventricular noncompaction in a community hospital cohort of patients with systolic dysfunction. *Echocardiography* **2008**, *25*, 8–12. [CrossRef] [PubMed]
43. Ritter, M.; Oechslin, E.; Sütsch, G.; Attenhofer, C.; Schneider, J.; Jenni, R. Isolated Noncompaction of the Myocardium in Adults. *Mayo Clin. Proc.* **1997**, *72*, 26–31. [CrossRef]
44. Ross, S.B.; Jones, K.; Blanch, B.; Puranik, R.; McGeechan, K.; Barratt, A.; Semsarian, C. A systematic review and meta-analysis of the prevalence of left ventricular non-compaction in adults. *Eur. Heart J.* **2020**, *41*, 1428–1436. [CrossRef]

45. Weir-McCall, J.R.; Yeap, P.M.; Papagiorcopulo, C.; Fitzgerald, K.; Gandy, S.J.; Lambert, M.; Belch, J.J.F.; Cavin, I.; Littleford, R.; Macfarlane, J.A.; et al. Left Ventricular Noncompaction Anatomical phenotype or distinct cardiomyopathy? *J. Am. Coll. Cardiol.* **2016**, *68*, 2157–2165. [CrossRef]
46. Engberding, R.; Stöllberger, C.; Schneider, B.; Nothnagel, D.; Fehske, W.; Gerecke, B.J. Heart failure in noncompaction cardiomyopathy—Data from the German noncompaction registry (ALKK). *Circulation* **2012**, *126*, A14769.
47. Gerecke, B.; Stoellberger, C.; Schneider, B.; Fehske, W.; Nothnagel, D.; Engberding, R. Arrhythmias in isolated noncompaction cardiomyopathy—Data form the German Noncompaction Registry (ALKK). *Circulation* **2011**, *124*, A11978.
48. Gerecke, B.; Engberding, R. Isolated noncompaction cardiomyopathy with special emphasis on arrhythmia complications. *Herzschr. Elektrophys.* **2012**, *23*, 201–210. [CrossRef]
49. Howard, T.S.; Valdes, S.O.; Hope, K.; Morris, S.A.; Landstrom, A.P.; Schneider, A.E.; Miyake, C.Y.; Denfield, S.W.; Pignatelli, R.H.; Wang, Y.; et al. Association of Wolff-Parkinson-White with Left Ventricular Noncompaction Cardiomyopathy in Children. *J. Card. Fail.* **2019**, *25*, 1004–1008. [CrossRef]
50. Stöllberger, C.; Blazek, G.; Dobias, C.; Hanafin, A.; Wegner, C.; Finsterer, J. Frequency of Stroke and Embolism in Left Ventricular Hypertrabeculation/Noncompaction. *Am. J. Cardiol.* **2011**, *108*, 1021–1023. [CrossRef]
51. Stöllberger, C.; Blazek, G.; Gessner, M.; Bichler, K.; Wegner, C.; Finsterer, J. Neuromuscular comorbidity, heart failure, and atrial fibrillation as prognostic factors in left ventricular hypertrabeculation/noncompaction. *Herz* **2015**, *40*, 906–911. [CrossRef]
52. Stöllberger, C.; Wegner, C.; Finsterer, J. Left ventricular hypertrabeculation/noncompaction, cardiac phenotype, and neuromuscular disorders. *Herz* **2018**, *44*, 659–665. [CrossRef]
53. Moric-Janiszewska, E.; Markiewicz-Łoskot, G. Genetic Heterogeneity of Left-ventricular Noncompaction Cardiomyopathy. *Clin. Cardiol.* **2008**, *31*, 201–204. [CrossRef]
54. Stähli, B.E.; Gebhard, C.; Biaggi, P.; Klaassen, S.; Buechel, E.V.; Jost, C.H.A.; Jenni, R.; Tanner, F.C.; Greutmann, M. Left ventricular non-compaction: Prevalence in congenital heart disease. *Int. J. Cardiol.* **2013**, *167*, 2477–2481. [CrossRef] [PubMed]
55. Jost, C.H.A.; Connolly, H.M.; O'Leary, P.W.; Warnes, C.A.; Tajik, A.J.; Seward, J.B. Left Heart Lesions in Patients With Ebstein Anomaly. *Mayo Clin. Proc.* **2005**, *80*, 361–368. [CrossRef]
56. Friedberg, M.K.; Ursell, P.C.; Silverman, N.H. Isomerism of the Left Atrial Appendage Associated With Ventricular Noncompaction. *Am. J. Cardiol.* **2005**, *96*, 985–990. [CrossRef]
57. Lilje, C.; Porciani, M.C.; Lilli, A.; Macioce, R.; Cappelli, F.; Demarchi, G.; Pappone, A.; Ricciardi, G.; Padeletti, L. Complications of non-compaction of the left ventricular myocardium in a paediatric population: A prospective study. *Eur. Heart J.* **2006**, *27*, 1855–1860. [CrossRef] [PubMed]
58. Finsterer, J. Barth syndrome: Mechanisms and management. *Appl. Clin. Genet.* **2019**, *12*, 95–106. [CrossRef] [PubMed]
59. Panduranga, P.; Mukhaini, M.K. Left-ventricular non-compaction with coronary artery disease. *Int. J. Cardiol.* **2011**, *150*, e37–e39. [CrossRef] [PubMed]
60. Toufan, M.; Shahvalizadeh, R.; Khalili, M. Myocardial infarction in a patient with left ventricular noncompaction: A case report. *Int. J. Gen. Med.* **2012**, *5*, 661–665. [CrossRef] [PubMed]
61. Yavuzgil, O.; Gurgun, C.; Çinar, C.S.; Yüksel, A. Anterior myocardial infarction in an adult patient with left ventricular hypertrabeculation/noncompaction. *Int. J. Cardiol.* **2006**, *106*, 394–395. [CrossRef] [PubMed]
62. Engberding, R.; Stöllberger, C.; Ong, P.; Yelbuz, T.M.; Gerecke, B.J.; Breithardt, G. Isolated Non-Compaction Cardiomyopathy. *Dtsch. Aerzteblatt Online* **2010**, *107*, 206–213. [CrossRef] [PubMed]
63. Paterick, T.E.; Tajik, A.J. Left ventricular noncompaction—A diagnostically challenging cardiomyopathy. *Circ. J.* **2012**, *76*, 1556–1562. [CrossRef]
64. Senior, R.; Becher, H.; Monaghan, M.; Agati, L.; Zamorano, J.; Vanoverschelde, J.L.; Nihoyannopoulos, P.; Edvardsen, T.; Lancellotti, P.; Delgado, V.; et al. Clinical practice of contrast echocardiography: Recommendation by the European Association of Cardiovascular Imaging (EACVI) 2017. *Eur. Heart J. Cardiovasc. Imaging* **2017**, *18*, 1205–1205af. [CrossRef]
65. Bhat, T.; Lafferty, J.; Teli, S.; Rjaili, G.A.; Olkovsky, Y.; Costantino, T. Isolated left ventricular noncompaction cardiomyo-pathy diagnosed by transesophageal echocardiography. *Clin. Med. Insights Cardiol.* **2011**, *5*, 23–27. [CrossRef]
66. Soliman, O.I.; McGhie, J.; ten Cate, F.J.; Paelinck, B.P.; Caliskan, K. Multimodality Imaging, Diagnostic Challenges and Proposed Diagnostic Algorithm for Noncompaction Cardiomyopathy. In *Noncompaction Cardiomyopathy*; Caliskan, K., Soliman, O.I., ten Cate, F.J., Eds.; Springer Nature: Cham, Switzerland, 2019; pp. 17–40.
67. Engberding, R.; Stöllberger, C.; Gerecke, B.J. Left ventricular noncompaction: Affected regions in respect to LV function—Data from the German Noncompaction Registry (ALKK). *Circulation* **2012**, *126*, A14830.
68. Engberding, R.; Gerecke, B. Noncompaction Cardiomyopathy, a Novel Clinical Entity (Historical Perspective). In *Noncompaction Cardiomyopathy*; Caliskan, K., Soliman, O.I., ten Cate, F.J., Eds.; Springer Nature: Cham, Switzerland, 2019; pp. 1–16. [CrossRef]
69. Engberding, R.; Yelbuz, T.M.; Breithardt, G. Isolated noncompaction of the left ventricular myocardium—A review of the literature two decades after the initial case description. *Clin. Res. Cardiol.* **2007**, *96*, 481–488. [CrossRef]
70. Paterick, T.E.; Umland, M.M.; Jan, M.F.; Ammar, K.A.; Kramer, C.; Khandheria, B.K.; Seward, J.B.; Tajik, A.J. Left Ventricular Noncompaction: A 25-Year Odyssey. *J. Am. Soc. Echocardiogr.* **2012**, *25*, 363–375. [CrossRef]
71. Frischknecht, B.S.; Attenhofer Jost, C.H.; Oechslin, E.N.; Seifert, B.; Hoigné, P.; Roos, M.; Jenni, R. Validation of noncompaction criteria in dilated cardiomyopathy, and valvular and hypertensive heart disease. *J. Am. Soc. Echocardiogr.* **2005**, *18*, 865–872. [CrossRef]

72. Belanger, A.R.; Miller, M.A.; Donthireddi, U.R.; Najovits, A.J.; Goldman, M.E. New Classification Scheme of Left Ventricular Noncompaction and Correlation with Ventricular Performance. *Am. J. Cardiol.* **2008**, *102*, 92–96. [CrossRef]
73. Gebhard, C.; Stähli, B.E.; Greutmann, M.; Biaggi, P.; Jenni, R.; Tanner, F.C. Reduced Left Ventricular Compacta Thickness: A Novel Echocardiographic Criterion for Non-Compaction Cardiomyopathy. *J. Am. Soc. Echocardiogr.* **2012**, *25*, 1050–1057. [CrossRef]
74. Sabatino, J.; Di Salvo, G.; Krupickova, S.; Fraisse, A.; Prota, C.; Bucciarelli, V.; Josen, M.; Paredes, J.; Sirico, D.; Voges, I.; et al. Left Ventricular Twist Mechanics to Identify Left Ventricular Noncompaction in Childhood. *Circ. Cardiovasc. Imaging* **2019**, *12*, e007805. [CrossRef]
75. Van Dalen, B.M.; Caliskan, K.; Soliman, O.I.; Nemes, A.; Vletter, W.B.; Cate, F.J.T.; Geleijnse, M.L. Left ventricular solid body rotation in non-compaction cardiomyopathy: A potential new objective and quantitative functional diagnostic criterion? *Eur. J. Heart Fail.* **2008**, *10*, 1088–1093. [CrossRef] [PubMed]
76. Caliskan, K.; Soliman, O.; Nemes, A.; Van Domburg, R.T.; Simoons, M.L.; Geleijnse, M.L. No relationship between left ventricular radial wall motion and longitudinal velocity and the extent and severity of noncompaction cardiomyopathy. *Cardiovasc. Ultrasound* **2012**, *10*, 9. [CrossRef] [PubMed]
77. Rudolecká, J.; Veiser, T.; Plášek, J.; Homza, M.; Fürstová, J. Ventricular twist in isolated left ventricular noncompaction. *Cor. Vasa* **2014**, *56*, e471–e477. [CrossRef]
78. Jenni, R.; Oechslin, E.; Schneider, J.; Attenhofer Jost, J.; Kaufmann, P.A. Echocardiographic and pathoanatomical characteristics of isolated left ventricular non-compaction: A step towards classification as a distinct cardiomyopathy. *Heart* **2001**, *86*, 666–671. [CrossRef]
79. Arunamata, A.; Stringer, J.; Balasubramanian, S.; Tacy, T.A.; Silverman, N.H.; Punn, R. Cardiac Segmental Strain Analysis in Pediatric Left Ventricular Noncompaction Cardiomyopathy. *J. Am. Soc. Echocardiogr.* **2019**, *32*, 763–773. [CrossRef]
80. Huttin, O.; Venner, C.; Frikha, Z.; Voilliot, D.; Marie, P.-Y.; Aliot, E.; Sadoul, N.; Juillière, Y.; Brembilla-Perrot, B.; Selton-Suty, C. Myocardial deformation pattern in left ventricular non-compaction: Comparison with dilated cardiomyopathy. *IJC Heart Vasc.* **2014**, *5*, 9–14. [CrossRef] [PubMed]
81. Stöllberger, C.; Gerecke, B.; Finsterer, J.; Engberding, R. Refinement of echocardiographic criteria for left ventricular noncompaction. *Int. J. Cardiol.* **2013**, *165*, 463–467. [CrossRef]
82. Stöllberger, C.; Gerecke, B.; Engberding, R.; Grabner, B.; Wandaller, C.; Finsterer, J.; Gietzelt, M.; Balzereit, A. Interobserver Agreement of the Echocardiographic Diagnosis of LV Hypertrabeculation/Noncompaction. *JACC Cardiovasc. Imaging* **2015**, *8*, 1252–1257. [CrossRef]
83. Joong, A.; Hayes, D.A.; Anderson, B.R.; Zuckerman, W.A.; Carroll, S.J.; Lai, W.W. Comparison of Echocardiographic Diagnostic Criteria of Left Ventricular Noncompaction in a Pediatric Population. *Pediatr. Cardiol.* **2017**, *38*, 1493–1504. [CrossRef] [PubMed]
84. Kohli, S.K.; Pantazis, A.A.; Shah, J.S.; Adeyemi, B.; Jackson, G.; McKenna, W.J.; Sharma, S.; Elliott, P.M. Diagnosis of left-ventricular non-compaction in patients with left-ventricular systolic dysfunction: Time for a reappraisal of diagnostic criteria? *Eur. Heart J.* **2007**, *29*, 89–95. [CrossRef]
85. Petersen, S.E.; Selvanayagam, J.B.; Wiesmann, F.; Robson, M.D.; Francis, J.M.; Anderson, R.H.; Watkins, H.; Neubauer, S. Left Ventricular Non-Compaction. Insights from cardiovascular magnetic resonance imaging. *J. Am. Coll. Cardiol.* **2005**, *46*, 101–105. [CrossRef] [PubMed]
86. Stacey, R.B.; Andersen, M.M.; Clair, M.S.; Hundley, W.G.; Thohan, V. Comparison of Systolic and Diastolic Criteria for Isolated LV Noncompaction in CMR. *JACC Cardiovasc. Imaging* **2013**, *6*, 931–940. [CrossRef] [PubMed]
87. Jacquier, A.; Thuny, F.; Jop, B.; Giorgi, R.; Cohen, F.; Gaubert, J.-Y.; Vidal, V.; Bartoli, J.M.; Habib, G.; Moulin, G. Measurement of trabeculated left ventricular mass using cardiac magnetic resonance imaging in the diagnosis of left ventricular non-compaction. *Eur. Heart J.* **2010**, *31*, 1098–1104. [CrossRef]
88. Captur, G.; Zemrak, F.; Muthurangu, V.; Petersen, S.E.; Chumming, L.; Bassett, P.; Kawel-Boehm, N.; McKenna, W.J.; Elliott, P.M.; Lima, J.A.; et al. Fractal analysis of myocardial trabeculations in 2547 study participants: Multi-ethnic study of atherosclerosis. *Radiology* **2015**, *277*, 707–715. [CrossRef]
89. Grothoff, M.; Pachowsky, M.; Hoffmann, J.; Posch, M.; Klaassen, S.; Lehmkuhl, L.; Gutberlet, M. Value of cardiovascular MR in diagnosing left ventricular non-compaction cardiomyopathy and in discriminating between other cardiomyopathies. *Eur. Radiol.* **2012**, *22*, 2699–2709. [CrossRef]
90. Dreisbach, J.G.; Mathur, S.; Houbois, C.P.; Oechslin, E.; Ross, H.; Hanneman, K.; Wintersperger, B.J. Cardiovascular magnetic resonance based diagnosis of left ventricular non-compaction cardiomyopathy: Impact of cine bSSFP strain analysis. *J. Cardiovasc. Magn. Reson.* **2020**, *22*, 1–14. [CrossRef]
91. Dodd, J.D.; Holmvang, G.; Hoffmann, U.; Ferencik, M.; Abbara, S.; Brady, T.J.; Cury, R.C. Quantification of Left Ventricular Noncompaction and Trabecular Delayed Hyperenhancement with Cardiac MRI: Correlation with Clinical Severity. *Am. J. Roentgenol.* **2007**, *189*, 974–980. [CrossRef]
92. Choi, Y.; Kim, S.M.; Lee, S.-C.; Chang, S.-A.; Jang, S.Y.; Choe, Y.H. Quantification of left ventricular trabeculae using cardiovascular magnetic resonance for the diagnosis of left ventricular non-compaction: Evaluation of trabecular volume and refined semi-quantitative criteria. *J. Cardiovasc. Magn. Reson.* **2016**, *18*, 1–13. [CrossRef]
93. Miller, E.M.; Hinton, R.B.; Czosek, R.; Lorts, A.; Parrott, A.; Shikany, A.R.; Ittenbach, R.F.; Ware, S.M. Genetic Testing in Pediatric Left Ventricular Noncompaction. *Circ. Cardiovasc. Genet.* **2017**, *10*, e001735. [CrossRef]

94. Donal, E.; Delgado, V.; Bucciarelli-Ducci, C.; Galli, E.; Haugaa, K.H.; Charron, P.; Voigt, J.-U.; Cardim, N.; Masci, P.G.; Galderisi, M.; et al. Multimodality imaging in the diagnosis, risk stratification, and management of patients with dilated cardiomyopathies: An expert consensus document from the European Association of Cardiovascular Imaging. *Eur. Heart J. Cardiovasc. Imaging* **2019**, *20*, 1075–1093. [CrossRef]
95. Conces, D.J.; Ryan, T.; Tarver, R.D. Noncompaction of ventricular myocardium: CT appearance. *Am. J. Roentgenol.* **1991**, *156*, 717–718. [CrossRef] [PubMed]
96. Meléndez-Ramírez, G.; Castillo-Castellon, F.; Espínola-Zavaleta, N.; Meave, A.; Kimura-Hayama, E.T. Left ventricular noncompaction: A proposal of new diagnostic criteria by multidetector computed tomography. *J. Cardiovasc. Comput. Tomogr.* **2012**, *6*, 346–354. [CrossRef]
97. Fuchs, T.A.; Erhart, L.; Ghadri, J.R.; Herzog, B.A.; Giannopoulos, A.; Buechel, R.R.; Stämpfli, S.F.; Gruner, C.; Pazhenkottil, A.P.; Niemann, M.; et al. Diagnostic criteria for left ventricular non-compaction in cardiac computed tomography. *PLoS ONE* **2020**, *15*, e0235751. [CrossRef]
98. Stöllberger, C.; Winkler-Dworak, M.; Blazek, G.; Finsterer, J. Association of Electrocardiographic Abnormalities with Cardiac Findings and Neuromuscular Disorders in Left Ventricular Hypertrabeculation/Non-Compaction. *Cardiology* **2007**, *107*, 374–379. [CrossRef] [PubMed]
99. Rapatz, K.; Finsterer, J.; Voill-Glaninger, A.; Wilfinger-Lutz, N.; Winkler-Dworak, M.; Stöllberger, C. NT-pro-BNP in patients with left ventricular hypertrabeculation/non-compaction. *ESC Heart Fail.* **2020**, *7*, 4126–4133. [CrossRef] [PubMed]
100. Finsterer, J.; Stöllberger, C.; Krugluger, W. Positive troponin-T in noncompaction is associated with neuromuscular disorders and poor outcome. *Clin. Res. Cardiol.* **2006**, *96*, 109–113. [CrossRef]
101. Biagini, E.; Ragni, L.; Ferlito, M.; Pasquale, F.; Lofiego, C.; Leone, O.; Rocchi, G.; Perugini, E.; Zagnoni, S.; Branzi, A.; et al. Different Types of Cardiomyopathy Associated with Isolated Ventricular Noncompaction. *Am. J. Cardiol.* **2006**, *98*, 821–824. [CrossRef]
102. Stollberger, C.; Finsterer, J. Pitfalls in the diagnosis of left ventricular hypertrabeculation/non-compaction. *Postgrad. Med. J.* **2006**, *82*, 679–683. [CrossRef] [PubMed]
103. Schaufelberger, M. Cardiomyopathy and pregnancy. *Heart* **2019**, *105*, 1543–1551. [CrossRef]
104. Reimold, S.C. Reversible left ventricular trabeculations in pregnancy. Is this sufficient to make the diagnosis of left ventricular noncompaction? *Circulation* **2014**, *130*, 453–456. [CrossRef]
105. Rajagopalan, N.; Attili, A.K.; Bodiwala, K.; Bailey, A.L. Features of left ventricular noncompaction in peripartum cardiomyopathy: A case series. *Int. J. Cardiol.* **2013**, *165*, e13–e14. [CrossRef]
106. Luijkx, T.; Cramer, M.J.; Zaidi, A.; Rienks, R.; Senden, P.J.; Sharma, S.; Van Hellemondt, F.J.; Buckens, C.F.; Mali, W.P.; Velthuis, B.K. Ethnic differences in ventricular hypertrabeculation on cardiac MRI in elite football players. *Neth. Heart J.* **2012**, *20*, 389–395. [CrossRef]
107. de la Chica, J.A.; Gómez-Talavera, S.; García-Ruiz, J.M.; García-Lunar, I.; Oliva, B.; Fernández-Alvira, J.M.; López-Melgar, B.; Sánchez-González, J.; de la Pompa, J.L.; Mendiguren, J.M.; et al. Association Between Left Ventricular Noncompaction and Vigorous Physical Activity. *J. Am. Coll. Cardiol.* **2020**, *76*, 1723–1733. [CrossRef]
108. Loria, V.; Colizzi, C.; Vaccarella, M.; Franceschi, F.; Aspromonte, N. Left Ventricular Noncompaction: Cause or Consequence of Myocardial Disease? A Case Report and Literature Review. *Cardiology* **2019**, *143*, 100–104. [CrossRef] [PubMed]
109. Luckie, M.; Irwin, B.; Nair, S.; Greenwood, J.; Khattar, R. Left ventricular non-compaction in identical twins with thalassaemia and cardiac iron overload. *Eur. J. Echocardiogr.* **2009**, *10*, 509–512. [CrossRef] [PubMed]
110. Harvey, R.P. Patterning the vertebrate heart. *Nat. Rev. Genet.* **2002**, *3*, 544–556. [CrossRef]
111. Srivastava, D.; Olson, E.N. A genetic blueprint for cardiac development. *Nat. Cell Biol.* **2000**, *407*, 221–226. [CrossRef] [PubMed]
112. Sedmera, D.; Pexieder, T.; Vuillemin, M.; Thompson, R.P.; Anderson, R.H. Developmental patterning of the myocardium. *Anat. Rec.* **2000**, *258*, 319–337. [CrossRef]
113. Agmon, Y.; Connolly, H.M.; Olson, L.J.; Khandheria, B.K.; Seward, J.B. Noncompaction of the Ventricular Myocardium. *J. Am. Soc. Echocardiogr.* **1999**, *12*, 859–863. [CrossRef]
114. Bernanke, D.H.; Velkey, J.M. Development of the coronary blood supply: Changing concepts and current ideas. *Anat. Rec. Adv. Integr. Anat. Evol. Biol.* **2002**, *269*, 198–208. [CrossRef]
115. Freedom, R.M.; Yoo, S.-J.; Perrin, D.; Taylor, G.; Petersen, S.; Anderson, R.H. The morphological spectrum of ventricular noncompaction. *Cardiol. Young* **2005**, *15*, 345–364. [CrossRef] [PubMed]
116. Henderson, D.J.; Anderson, R.H. The Development and Structure of the Ventricles in the Human Heart. *Pediatr. Cardiol.* **2009**, *30*, 588–596. [CrossRef] [PubMed]
117. MacGrogan, D.; Münch, J.; De La Pompa, J.L. Notch and interacting signalling pathways in cardiac development, disease, and regeneration. *Nat. Rev. Cardiol.* **2018**, *15*, 685–704. [CrossRef]
118. Luxán, G.; Casanova, J.C.; Martínez-Poveda, B.; Prados, B.; D'Amato, G.; MacGrogan, D.; Gonzalez-Rajal, A.; Dobarro, D.; Torroja, C.; Martinez, F.; et al. Mutations in the NOTCH pathway regulator MIB1 cause left ventricular noncompaction cardiomyopathy. *Nat. Med.* **2013**, *19*, 193–201. [CrossRef]
119. Meyer, D.; Birchmeier, C. Multiple essential functions of neuregulin in development. *Nat. Cell Biol.* **1995**, *378*, 386–390. [CrossRef]
120. Gassmann, M.; Casagranda, F.; Orioli, D.; Simon, H.; Lai, C.; Klein, R.; Lemke, G. Aberrant neural and cardiac development in mice lacking the ErbB4 neuregulin receptor. *Nat. Cell Biol.* **1995**, *378*, 390–394. [CrossRef]

121. Choquet, C.; Kelly, R.; Miquerol, L. Defects in Trabecular Development Contribute to Left Ventricular Noncompaction. *Pediatr. Cardiol.* **2019**, *40*, 1331–1338. [CrossRef]
122. Allenby, P.A.; Gould, N.S.; Schwartz, M.F.; Chiemmongkoltip, P. Dysplastic cardiac development presenting as cardiomyopathy. *Arch Pathol. Lab Med.* **1988**, *122*, 1255–1258.
123. Boyd, M.T.; Seward, J.B.; Tajik, A.J.; Edwards, W.D. Frequency and location of prominent left ventricular trabeculations at autopsy in 474 normal human hearts: Implications for evaluation of mural thrombi by two-dimensional echocardiography. *J. Am. Coll. Cardiol.* **1987**, *9*, 323–326. [CrossRef]
124. Stöllberger, C.; Finsterer, J. Left ventricular hypertrabeculation/noncompaction. *J. Am. Soc. Echocardiogr.* **2004**, *17*, 91–100. [CrossRef]
125. Burke, A.; Mont, E.; Kutys, R.; Virmani, R. Left ventricular noncompaction: A pathological study of 14 cases. *Hum. Pathol.* **2005**, *36*, 403–411. [CrossRef] [PubMed]
126. Finsterer, J.; Stöllberger, C. Ultrastructural Findings in Noncompaction Prevail with Neuromuscular Disorders. *Cardiology* **2013**, *126*, 219–223. [CrossRef] [PubMed]
127. Prentice, H. Studies on Left Ventricular Hypertrabeculation/Noncompaction: The Need for In-Depth Ultrastructural Investigations. *Cardiology* **2013**, *126*, 255–257. [CrossRef] [PubMed]
128. Bleyl, S.B.; Mumford, B.R.; Thompson, V.; Carey, J.C.; Pysher, T.J.; Chin, T.K.; Ward, K. Neonatal, Lethal Noncompaction of the Left Ventricular Myocardium Is Allelic with Barth Syndrome. *Am. J. Hum. Genet.* **1997**, *61*, 868–872. [CrossRef]
129. Bozkurt, B.; Colvin, M.; Cook, J.; Cooper, L.T.; Deswal, A.; Fonarow, G.; Francis, G.S.; Lenihan, D.; Lewis, E.F.; McNamara, D.M.; et al. Current Diagnostic and Treatment Strategies for Specific Dilated Cardiomyopathies: A Scientific Statement from the American Heart Association. *Circulation* **2016**, *134*, e579–e646. [CrossRef] [PubMed]
130. Corrado, G.; Checcarelli, N.; Santarone, M.; Stöllberger, C.; Finsterer, J. Left Ventricular Hypertrabeculation/Noncompaction with PMP22 Duplication-Based Charcot-Marie-Tooth Disease Type 1A. *Cardiology* **2006**, *105*, 142–145. [CrossRef]
131. Johnson, M.T.; Zhang, S.; Gilkeson, R.; Ameduri, R.; Siwik, E.; Patel, C.R.; Chebotarev, O.; Kenton, A.B.; Bowles, K.R.; Towbin, J.A.; et al. Intrafamilial variability of noncompaction of the ventricular myocardium. *Am. Heart J.* **2006**, *151*, 1012–e7. [CrossRef]
132. Klaassen, S.; Probst, S.; Oechslin, E.; Gerull, B.; Krings, G.; Schuler, P.; Greutmann, M.; Hurlimann, D.; Yegitbasi, M.; Pons, L.; et al. Mutations in Sarcomere Protein Genes in Left Ventricular Noncompaction. *Circulation* **2008**, *117*, 2893–2901. [CrossRef]
133. Vio, R.; Angelini, A.; Basso, C.; Cipriani, A.; Zorzi, A.; Melacini, P.; Thiene, G.; Rampazzo, A.; Corrado, D.; Calore, C. Hypertrophic Cardiomyopathy and Primary Restrictive Cardiomyopathy: Similarities, Differences and Phenocopies. *J. Clin. Med.* **2021**, *10*, 1954. [CrossRef]
134. van Waning, J.I.; Caliskan, K.; Michels, M.; Schinkel, A.F.; Hirsch, A.; Dalinghaus, M.; Hoedemaekers, Y.M.; Wessels, M.W.; IJpma, A.S.; Hofstra, R.M.; et al. Cardiac Phenotypes, Genetics, and Risks in Familial Noncompaction Cardiomyopathy. *J. Am. Coll. Cardiol.* **2019**, *73*, 1601–1611. [CrossRef] [PubMed]
135. Shan, L.; Makita, N.; Xing, Y.; Watanabe, S.; Futatani, T.; Ye, F.; Saito, K.; Ibuki, K.; Watanabe, K.; Hirono, K. SCN5A variants in Japanese patients with left ventricular noncompaction and arrhythmia. *Mol. Genet. Metab.* **2008**, *93*, 468–474. [CrossRef] [PubMed]
136. Kolokotronis, K.; Kühnisch, J.; Klopocki, E.; Dartsch, J.; Rost, S.; Huculak, C.; Mearini, G.; Störk, S.; Carrier, L.; Klaassen, S.; et al. Biallelic mutation in MYH7 and MYBPC3 leads to severe cardiomyopathy with left ventricular noncompaction phenotype. *Hum. Mutat.* **2019**, *40*, 1101–1114. [CrossRef]
137. Ichida, F. Left ventricular noncompaction—risk stratification and genetic consideration. *J. Cardiol.* **2019**, *75*, 1–9. [CrossRef] [PubMed]
138. Mazzarotto, F.; Hawley, M.H.; Beltrami, M.; Beekman, L.; de Marvao, A.; McGurk, K.A.; Statton, B.; Boschi, B.; Girolami, F.; Roberts, A.M.; et al. Systematic large-scale assessment of the genetic architecture of left ventricular noncompaction reveals diverse etiologies. *Genet. Med.* **2021**, *23*, 856–864. [CrossRef] [PubMed]
139. Ross, S.B.; Singer, E.S.; Driscoll, E.; Nowak, N.; Yeates, L.; Puranik, R.; Sy, R.W.; Rajagopalan, S.; Barratt, A.; Ingles, J.; et al. Genetic architecture of left ventricular noncompaction in adults. *Hum. Genome Var.* **2020**, *7*, 33. [CrossRef]
140. Hershberger, R.E.; Givertz, M.M.; Ho, C.Y.; Judge, D.P.; Kantor, P.F.; McBride, K.L.; Morales, A.; Taylor, M.R.; Vatta, M. Genetic evaluation of cardiomyopathy: A clinical practice resource of the American College of Medical Genetics and Genomics (ACMG). *Genet. Med.* **2018**, *20*, 899–909. [CrossRef]
141. Ackerman, M.J.; Priori, S.G.; Willems, S.; Berul, C.; Brugada, R.; Calkins, H.; Camm, J.; Ellinor, P.T.; Gollob, M.; Hamilton, R.; et al. HRS/EHRA Consensus statement on the state of genetic testing for the channelopathies and cardiomyopathies. *Europace* **2011**, *13*, 1077–1109. [CrossRef] [PubMed]
142. Schulze-Bahr, E.; Klaassen, S.; Abdul-Khaliq, H.; Schunkert, H. Gendiagnostik bei kardiovaskulären Erkrankungen. Positionspapier der Deutschen Gesellschaft für Kardiologie (DGK) und der Deutschen Gesellschaft für Pädiatrische Kardiologie (DGPK). *Kardiologe* **2015**, *9*, 213–243. [CrossRef]
143. Musunuru, K.; Hershberger, R.E.; Day, S.M.; Klinedinst, N.J.; Landstrom, A.P.; Parikh, V.N.; Prakash, S.; Semsarian, C.; Sturm, A.C. on behalf of the American Heart Association Council on Genomic and Precision Medicine; Council on Arteriosclerosis, Thrombosis and Vascular Biology; Council on Cardiovascular and Stroke Nursing; and Council on Clinical Cardiology. Genetic Testing for inherited cardiovascular diseases. *Circ. Genom. Precis. Med.* **2020**, *13*, e000067. [CrossRef]

144. Zemrak, F.; Raisi-Estabragh, Z.; Khanji, M.Y.; Mohiddin, S.A.; Bruder, O.; Wagner, A.; Lombardi, M.; Schwitter, J.; Van Rossum, A.C.; Pilz, G.; et al. Left Ventricular Hypertrabeculation Is Not Associated With Cardiovascular Morbity or Mortality: Insights From the Eurocmr Registry. *Front. Cardiovasc. Med.* **2020**, *7*, 158. [CrossRef]
145. Petersen, S.; Neubauer, S. Excessive trabeculations and prognosis. The plot thickens. *Circ. Cardiovasc. Imaging* **2017**, *10*, e006908. [CrossRef]
146. Lofiego, C.; Biagini, E.; Ferlito, M.; Pasquale, F.; Rocchi, G.; Perugini, E.; Leone, O.; Bracchetti, G.; Caliskan, K.; Branzi, A.; et al. Paradoxical Contributions of Non-Compacted and Compacted Segments to Global Left Ventricular Dysfunction in Isolated Left Ventricular Noncompaction. *Am. J. Cardiol.* **2006**, *97*, 738–741. [CrossRef]
147. Gerecke, B.J.; Stoellberger, C.; Gietzelt, M.; Haux, R.; Engberding, R. Risk factors in noncompaction cardiomyopathy—Data form the German Noncompaction Registry (ALKK). *Eur. Heart J.* **2013**, *34* (Suppl. 1), 166. [CrossRef]
148. Pignatelli, R.H.; MacMahon, C.J.-; Dreyer, W.J.; Denfield, S.W.; Price, J.; Belmont, J.W.; Craigen, W.J.; Wu, J.; El Said, H.; Bezold, L.I.; et al. Clinical characterization of left ventricular noncompaction in children. A relatively common form of cardiomyopathy. *Circulation* **2003**, *108*, 2672–2678. [CrossRef] [PubMed]
149. Al-Wakeel-Marquard, N.; Degener, F.; Herbst, C.; Kühnisch, J.; Dartsch, J.; Schmitt, B.; Kuehne, T.; Messroghli, D.; Berger, F.; Klaassen, S. RIKADA Study Reveals Risk Factors in Pediatric Primary Cardiomyopathy. *J. Am. Heart Assoc.* **2019**, *8*, e012531. [CrossRef] [PubMed]
150. Van Waning, J.I.; Caliskan, K.; Hoedemaekers, Y.M.; Van Spaendonck-Zwarts, K.Y.; Baas, A.F.; Boekholdt, S.M.; Van Melle, J.P.; Teske, A.J.; Asselbergs, F.W.; Backx, P.C.M.; et al. Genetics, Clinical Features, and Long-Term Outcome of Noncompaction Cardiomyopathy. *J. Am. Coll. Cardiol.* **2018**, *71*, 711–722. [CrossRef] [PubMed]
151. Sedaghat-Hamedani, F.; Haas, J.; Zhu, F.; Geier, C.; Kayvanpour, E.; Liss, M.; Lai, A.; Frese, K.; Pribe-Wolferts, R.; Amr, A.; et al. Clinical genetics and outcome of left ventricular non-compaction cardiomyopathy. *Eur. Heart J.* **2017**, *38*, 3449–3460. [CrossRef]
152. Aung, N.; Doimo, S.; Ricci, F.; Sanghvi, M.M.; Pedrosa, C.; Woodbridge, S.P.; Al-Balah, A.; Zemrak, F.; Khanji, M.Y.; Naci, H.; et al. Prognostic significance of left ventricular noncompaction. Systematic review and meta-analysis of observational studies. *Circ. Cardiovasc. Imaging* **2020**, *13*, e009712. [CrossRef] [PubMed]
153. Amzulescu, M.S.; Rousseau, M.F.; Ahn, S.A.; Boileau, L.; de Mester de Ravenstein, C.; Vancraeynest, D.; Pasquet, A.; Vanoverschelde, J.L.; Pouleur, A.C.; Gerber, B.L. Prognostic impact of hypertrabeculation and noncompaction phenotype in dilated cardiomyopathy. A CMR study. *J. Am. Coll. Cardiol. Imging* **2015**, *8*, 934–946. [CrossRef] [PubMed]
154. Romano, S.; Judd, R.M.; Kim, R.J.; Kim, H.W.; Klem, I.; Heitner, J.F.; Shah, D.J.; Jue, J.; White, B.E.; Indorkar, R.; et al. Feature-Tracking Global Longitudinal Strain Predicts Death in a Multicenter Population of Patients with Ischemic and Nonischemic Dilated Cardiomyopathy Incremental to Ejection Fraction and Late Gadolinium Enhancement. *JACC Cardiovasc. Imaging* **2018**, *11*, 1419–1429. [CrossRef]
155. Grigoratos, C.; Barison, A.; Ivanov, A.; Andreini, D.; Amzulescu, M.S.; Mazurkiewicz, L.; de Luca, A.; Grzybowski, J.; Masci, P.G.; Marczak, M.; et al. Meta-analysis of the prognostic role of late gadolinium enhancement and global systolic impairment in left ventricular noncompaction. *J. Am. Coll. Cardiol. Imag* **2019**, *12*, 2141–2151. [CrossRef]
156. Ashrith, G.; Gupta, D.; Hanmer, J.; Weiss, R.M. Cardiovascular magnetic resonance characterization of left ventricular non-compaction provides independent prognostic information in patients with incident heart failure or suspected cardiomyopathy. *J. Cardiovasc. Magn. Reson.* **2014**, *16*, 64. [CrossRef]
157. Minamisawa, M.; Koyama, J.; Kozuka, A.; Miura, T.; Ebisawa, S.; Motoki, H.; Okada, A.; Izawa, A.; Ikeda, U.; Information, P.E.K.F.C. Regression of left ventricular hypertrabeculation is associated with improvement in systolic function and favorable prognosis in adult patients with non-ischemic cardiomyopathy. *J. Cardiol.* **2016**, *68*, 431–438. [CrossRef] [PubMed]
158. Bertini, M.; Ziacchi, M.; Biffi, M.; Biagini, E.; Rocchi, G.; Martignani, C.; Ferlito, M.; Pasquale, F.; Cervi, E.; Branzi, A.; et al. Effects of cardiac resynchronisation therapy on dilated cardiomyopathy with isolated ventricular non-compaction. *Heart* **2010**, *97*, 295–300. [CrossRef] [PubMed]
159. Uribarri, A.; Rojas, S.V.; Avsar, M.; Hanke, J.S.; Napp, L.C.; Berliner, D.; Bavendiek, U.; Bauersachs, J.; Bara, C.; Sanchez, P.L.; et al. First series of mechanical circulatory support in non-compaction cardiomyopathy: Is LVAD implantation a safe alternative? *Int. J. Cardiol.* **2015**, *197*, 128–132. [CrossRef]
160. Kovacevic-Preradovic, T.; Jenni, R.; Oechslin, E.; Noll, G.; Seifert, B.; Jost, C.A. Isolated Left Ventricular Noncompaction as a Cause for Heart Failure and Heart Transplantation: A Single Center Experience. *Cardiology* **2009**, *112*, 158–164. [CrossRef] [PubMed]
161. Gerecke, B.; Stöllberger, C.; Gradaus, F.; Andresen, H.; Engberding, R. ICD therapy in noncompaction cardiomyopathy: Data from the German left ventricular noncompaction registry (ALKK). *Circulation* **2009**, *120*, A2342.
162. Sohns, C.; Ouyang, F.; Volkmer, M.; Metzner, A.; Nürnberg, J.H.; Ventura, R.; Gerecke, B.; Jansen, H.; Reinhardt, A.; Kuck, K.-H.; et al. Therapy of ventricular arrhythmias in patients suffering from isolated left ventricular non-compaction cardiomyopathy. *Europace* **2019**, *21*, 961–969. [CrossRef] [PubMed]

163. Hindricks, G.; Potpara, T.; Dagres, N.; Arbelo, E.; Bax, J.J.; Blomström-Lundqvist, C.; Boriani, G.; Castella, M.; Dan, G.A.; Dilaveris, P.E.; et al. 2020 ESC Guidelines for the diagnosis and management of atrial fibrillation developed in collaboration with the European Association for Cardio-Thoracic Surgery (EACTS): The Task Force for the diagnosis and management of atrial fibrillation of the European Society of Cardiology (ESC) Developed with the special contribution of the European Heart Rhythm Association (EHRA) of the ESC. *Eur. Heart J.* **2020**, 1125. [CrossRef]
164. Epstein, A.E.; DiMarco, J.P.; Ellenbogen, K.A.; Estes, N.A.M.; Freedman, R.A.; Gettes, L.S.; Gillinov, A.M.; Gregoratos, G.; Hammill, S.C.; Hayes, D.L.; et al. ACC/AHA/HRS 2008 Guidelines for device-based therapy of cardiac rhythm abnormalities. *J. Am. Coll. Cardiol.* **2008**, *51*, e1–e61. [CrossRef]
165. Priori, S.G.; Blomström-Lundqvist, C.; Mazzanti, A.; Blom, N.; Borggrefe, M.; Camm, J.; Elliott, P.M.; Fitzsimons, D.; Hatala, R. 2015 ESC Guidelines for the management of patients with ventricular arrhythmias and the prevention of sudden cardiac death. *Eur. Heart J.* **2015**, *36*, 2793–2867. [CrossRef] [PubMed]
166. Al-Khatib, S.; Stevenson, W.G.; Ackerman, M.J.; Bryant, W.J.; Callans, D.J.; Curtis, A.B.; Deal, B.J.; Dickfeld, T.; Field, M.E.; Fonarow, G.C.; et al. 2017 AHA/ACC/HRS Guideline for management of patients with ventricular arrhythmias and the prevention of sudden cardia death. *Circulation* **2018**, *138*, e272–e391. [CrossRef] [PubMed]
167. Takamatsu, M.; Kamohara, K.; Sato, M.; Koga, Y. Effect of Noncompacted Myocardial Resection on Isolated Left Ventricular Noncompaction. *Ann. Thorac. Surg.* **2020**, *110*, e387–e389. [CrossRef]
168. Sharma, S.; Gati, S.; Back, M.; Börjesson, M.; Caselli, S.; Collet, J.P.; Corrado, D.; Drezner, J.A.; Halle, M.; Hansen, D.; et al. 2020 ESC Guidelines on sports cardiology and exercise in patients with cardiovascular disease. *Eur. Heart J.* **2021**, *41*, 17–96. [CrossRef] [PubMed]

Journal of
Clinical Medicine

MDPI

Review

Arrhythmogenic Cardiomyopathy—Current Treatment and Future Options

Federico Migliore †, Giulia Mattesi †, Alessandro Zorzi , Barbara Bauce, Ilaria Rigato, Domenico Corrado * and Alberto Cipriani

Department of Cardiac, Thoracic and Vascular Sciences and Public Health, University of Padova, Via Giustiniani 2, 35128 Padova, Italy; federico.migliore@unipd.it (F.M.); g.mattesi17@gmail.com (G.M.); alessandro.zorzi@unipd.it (A.Z.); barbara.bauce@unipd.it (B.B.); ilaria.rigato@unipd.it (I.R.); alberto.cipriani@unipd.it (A.C.)

* Correspondence: domenico.corrado@unipd.it; Tel.: +39-049-821-2322; Fax: +39-049-821-2309

† These authors contributed equally as first authors.

Abstract: Arrhythmogenic cardiomyopathy (ACM) is an inheritable heart muscle disease characterised pathologically by fibrofatty myocardial replacement and clinically by ventricular arrhythmias (VAs) and sudden cardiac death (SCD). Although, in its original description, the disease was believed to predominantly involve the right ventricle, biventricular and left-dominant variants, in which the myocardial lesions affect in parallel or even mostly the left ventricle, are nowadays commonly observed. The clinical management of these patients has two main purposes: the prevention of SCD and the control of arrhythmic and heart failure (HF) events. An implantable cardioverter defibrillator (ICD) is the only proven lifesaving treatment, despite significant morbidity because of device-related complications and inappropriate shocks. Selection of patients who can benefit the most from ICD therapy is one of the most challenging issues in clinical practice. Risk stratification in ACM patients is mostly based on arrhythmic burden and ventricular dysfunction severity, although other clinical features resulting from electrocardiogram and imaging modalities such as cardiac magnetic resonance may have a role. Medical therapy is crucial for treatment of VAs and the prevention of negative ventricular remodelling. In this regard, the efficacy of novel anti-HF molecules and drugs acting on the inflammatory pathway in patients with ACM is, to date, unknown. Catheter ablation represents an effective strategy to treat ventricular tachycardia relapses and recurrent ICD shocks. The present review will address the current strategies for prevention of SCD and treatment of VAs and HF in patients with ACM.

Keywords: arrhythmogenic cardiomyopathy; risk stratification; drug therapy; implantable cardioverter defibrillator; catheter ablation; treatment

Citation: Migliore, F.; Mattesi, G.; Zorzi, A.; Bauce, B.; Rigato, I.; Corrado, D.; Cipriani, A. Arrhythmogenic Cardiomyopathy—Current Treatment and Future Options. *J. Clin. Med.* **2021**, *10*, 2750. https://doi.org/10.3390/jcm10132750

Academic Editor: Stefan Peters

Received: 30 April 2021
Accepted: 14 June 2021
Published: 22 June 2021

1. Introduction

1.1. Definition and Classification

Arrhythmogenic cardiomyopathy (ACM) is a genetically determined heart muscle disease characterised pathologically by fibrofatty replacement of right and left ventricular myocardium and clinically by ventricular arrhythmias (VAs) and arrhythmic sudden cardiac death (SCD) [1].

Although the fibrofatty tissue is usually considered the hallmark lesion of ACM, it should be more properly regarded as a marker of advanced stages of the disease [2]. Experimental studies on transgenic animal models showed a histologic pattern consistent with acute myocarditis in the early stages of the disease [3]. The pathological process progresses from the epicardium to the endocardium, leading to wall thinning and aneurysm formation, typically localised at the inferior wall, apex, and infundibulum of the right ventricle (RV) (the so called "triangle of dysplasia") [2,4]. Indeed, in its original description, the disease was characterised by a predominant involvement of the RV ("Arrhythmogenic right ventricular cardiomyopathy, ARVC"), with left ventricular deterioration occurring later in the history of the disease. However, autopsy investigations, genotype–phenotype correlation studies, and the increasing use of contrast-enhanced cardiac magnetic resonance (CMR) led to the discovery of biventricular and left-dominant variants, in which the myocardial lesions do not remain confined to the RV, but affect in parallel or even predominantly the left ventricle (LV) [5]. When the LV, whose wall is thicker than that of the RV, is involved in the disease process, the fibrofatty scar tends to remain confined to the subepicardial layers, sparing the sub-endocardium, which mostly contribute to myocardial thickening [6]. Indeed, LV lesions do not determine wall thinning nor wall motion abnormalities, making the diagnosis more challenging (Figure 1).

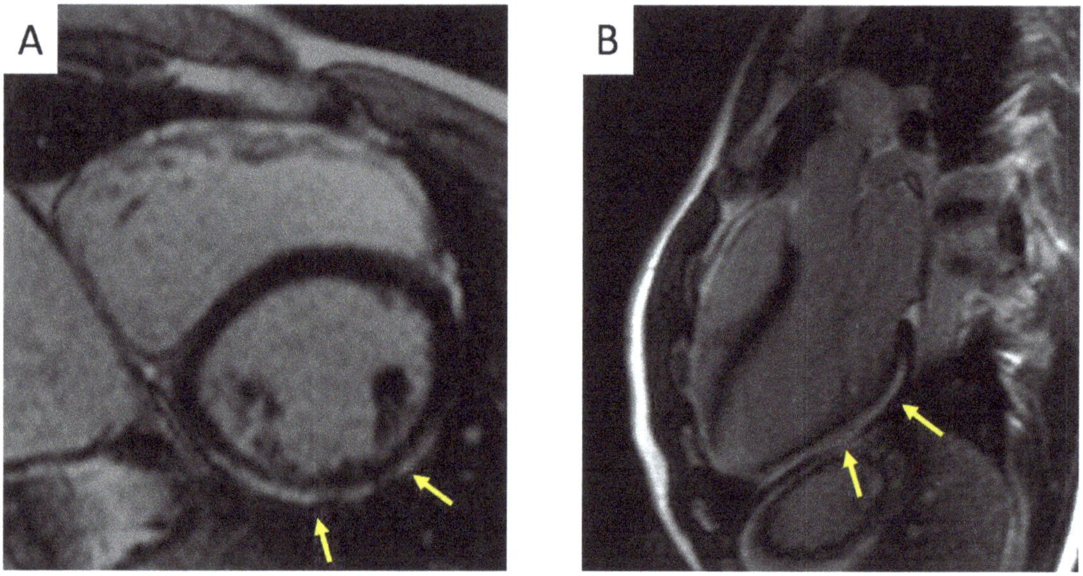

Figure 1. Cardiac magnetic resonance in a patient with a desmosomal gene related biventricular ACM showing the typical LV LGE pattern. (**A**) Short axis view demonstrating subepicardial LGE at the LV mid-inferolateral segments. (**B**) Three-chamber view exhibiting extensive LGE stria at the LV posterolateral wall. ACM = arrhythmogenic cardiomyopathy; LGE = late gadolinium enhancement; LV = left ventricle.

The disease is phenotypically classified in three variants: "right dominant", characterised by the predominant RV involvement, with no LV abnormalities; "biventricular" with involvement of both the RV and LV; and "left dominant" (also referred to as "Arrhythmogenic left ventricular cardiomyopathy, ALVC") characterised by a predominant LV involvement, with no RV abnormalities. The broader term "Arrhythmogenic cardiomyopathy, ACM" is currently used to encompass the whole spectrum of the abovementioned disease phenotypic expressions [7]. This term should not be confused with the one of "arrhythmogenic cardiomyopathies", which has been proposed to comprise a series of different conditions that share non-ischemic myocardial scarring and the propensity to scar-related VAs [7]. In the present review, the term ACM refers to the phenotypic variants of a genetically determined cardiomyopathy whose hallmark lesion is the fibrofatty replacement, which can localise in the RV (ARVC), LV (ALVC) or both ventricles (biventricular ACM).

1.2. Genetic Background

Arrhythmogenic cardiomyopathy is generally transmitted as an autosomal dominant trait that is age-related, with incomplete penetrance and variable expressivity. For the classic right-dominant variant, the mutant genes are those encoding for desmosomal proteins, such as plakoglobin (*JUP*), plakophilin-2 (*PKP2*), desmoplakin (*DSP*), desmoglein (*DSG2*), and desmocollin (*DSC2*) [8–12]. In addition, genes encoding for adherent junctional proteins, such as α-T-catenin (*CTNNA3*) and N-cadherin (*CDH2*), have also arose as potentially relevant in the pathogenesis of ACM [13,14]. Desmosomes and adherens junctions provide cellular–mechanical integration, the sodium channels facilitate the initiation of the electrical impulse, and gap junctions mediate the impulse propagations. Altogether, these protein complexes compose structures known as intercalated discs, which ultimately interconnect cardiomyocytes to each other, being responsible for both intercellular electromechanical connections and intracellular signalling cascades (Wnt-β catenin signalling pathway) [15]. A disturbed desmosomal organisation ends in cell death and scarring. However, VAs and SCD can occur before the overt disease [16], as a consequence of purely electrical changes. Indeed, because of a mutation-induced gap junction remodelling, the sodium current can be reduced and cause polymorphic VAs by a mechanism similar to that observed in Brugada Syndrome [17]. Besides the mentioned genes, biventricular and left-dominant forms are usually associated with mutations in non-desmosomal genes encoding for transmembrane protein 43 (*TMEM 43*), lamin A/C (*LMNA*), desmin (*DES*), filamin C (*FLNC*), titin (*TTN*), sodium voltage-gated channel alpha subunit 5 (*SCN5A*), phospholamban (*PLN*), the cardiac ryanodine receptor-2 (*RYR2*) and transforming growth factor beta-3 (*TGFβ-3*) [18–23]. Genotyping is not only useful for diagnostic purposes, but also for prognostic reasons. Indeed, some mutant genes in ACM have been associated with a higher risk of SCD and heart failure (HF). In particular, mutations of *TMEM43* p.S358L are characterised by higher disease penetrance and risk of SCD. *FLNC, DES* and *PLN* mutations have been associated with peculiar patterns of LV fibrosis and arrhythmic propensity, with higher risk of VAs and SCD [24–31].

1.3. Role of Inflammation in Arrhythmogenic Cardiomyopathy

The presence of inflammatory infiltrates (mainly T-cells) among dying myocytes has been demonstrated in histopathologic analysis of ventricular myocardium at postmortem or in experimental studies on transgenic animals, raising questions about the role of the immune system in the pathogenesis of the disease [2,3]. Arrhythmogenic cardiomyopathy in its early stages may present with acute chest pain and troponins release ("hot phase"), which resembles the infarct-like manifestation of some clinically suspected myocarditis [2,32–34]. The presence of autoantibodies has been reported in ACM patients and in their relatives, with a positive status being more frequent in a familial than in a sporadic pattern [35,36]. Whether inflammation is the cause or a consequence of cardiomyocytes apoptosis in ACM remains to be established. The increasing interest in the role of the immune system in the pathogenesis of the disease has translated into pharmacologic research targeting the biologic pathway involved in myocardial inflammation.

1.4. Diagnosis

It is important to underline that in ACM the diagnosis is multiparametric. In 1994, an International Task Force (TF) developed the first diagnostic scoring system for the disease, consisting of major and minor criteria grouped into different categories. A "definite" ACM diagnosis was made when multiple criteria (two major criteria, or one major and two minor criteria, or four minor criteria from different categories) were met because no diagnostic test was considered specific enough to reach a final diagnosis. If the number of criteria was not sufficient to satisfy a "Definitive" diagnosis, the disease diagnosis could be downgraded as "borderline" (one major criterion and one minor criterion, or three minor criteria), or "possible" (one major criterion alone, or two minor criteria) [37]. In later years, clinical studies demonstrated that these criteria were highly specific, but lacked sensitivity in mild forms of the disease (for example, in the early diagnosis of family members). Consequently, the revised 2010 TF criteria included new electrocardiographic parameters and quantitative measurements in echocardiogram and CMR imaging to increase this scarce diagnostic sensitivity. Notably, the demonstration of a pathogenic variant in ACM-related genes became a major diagnostic criterion [38]. However, the 2010 TF criteria still had limitations. In 2019, an International Expert Report provided an extensive critical review of their clinical performance, pointing out that the main limitation of the 2010 TF criteria was the absence of specific criteria for the diagnosis of ALVC. In particular, tissue characterisation provided by CMR, which allows the identification of the fibrofatty scar at the LV level to increase the diagnostic sensitivity, was not included [39]. Starting from 2010, there has been growing knowledge of biventricular and left-dominant variants, and in 2017, the term "Arrhythmogenic Cardiomyopathy" was used to give a new definition of the disease [1]. In this context, the 2020 International Expert consensus document provided upgraded criteria ("the Padua Criteria") for the diagnosis of the entire spectrum of ACM phenotypes, especially the left-sided forms, emphasising the use of myocardial tissue characterisation by CMR for diagnosis [40,41].

2. Management

Sudden cardiac death, due to ventricular electrical instability, and HF, as a result of progressive ventricular dilatation and dysfunction, represent the most feared outcomes in ACM. The main objectives in ACM management are: the management of VAs, the prevention of SCD, the attenuation of arrhythmic and HF symptoms, and the slowdown of disease progression. To reach these goals, the patient's risk profile and symptoms must be assessed, and the most appropriate therapy should be chosen accordingly.

2.1. Prevention of Sudden Cardiac Death

2.1.1. Risk Stratification

Because ACM patients are often young with a life expectancy of many years, it is of utmost importance to decide whether the patient's risk of SCD is sufficiently high to justify aggressive therapy, including the insertion of an implantable cardioverter defibrillator (ICD).

Risk stratification in ACM patients is mostly based on the severity of arrhythmias and ventricular dysfunction. Several clinical predictors of poor outcome have been described over the years. Independent predictors of poor prognosis, found in at least one published multivariable analysis, referred as "major" risk factors, are the following: malignant arrhythmic events including SCD, cardiac arrest (CA) due to ventricular tachycardia (VT)/fibrillation (VF), appropriate ICD interventions, or ICD therapy on fast VT/VF; unexplained syncope; non-sustained VT on 24-h Holter monitoring; and RV/LV systolic dysfunction, either severe (RV fractional area change $\leq$17% or RV EF $\leq$ 35% for the RV and LV EF $\leq$ 35% for the LV) or moderate (RV fractional area change between 24 and 17% or RV EF between 40 and 36% for the RV and LV EF between 45 and 36% for the LV). "Minor" risk factors associated with adverse events include: male gender; compound genotype; young age at the time of diagnosis; proband status; inducible VT/VF at programmed ventricular stimulation (PVS); extent of electroanatomic scar and fragmented electrograms on RV voltage mapping; extent of T-wave inversion across precordial and inferior leads; low QRS amplitude and QRS fragmentation, [42]. Some genetic defects have also been associated with a worse arrhythmic outcome. The *TMEM43* p.S358L founder mutation has an almost complete disease penetrance and a high risk of SCD among male carriers [18]. Digenic and compound genotypes are independent predictors of life-threatening VAs and SCD [43].

A flow chart of the treatment of patients with ACM is reported in Figure 2.

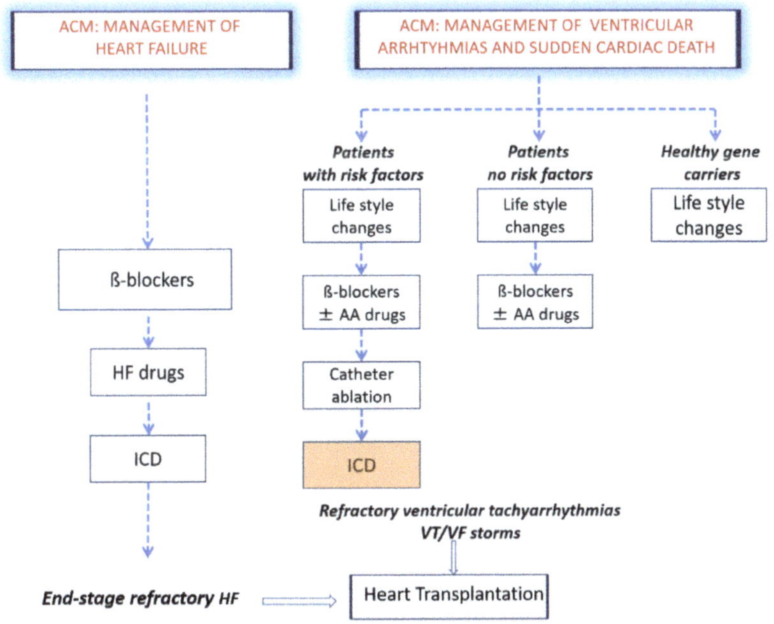

Figure 2. Flow chart of treatment of patients with ACM. Both healthy gene carriers and ACM patients should avoid intense sport activity, to prevent exercise-induced arrhythmic events and disease development or progression. Betablockers, since they prevent arrhythmic events and lower right ventricular wall stress, are essential drugs to be used in all clinically affected individuals. In patients suffering from VAs, AA drugs give the opportunity to improve symptoms. Catheter ablation is an interventional option for patients with episodes of sustained monomorphic VT. Patients for whom the implantation of an ICD is most often indicated are those with history of VF or sustained VT. In advanced stages of the disease, when HF occurs, betablockers and other HF drugs are indicated. AA drugs = antiarrhythmic drugs; ACM = arrhythmogenic cardiomyopathy; HF = heart failure; ICD = implantable cardioverter defibrillator; Vas = ventricular arrhythmias; VT = ventricular tachycardia; VF = ventricular fibrillation.

Three categories of arrhythmic risk ("high", "moderate" and "low" risk) have been identified by the 2015 Task Force consensus document on treatment of ACM (Figure 3). The "high-risk" category comprises patients with a history of CA or hemodynamically unstable VT or those with severe ventricular dysfunction, either right (RV fractional area change $\leq$17% or RV ejection fraction $\leq$35%) or left (LV ejection fraction $\leq$35%). The "intermediate risk" category includes patients with $\geq$1 "major" risk factors, such as syncope, non-sustained VT, or moderate right (RV fractional area change 17–24% or RV ejection fraction 36–40%) and/or left (LV ejection fraction 36–45%) ventricular dysfunction and patients with $\geq$1 "minor" risk factors. Asymptomatic patients with no risk factors and healthy gene carriers have a low risk of malignant VAs ("low-risk" category) [42]. Figure 3 illustrates risk categories in patients affected by ACM [44].

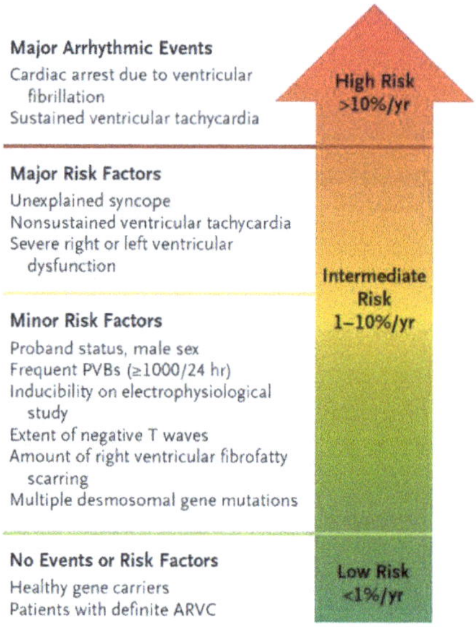

Figure 3. Risk stratification in patients affected by ACM. Risk of major arrhythmic events is based on previous events and specific risk factors. ACM= arrhythmogenic cardiomyopathy. From The New England Journal of Medicine, Domenico Corrado, Mark S. Link, Hugh Calkins, Arrhythmogenic Right Ventricular Cardiomyopathy. New Engl. J. Med. 2017, 376, 61–72. Copyright © 2021 Massachusetts Medical Society. Reprinted with permission [44].

Recently, a calculator has been proposed for "primary" risk stratification of patients with ACM [45]. However, this calculator shows significant limitations due to the important selection biases and inhomogeneous study population of the original Cadrin-Tourigny investigation used to predict outcome. Indeed, the outcome predictors were the same factors, such as syncope, non-sustained ventricular VT, and RV (but no LV) systolic dysfunction, which led to ICD implantation. The arrhythmic outcome was assessed using a combined endpoint including appropriate ICD intervention on VT, which is a poor surrogate of SCD because the majority of episodes in ACM patients are self-terminating and even short episodes of fast (>180/min) VT are hemodynamically well tolerated and most often asymptomatic, because the systolic function of the LV is usually preserved or slightly depressed. Since only one-fourth of the total study population had an ICD, 60% of the study patients (without an ICD) were prevented from experiencing an appropriate ICD intervention, which accounted for 70% of outcomes during the follow-up.

The same authors recently developed a new calculator for the prediction of life-threatening VAs (i.e., fast VT/VF, or sudden CA) using the same study design of the previous study [46]. Surprisingly, classic major risk factors such as a history of sustained VT or VF and the severity of ventricular systolic dysfunction did not predict the occurrence of life-threatening VAs. Conversely, malignant arrhythmic events were associated with younger age, male sex, the burden of ectopic ventricular beats and the extent of T-wave inversion in the inferior and precordial leads. The use of the calculator may be associated with overestimation of the risk of VT and VF, which may translate into overtreatment with ICD of asymptomatic ACM patients. Hence, before this calculator can be recommended for clinical use, validation studies are needed to confirm its predictive accuracy among the "real world" ACM patient population (www.arvcrisk.com; accessed on 21 June 2021).

2.1.2. New Risk Predictors

Novel biomarkers are currently emerging as useful tools for risk prediction [47]. Testosterone, plasma bridging integrator 1, soluble ST2, miRNAs, anti-DSG2 antibodies, correlate with disease severity and arrhythmias incidence [35,48–60]. Rearrangement at the intercalated disk (remodelling of connexin 43 gap junction proteins, sodium channels, and desmosomal proteins, particularly plakoglobin) determined by immunohistochemistry may predict arrhythmic events [61]. Ajmaline challenge can show ST elevation, which is also indicative of sodium channel remodelling [62,63]. Conduction delays, undetectable on 12-lead ECG and associated with a higher risk of arrhythmias, can be unmasked by cardiac activation imaging [64] or by echocardiography deformation imaging [65]. Contrast-enhanced CMR with late gadolinium enhancement (LGE) technique can provide a non-invasive assessment of myocardial fibrosis [66].

2.1.3. Indications for ICD Implantation

Although randomised trials of ICD therapy have not been performed, data from observational studies have consistently shown that it is effective and safe. The 2015 TF consensus conference on treatment of ACM provided recommendations for ICD implantation with the aim to optimise the prevention of SCD and avoid overtreatment of patients at low risk (Figure 4). Patients who benefit most from ICD are those who have had an episode of VF or sustained VT. It remains uncertain whether ICD therapy is appropriate for primary prevention of SCD among patients with one or more risk factors and no prior major arrhythmic events [63,64].

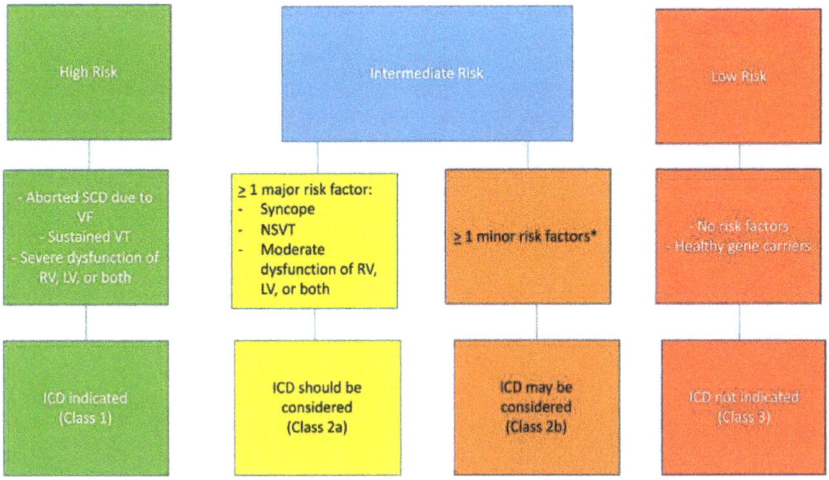

Figure 4. Flow chart of risk stratification and indications of ICD implantation in ACM. Based on the available data on annual mortality rates associated with specific risk factors, the estimated risk of major arrhythmic events in the high-risk category is >10%/year; in the intermediate category, it ranges from 1 to 10%/year; and in the low-risk category, <1%/year. Indications of ICD implantation were determined by consensus considering not only the statistical risk, but also general health, socioeconomic factors, the psychological impact and the adverse effects of the device. * See the text for distinction between major and minor risk factors. ACM = arrhythmogenic cardiomyopathy; ICD = implantable cardioverter defibrillator; LV = left ventricle; NSVT = non sustained ventricular tachycardia; RV = right ventricle; SCD = sudden cardiac death; VF = ventricular fibrillation; VT = ventricular tachycardia. Modified with permission from Corrado et al. [42].

In asymptomatic patients with no risk factors and in healthy gene carriers, there is generally no indication of prophylactic ICD implantation because of the low risk of arrhythmias and the significant risk of device- and electrode-related complications during long-term follow-up [46].

2.1.4. Transvenous Versus Subcutaneous ICD

ACM patients are usually young and receive an ICD for primary prevention. Thus, it is of utmost importance to prevent SCD whilst avoiding complications such as lead failure, device infections, and inappropriate shocks, frequently associated with the transvenous ICD (TV-ICD) (estimated rate—3.7% per year).

Subcutaneous ICD (S-ICD), thanks to its entirely subcutaneous position, is progressively establishing itself in clinical practice as a valid alternative to the TV-ICD, especially among patients with limited vascular access, increased risk of infection and a structurally normal heart with no need for pacing [67]. In ACM patients, the matter of its use has been more complicated because of the intrinsic characteristics of the disease, which is progressive and associated with the possibility of electrocardiographic depolarisation/repolarisation changes, leading to double QRS counting and P- or T-wave oversensing and potential inappropriate shock delivery [68]. Migliore et al., in a multicentre study enrolling ACM patients receiving S-ICD, demonstrated that S-ICD was a safe and effective therapy for treatment of both induced and spontaneous VAs (Figure 5). However, the use of S-ICD in this population still has some limitations [68]. First, S-ICD cannot deliver anti-tachycardia pacing (ATP) therapy, which may be a "pain-free" solution for VT. However, it has been demonstrated that many of these episodes are self-limiting and haemodynamically well tolerated, thus not needing interruption [69]. Moreover, while re-entrant VTs characterise the advanced stages of the disease, young patients usually suffer VF episodes, reflecting the acute electrical instability of the early phases of the disease [16]. The second issue relies on the higher incidence of inappropriate shocks in ACM patients, which can be triggered by the type of population, mostly of young and active patients, and the higher prevalence of electrocardiographic abnormalities. The latter include: reduced QRS voltages amplitude; negative T-waves; right atrial enlargement with peaked P waves; repolarisation abnormalities depending on the heart rate [69]; and R-wave amplitude decline during follow-up. These electrocardiographic features predispose this population to possible cardiac and/or non-cardiac oversensing and subsequent inappropriate therapy. This is why strategies which aim to reduce inappropriate shocks are based on careful electrocardiographic screening [70], device programming (single vs. dual-zone programming), new implantation techniques [71], and software upgrades such as "SMART Pass" to reduce oversensing [72].

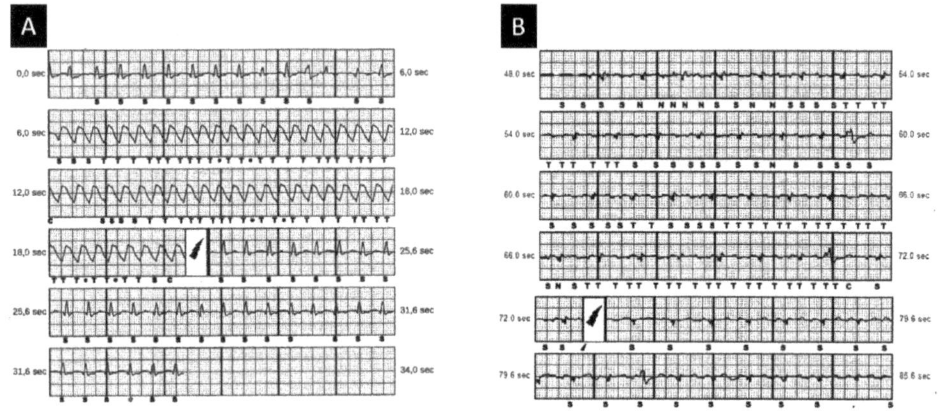

Figure 5. Appropriate and inappropriate S-ICD shocks. (**A**) S-ICD stored electrogram showing appropriately detected and treated ventricular arrhythmia episode. (**B**) S-ICD stored electrogram of inappropriate shock due to P/T-wave oversensing during effort. S-ICD = subcutaneous implantable cardioverter defibrillator. Modified with permission from Migliore et al. [68].

2.2. Improvement of Symptoms and Quality of Life

The implant of an ICD is the only therapeutic option of proven efficacy for the prevention of SCD by interruption of otherwise lethal VAs. However, ACM patients often complain of arrhythmic (palpitations, VT recurrences, or ICD discharges) and HF symptoms that affect their quality of life. Currently available treatment options include either pharmacologic or non-pharmacologic therapy.

2.2.1. Traditional Pharmacologic Therapy

Traditional pharmacological therapy includes the use of betablockers, antiarrhythmic drugs (AADs), and HF drugs.

Adrenergic stimulation in ACM patients promotes VAs and SCD, which typically occur during or soon after a physical effort. By preventing effort-induced VAs, betablockers find their ideal location in this setting. Indeed, they receive a class I recommendation for ACM patients symptomatic for frequent premature ventricular beats (PVBs) and non-sustained VT, patients with recurrent VT, appropriate ICD therapies, or inappropriate ICD interventions resulting from sinus tachycardia, supraventricular tachycardia, or atrial fibrillation/flutter with a high ventricular rate. Moreover, they reduce the ventricular wall stress, lowering disease progression. Therefore, there is a class IIa for recommendation of their use in all patients with a definite diagnosis of ACM, irrespective of arrhythmias. Instead, in phenotype-negative gene carriers, prophylactic use of these drugs is not justified [42,73].

Among AADs, amiodarone and sotalol are the most effective drugs with a relatively low proarrhythmic risk. They are recommended in ACM patients with frequent appropriate ICD discharges (class I) to improve symptoms in patients with frequent PVBs and/or non-sustained VT (class IIa) and as an adjunctive therapy when betablockers alone are not sufficient to control the arrhythmic burden in symptomatic patients with frequent PVBs and/or non-sustained VT [42,73].

When right and/or left HF occurs, the standard HF pharmacological treatment including angiotensin-converting enzyme inhibitors, angiotensin II receptor blockers, (betablockers), and diuretics is recommended (class I) [42].

Left-ventricle assist devices and heart transplantation represent the final treatment options when the disease progresses to an end-stage phase. The largest assembled cohort of ACM patients undergoing heart transplant showed high post-transplantation survival rates (94% and 88% at 1 and 6 years, respectively) [74–76].

Another not uncommon issue in severely dilated ventricles with aneurysms and sacculations is represented by thrombus formation and related thromboembolic complications. There is no indication for primary prevention with anticoagulants; however, when a thrombus is documented or a thromboembolic event occurs, long-term anticoagulants should be started (class I) [42].

2.2.2. New Pharmacological Options

Heart Failure Drugs

The PARADIGM-HF study established the favourable impact of therapy with sacubitril/valsartan (LCZ696) on the outcomes of patients with HF [77]. Whether this treatment is effective in ACM patients with RV, LV or biventricular systolic dysfunction remains to be established. Studies validating the role of these neurohormonal antagonists in ACM represent a major research priority.

Anti-Inflammatory Drugs

Glycogen synthase kinase-3β (GSK3 β) and the nuclear factor-kB (NFkB) signalling pathways are abnormally activated in cardiac myocytes in ACM. A small molecule, SB216763 (SB2), a GSK3β inhibitor, appears to prevent or reverse the disease in animal models by reducing the Wtn-β catenin signalling pathway (which is enhanced by GSK3β) [78,79]. However, long-term use of GSK3β antagonists and its effects on the Wtn-β catenin signalling pathway carry an unacceptable risk of developing cancer, limiting their clinical applicability. Thus, subsequent research focused on a downstream level and on inflammatory signalling. NFκB promotes inflammatory responses and interacts with GSK3β. Bay 11-7082, an inhibitor of NFκB, has been demonstrated to reduce the development of disease features [80]. On the same line, the inhibition of the TNFα, IL-1 and NLRP3 inflammasome in experimental models has been shown to have a potential benefit in ACM treatment by reducing inflammation and fibrosis [81–83]. These findings gave evidence of the efficacy of targeting the inflammatory pathway as a potential therapeutic option in ACM patients.

Another signalling pathway that is altered, causing LMNA-associated cardiomyopathy, is that of MAP kinase (p38α branch). ARRY-797, a p38 MAPK inhibitor, has been shown to reverse cardiac dysfunction in animal models of *LMNA* and important results are expected from a clinical trial (ClinicalTrials.gov Identifier: NCT03439514) currently underway in patients with dilated cardiomyopathy due to *LMNA* mutations [84].

2.2.3. Non-Pharmacologic Therapy by Catheter Ablation

When pharmacological therapy confers only a partial control of arrhythmias or are poorly tolerated, catheter ablation can represent a potentially effective treatment for recurrent sustained VT episodes and ICD shocks in ACM patients. Therefore, it is recommended in cases of incessant VT or frequent appropriate ICD interventions on VT, despite maximal pharmacological therapy, and may be considered in patients who do not desire or cannot tolerate pharmacological therapies [42]. Since catheter ablation does not prevent SCD, it should not be considered as an alternative to ICD implantation in ACM patients with a history of sustained VT, with the possible exception of selected cases with a drug refractory, haemodynamically stable, single morphology VT [42].

Myocardial scars are imaged as low-voltage regions (areas $\geq$1 cm^2 with low bipolar voltages (<1.5 mV), and fractionated potentials (i.e., >3 deflections, amplitude $\leq$1.5 mV, duration >70 ms)) by bipolar three-dimensional electroanatomic voltage mapping (3D-EVM). As mentioned above, these alterations not only have a diagnostic value but also carry a prognostic significance as they correlate with arrhythmic events. However, 3D-EVM can miss low-voltage areas in about 25–30% of cases and the success rate of the endocardial approach is still modest because of the epicardial location of the majority of VT circuits [85]. This epicardial substrate can be evidenced as abnormal epicardial bipolar low-voltage areas (amplitude < 1.0 mV) by epicardial voltage mapping [86] or, as an alternative to this invasive approach, by using a threshold of <5.5 mV at unipolar endocardial mapping [87].

The catheter ablation technique includes patient sedation, mapping, electrophysiological study, and ablation itself. For the endocardial approach, conscious sedation is favoured, while for the epicardial approach, general anaesthesia is preferred. The endocardial approach relies on a standard transfemoral access, whereas a pericardial access is employed in the epicardial approach (Figure 6). The following steps are similar for both the approaches: use of irrigated-tip catheters with contact force sensors to detect fractionated signals and late potentials, pace mapping to identify additional sites, PVS to induce VT, activation, and entrainment VT mapping to identify the tachycardia circuit or, as an alternative, a substrate-based ablation targeting "channels" and delayed/fractioned potentials within low voltages areas.

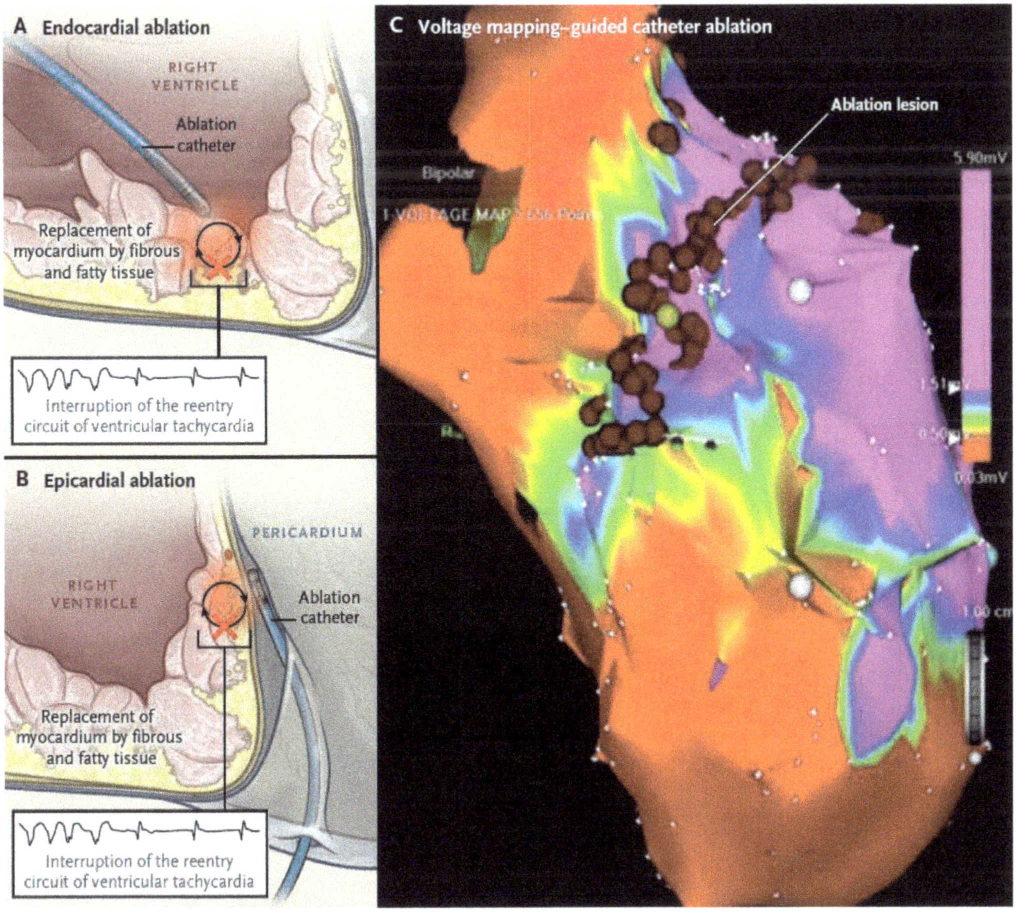

Figure 6. Catheter ablation in ACM patients. Panel (**A**) shows the subendocardial approach. Panel (**B**) shows the subepicardial approach. Panel (**C**) shows three-dimensional electro-anatomical voltage mapping to reconstruct regions of right ventricular scarring. ACM = arrhythmogenic cardiomyopathy. From The New England Journal of Medicine, Domenico Corrado, Mark S. Link, Hugh Calkins, Arrhythmogenic Right Ventricular Cardiomyopathy. New Engl. J. Med. 2017, 376, 61–72. Copyright © 2021 Massachusetts Medical Society. Reprinted with permission [44].

Patients with end-stage ACM require more extensive radiofrequency applications be delivered at the endocardium because of a wider endocardial than epicardial involvement. However, even in these cases, the epicardial approach (combined with endocardial) may be useful to achieve complete substrate elimination and decrease VT episodes during follow-up. Because recent studies demonstrated good long-term outcomes in patients showing no VT inducibility after endocardial-only ablation, the epicardial approach should be reserved only for when spontaneous or inducible VT persists after extensive previously performed endocardial ablation [88,89] (Table 1). Therefore, a stepwise method with a first attempt with endocardial-only ablation followed eventually by epicardial ablation in those patients exhibiting a bipolar vs. unipolar low-voltage areas may be preferred.

Table 1. Major series of ventricular tachycardia ablation outcomes in arrhythmogenic cardiomyopathy.

Author (Year)	Patients n (Men)	Ablation Technique			Complete Acute Success (%)	Procedure-Related Complications	Follow-up		
		Electro-Anatomic Map	Irrigated Tip	Epicardial Map/abl (%)			Mean (Months)	VT Recurrences (%)	Deaths or HT
Santangeli 2019	32 (23)	Yes	Yes	72%	100	1 (RV laceration)	46	19	N/A
Berruezo 2017	41 (36)	Yes	Yes	100%	90	2 (tamponade, death)	32	26.8	N/A
Mussigbrodt 2017	45 (30)	Yes	Yes	48.9%	84	5 (TIA, tamponade x2, PE x2 1 fatal)	31	44 *	N/A
Souissi 2018	49 (44)	Yes	Yes	100%	71	3 (tamponade, femoral AV fistula, intestinal perforation)	64	81 at 5 years 31 at 1 years *	6 deaths, 2 HT
Santangeli 2015	62 (45)	Yes	Yes	63%	77	5 (PE x2, pericardial effusion, RV puncture, CT)	56	29 *	5 NC, 5HT
Philips 2012	87 (45)	Yes	Yes	26.4%	82	2 (death, MI)	88	85	N/A
Berruezo 2012	11 (9)	Yes	Yes	100%	100	1 (tamponade)	11	9	0
Garcia 2009	13 (10)	Yes	Yes	Yes	92	0	18	23	1 HT
Nogami 2008	18 (13)	Yes	No	No	72	0	61	33	2 HF, 1 NC
Dalal, 2007	24 (11)	Yes	No	No	77	1 (death)	32	85	2 HT
Satomi 2006	17 (13)	Yes	No	No	88	0	26	24	0
Verma 2005	22 (15)	Yes	Yes	No	82	1 (tamponade)	37	36	0
Miljoen 2005	11 (8)	Yes	No	No	73	0	20	45	1 NC
Marchlinski 2004	19 (18)	Yes	Yes	No	74	0	27	11	0
Reithmann 2003	5 (3)	Yes	No	No	80	0	7	20	0
Ellison 1998	5 (4)	No	No	No	42	0	17	0	0

* The endpoint was freedom from ventricular tachycardia after the last ablation. AV = arterovenous, CT = constrictive pericarditis, HF = heart failure death, HT = heart transplantation, MI = myocardial infarction, NC = non-cardiac death, PE = pulmonary embolism, TIA = transient ischemic attack, RV = right ventricular.

3. Conclusions

Arrhythmogenic cardiomyopathy is characterised by progressive scarring of the ventricular myocardium and ventricular dilatation and dysfunction.

The clinical approach to the disease should embrace new concepts and awareness regarding the pathobiological basis and the role of the immune system in the development and progression of the disease. Risk stratification to guide ICD implantation remains a crucial point in the management of ACM patients for primary prevention of SCD. The emerging role of S-ICD offers the potential to revise the indications of ICD treatment. The significant advances of mapping and catheter ablation have led to effective non-pharmacologic therapy of sustained VT. Neurohormonal antagonists and drugs targeting the Wtn-β and NFκB pathways represent the major advances of pharmacological treatment.

Author Contributions: F.M., G.M. and D.C. contributed to the design of the work and drafted the manuscript. A.C., B.B., I.R., A.Z., and D.C. revised the manuscript. All authors gave final approval and agreed to be accountable for all aspects of work ensuring integrity and accuracy. All authors have read and agreed to the published version of the manuscript.

Funding: This research received no external funding.

Institutional Review Board Statement: Not applicable.

Informed Consent Statement: Not applicable.

Data Availability Statement: Data available in a publicly accessible repository.

Conflicts of Interest: The authors declare no conflict of interest.

References

1. Corrado, D.; Basso, C.; Judge, D. Arrhythmogenic Cardiomyopathy. *Circ. Res.* **2017**, *121*, 784–802. [CrossRef]
2. Basso, C.; Thiene, G.; Corrado, D.; Angelini, A.; Nava, A.; Valente, M. Arrhythmogenic Right Ventricular Cardiomyopathy: Dysplasia, dystrophy, or myocarditis? *Circulation* **1996**, *94*, 983–991. [CrossRef] [PubMed]
3. Pilichou, K.; Remme, C.A.; Basso, C.; Campian, M.E.; Rizzo, S.; Barnett, P.; Scicluna, B.; Bauce, B.; Hoff, M.J.B.V.D.; De Bakker, J.M.T.; et al. Myocyte necrosis underlies progressive myocardial dystrophy in mouse dsg2-related arrhythmogenic right ventricular cardiomyopathy. *J. Exp. Med.* **2009**, *206*, 1787–1802. [CrossRef]
4. Thiene, G.; Basso, C. Arrhythmogenic right ventricular cardiomyopathy: An update. *Cardiovasc. Pathol.* **2001**, *10*, 109–117. [CrossRef]
5. Sen-Chowdhry, S.; Syrris, P.; Prasad, S.K.; Hughes, S.E.; Merrifield, R.; Ward, D.; Pennell, D.; McKenna, W.J. Left-Dominant Arrhythmogenic Cardiomyopathy. *J. Am. Coll. Cardiol.* **2008**, *52*, 2175–2187. [CrossRef]
6. Te Riele, A.S.J.M.; James, C.A.; Philips, B.; Rastegar, N.; Bhonsale, A.; Groeneweg, J.A.; Murray, B.; Tichnell, C.; Judge, D.; Van Der Heijden, J.F.; et al. Mutation-Positive Arrhythmogenic Right Ventricular Dysplasia/Cardiomyopathy: The Triangle of Dysplasia Displaced. *J. Cardiovasc. Electrophysiol.* **2013**, *24*, 1311–1320. [CrossRef] [PubMed]
7. Corrado, D.; Van Tintelen, P.J.; McKenna, W.J.; Hauer, R.N.W.; Anastastakis, A.; Asimaki, A.; Basso, C.; Bauce, B.; Brunckhorst, C.; Bucciarelli-Ducci, C.; et al. International Experts. Arrhythmogenic right ventricular cardiomyopathy: Evaluation of the current diagnostic criteria and differential diagnosis. *Eur. Heart J.* **2020**, *41*, 1414–1429. [CrossRef] [PubMed]
8. McKoy, G.; Protonotarios, N.; Crosby, A.; Tsatsopoulou, A.; Anastasakis, A.; Coonar, A.; Norman, M.; Baboonian, C.; Jeffery, S.; McKenna, W.J. Identification of a deletion in plakoglobin in arrhythmogenic right ventricular cardiomyopathy with palmoplantar keratoderma and woolly hair (Naxos disease). *Lancet* **2000**, *355*, 2119–2124. [CrossRef]
9. Rampazzo, A.; Nava, A.; Malacrida, S.; Beffagna, G.; Bauce, B.; Rossi, V.; Zimbello, R.; Simionati, B.; Basso, C.; Thiene, G.; et al. Mutation in Human Desmoplakin Domain Binding to Plakoglobin Causes a Dominant Form of Arrhythmogenic Right Ventricular Cardiomyopathy. *Am. J. Hum. Genet.* **2002**, *71*, 1200–1206. [CrossRef]
10. Gerull, B.; Heuser, A.; Wichter, T.; Paul, M.; Basson, C.T.; A McDermott, D.; Lerman, B.B.; Markowitz, S.M.; Ellinor, P.T.; Macrae, C.A.; et al. Mutations in the desmosomal protein plakophilin-2 are common in arrhythmogenic right ventricular cardiomyopathy. *Nat. Genet.* **2004**, *36*, 1162–1164. [CrossRef]
11. Pilichou, K.; Nava, A.; Basso, C.; Beffagna, G.; Bauce, B.; Lorenzon, A.; Frigo, G.; Vettori, A.; Valente, M.; Towbin, J.; et al. Mutations in Desmoglein-2 Gene Are Associated with Arrhythmogenic Right Ventricular Cardiomyopathy. *Circulation* **2006**, *113*, 1171–1179. [CrossRef] [PubMed]
12. Syrris, P.; Ward, D.; Evans, A.; Asimaki, A.; Gandjbakhch, E.; Sen-Chowdhry, S.; McKenna, W.J. Arrhythmogenic Right Ventricular Dysplasia/Cardiomyopathy Associated with Mutations in the Desmosomal Gene Desmocollin-2. *Am. J. Hum. Genet.* **2006**, *79*, 978–984. [CrossRef] [PubMed]

13. Van Hengel, J.; Calore, M.; Bauce, B.; Dazzo, E.; Mazzotti, E.; De Bortoli, M.; Lorenzon, A.; Mura, I.E.L.; Beffagna, G.; Rigato, I.; et al. Mutations in the area composita protein αT-catenin are associated with arrhythmogenic right ventricular cardiomyopathy. *Eur. Hear. J.* **2013**, *34*, 201–210. [CrossRef] [PubMed]
14. Mayosi, B.M.; Fish, M.; Shaboodien, G.; Mastantuono, E.; Kraus, S.; Wieland, T.; Kotta, M.-C.; Chin, A.; Laing, N.; Ntusi, N.B.; et al. Identification of Cadherin 2 (CDH2) Mutations in Arrhythmogenic Right Ventricular Cardiomyopathy. *Circ. Cardiovasc. Genet.* **2017**, *10*. [CrossRef]
15. Gras, E.G.; Lombardi, R.; Giocondo, M.J.; Willerson, J.T.; Schneider, M.D.; Khoury, D.S.; Marian, A.J. Suppression of canonical Wnt/ -catenin signaling by nuclear plakoglobin recapitulates phenotype of arrhythmogenic right ventricular cardiomyopathy. *J. Clin. Investig.* **2006**, *116*, 2012–2021. [CrossRef]
16. Mattesi, G.; Zorzi, A.; Corrado, D.; Cipriani, A. Natural History of Arrhythmogenic Cardiomyopathy. *J. Clin. Med.* **2020**, *9*, 878. [CrossRef]
17. Corrado, D.; Zorzi, A.; Cerrone, M.; Rigato, I.; Mongillo, M.; Bauce, B.; Delmar, M. Relationship Between Arrhythmogenic Right Ventricular Cardiomyopathy and Brugada Syndrome. *Circ. Arrhythmia Electrophysiol.* **2016**, *9*, e003631. [CrossRef]
18. Merner, N.D.; Hodgkinson, K.A.; Haywood, A.F.; Connors, S.; French, V.M.; Drenckhahn, J.-D.; Kupprion, C.; Ramadanova, K.; Thierfelder, L.; McKenna, W.; et al. Arrhythmogenic Right Ventricular Cardiomyopathy Type 5 Is a Fully Penetrant, Lethal Arrhythmic Disorder Caused by a Missense Mutation in the TMEM43 Gene. *Am. J. Hum. Genet.* **2008**, *82*, 809–821. [CrossRef]
19. Quarta, G.; Syrris, P.; Ashworth, M.; Jenkins, S.; Alapi, K.Z.; Morgan, J.; Muir, A.; Pantazis, A.; McKenna, W.J.; Elliott, P.M. Mutations in the Lamin A/C gene mimic arrhythmogenic right ventricular cardiomyopathy. *Eur. Hear. J.* **2011**, *33*, 1128–1136. [CrossRef]
20. van Tintelen, J.P.; Van Gelder, I.C.; Asimaki, A.; Suurmeijer, A.J.; Wiesfeld, A.C.; Jongbloed, J.D.; Wijngaard, A.V.D.; Kuks, J.B.; van Spaendonck-Zwarts, K.Y.; Notermans, N.; et al. Severe cardiac phenotype with right ventricular predominance in a large cohort of patients with a single missense mutation in the DES gene. *Hear. Rhythm.* **2009**, *6*, 1574–1583. [CrossRef]
21. Taylor, M.; Graw, S.; Sinagra, G.; Barnes, C.; Slavov, D.; Brun, F.; Pinamonti, B.; Salcedo, E.E.; Sauer, W.; Pyxaras, S.; et al. Genetic Variation in Titin in Arrhythmogenic Right Ventricular Cardiomyopathy–Overlap Syndromes. *Circulation* **2011**, *124*, 876–885. [CrossRef] [PubMed]
22. Van Der Zwaag, P.A.; Van Rijsingen, I.A.; Asimaki, A.; Jongbloed, J.D.; Van Veldhuisen, D.J.; Wiesfeld, A.C.; Cox, M.G.; Van Lochem, L.T.; De Boer, R.A.; Hofstra, R.M.; et al. Phospholamban R14del mutation in patients diagnosed with dilated cardiomyopathy or arrhythmogenic right ventricular cardiomyopathy: Evidence supporting the concept of arrhythmogenic cardiomyopathy. *Eur. J. Hear. Fail.* **2012**, *14*, 1199–1207. [CrossRef]
23. Beffagna, G.; Occhi, G.; Nava, A.; Vitiello, L.; Ditadi, A.; Basso, C.; Bauce, B.; Carraro, G.; Thiene, G.; Towbin, J.A. Regulatory mutations in transforming growth factor-?3 gene cause arrhythmogenic right ventricular cardiomyopathy type 1. *Cardiovasc. Res.* **2005**, *65*, 366–373. [CrossRef] [PubMed]
24. Sen-Chowdhry, S.; Syrris, P.; Ward, D.; Asimaki, A.; Sevdalis, E.; McKenna, W.J. Clinical and Genetic Characterization of Families with Arrhythmogenic Right Ventricular Dysplasia/Cardiomyopathy Provides Novel Insights Into Patterns of Disease Expression. *Circulation* **2007**, *115*, 1710–1720. [CrossRef]
25. Bhonsale, A.; Groeneweg, J.A.; James, C.A.; Dooijes, D.; Tichnell, C.; Jongbloed, J.D.H.; Murray, B.; Riele, A.S.J.M.T.; Berg, M.P.V.D.; Bikker, H.; et al. Impact of genotype on clinical course in arrhythmogenic right ventricular dysplasia/cardiomyopathy-associated mutation carriers. *Eur. Hear. J.* **2015**, *36*, 847–855. [CrossRef]
26. Ortiz-Genga, M.F.; Cuenca, S.; Ferro, M.D.; Zorio, E.; Aranda, R.S.; Climent, V.; Padrón-Barthe, L.; Duro-Aguado, I.; Jiménez-Jáimez, J.; Hidalgo-Olivares, V.M.; et al. Truncating FLNC Mutations Are Associated With High-Risk Dilated and Arrhythmogenic Cardiomyopathies. *J. Am. Coll. Cardiol.* **2016**, *68*, 2440–2451. [CrossRef] [PubMed]
27. Dominguez, F.; Zorio, E.; Jimenez-Jaimez, J.; Salguero-Bodes, R.; Zwart, R.; Gonzalez-Lopez, E.; Molina, P.; Jiménez, F.J.B.; Delgado, J.F.; Braza-Boïls, A.; et al. Clinical characteristics and determinants of the phenotype in TMEM43 arrhythmogenic right ventricular cardiomyopathy type 5. *Hear. Rhythm.* **2020**, *17*, 945–954. [CrossRef]
28. Begay, R.; Graw, S.L.; Sinagra, G.; Asimaki, A.; Rowland, T.J.; Slavov, D.B.; Gowan, K.; Jones, K.L.; Brun, F.; Merlo, M.; et al. Filamin C Truncation Mutations Are Associated with Arrhythmogenic Dilated Cardiomyopathy and Changes in the Cell–Cell Adhesion Structures. *JACC Clin. Electrophysiol.* **2018**, *4*, 504–514. [CrossRef] [PubMed]
29. Augusto, J.B.; Eiros, R.; Nakou, E.; Moura-Ferreira, S.; Treibel, T.; Captur, G.; Akhtar, M.M.; Protonotarios, A.; Gossios, T.D.; Savvatis, K.; et al. Dilated cardiomyopathy and arrhythmogenic left ventricular cardiomyopathy: A comprehensive genotype-imaging phenotype study. *Eur. Hear. J. Cardiovasc. Imaging* **2019**, *21*, 326–336. [CrossRef]
30. Segura-Rodríguez, D.; Jiménez, F.J.B.; Carriel, V.; López-Fernández, S.; González-Molina, M.; Ramírez, J.M.O.; Fernández-Navarro, L.; García-Roa, M.D.; Cabrerizo, E.M.; Durand-Herrera, D.; et al. Myocardial fibrosis in arrhythmogenic cardiomyopathy: A genotype–phenotype correlation study. *Eur. Hear. J. Cardiovasc. Imaging* **2019**, *21*, 378–386. [CrossRef]
31. Mattesi, G.; Cipriani, A.; Bauce, B.; Rigato, I.; Zorzi, A.; Corrado, D. Arrhythmogenic Left Ventricular Cardiomyopathy: Genotype-Phenotype Correlations and New Diagnostic Criteria. *J. Clin. Med.* **2021**, *10*, 2212. [CrossRef] [PubMed]
32. Calabrese, F.; Angelini, A.; Thiene, G.; Basso, C.; Nava, A.; Valente, M. No detection of enteroviral genome in the myocardium of patients with arrhythmogenic right ventricular cardiomyopathy. *J. Clin. Pathol.* **2000**, *53*, 382–387. [CrossRef] [PubMed]
33. Thiene, G.; Corrado, D.; Nava, A.; Rossi, L.; Poletti, A.; Boffa, G.M.; Daliento, L.; Pennelli, N. Right ventricular cardiomyopathy: Is there evidence of an inflammatory aetiology? *Eur. Hear. J.* **1991**, *12*, 22–25. [CrossRef] [PubMed]

34. Bariani, R.; Cipriani, A.; Rizzo, S.; Celeghin, R.; Marinas, M.B.; Giorgi, B.; De Gaspari, M.; Rigato, I.; Leoni, L.; Zorzi, A.; et al. 'Hot phase' clinical presentation in arrhythmogenic cardiomyopathy. *Europace* **2021**, *23*, 907–917. [CrossRef] [PubMed]
35. Chatterjee, D.; Fatah, M.; Akdis, D.; A Spears, D.; Koopmann, T.T.; Mittal, K.; A Rafiq, M.; Cattanach, B.M.; Zhao, Q.; Healey, J.S.; et al. An autoantibody identifies arrhythmogenic right ventricular cardiomyopathy and participates in its pathogenesis. *Eur. Hear. J.* **2018**, *39*, 3932–3944. [CrossRef]
36. Caforio, A.L.; Re, F.; Avella, A.; Marcolongo, R.; Baratta, P.; Seguso, M.; Gallo, N.; Plebani, M.; Izquierdo-Bajo, A.; Cheng, C.-Y.; et al. Evidence From Family Studies for Autoimmunity in Arrhythmogenic Right Ventricular Cardiomyopathy. *Circulation* **2020**, *141*, 1238–1248. [CrossRef] [PubMed]
37. McKenna, W.J.; Thiene, G.; Nava, A.; Fontaliran, F.; Blomstrom-Lundqvist, C.; Fontaine, G.; Camerini, F. Diagnosis of arrhythmogenic right ventricular dysplasia/cardiomyopathy. Task Force of the Working Group Myocardial and Pericardial Disease of the European Society of Cardiology and of the Scientific Council on Cardiomyopathies of the International Society and Federation of Cardiology. *Br. Heart. J.* **1994**, *71*, 215–218. [CrossRef]
38. Marcus, F.I.; McKenna, W.J.; Sherrill, D.; Basso, C.; Bauce, B.; Bluemke, D.; Calkins, H.; Corrado, D.; Cox, M.G.; Daubert, J.P.; et al. Diagnosis of Arrhythmogenic Right Ventricular Cardiomyopathy/Dysplasia. *Circulation* **2010**, *121*, 1533–1541. [CrossRef]
39. Towbin, J.A.; McKenna, W.J.; Abrams, D.J.; Ackerman, M.J.; Calkins, H.; Darrieux, F.C.; Daubert, J.P.; De Chillou, C.; DePasquale, E.C.; Desai, M.Y.; et al. 2019 HRS expert consensus statement on evaluation, risk stratification, and management of arrhythmogenic cardiomyopathy. *Hear. Rhythm.* **2019**, *16*, e301–e372. [CrossRef]
40. Corrado, D.; Perazzolo Marra, M.; Zorzi, A.; Beffagna, G.; Cipriani, A.; Lazzari, M.; Migliore, F.; Pilichou, K.; Rampazzo, A.; Rigato, I.; et al. Diagnosis of arrhythmogenic cardiomyopathy: The Padua criteria. *Int. J. Cardiol.* **2020**, *319*, 106–114. [CrossRef]
41. Pontone, G.; Di Bella, G.; Castelletti, S.; Maestrini, V.; Festa, P.; Ait-Ali, L.; Masci, P.G.; Monti, L.; Di Giovine, G.; De Lazzari, M.; et al. Clinical recommendations of cardiac magnetic resonance, Part II. *J. Cardiovasc. Med.* **2017**, *18*, 209–222. [CrossRef] [PubMed]
42. Corrado, D.; Wichter, T.; Link, M.S.; Hauer, R.N.; Marchlinski, F.E.; Anastasakis, A.; Bauce, B.; Basso, C.; Brunckhorst, C.; Tsatsopoulou, A.; et al. Treatment of Arrhythmogenic Right Ventricular Cardiomyopathy/Dysplasia. *Circulation* **2015**, *132*, 441–453. [CrossRef] [PubMed]
43. Rigato, I.; Bauce, B.; Rampazzo, A.; Zorzi, A.; Pilichou, K.; Mazzotti, E.; Migliore, F.; Marra, M.P.; Lorenzon, A.; De Bortoli, M.; et al. Compound and Digenic Heterozygosity Predicts Lifetime Arrhythmic Outcome and Sudden Cardiac Death in Desmosomal Gene–Related Arrhythmogenic Right Ventricular Cardiomyopathy. *Circ. Cardiovasc. Genet.* **2013**, *6*, 533–542. [CrossRef] [PubMed]
44. Corrado, D.; Link, M.S.; Calkins, H. Arrhythmogenic Right Ventricular Cardiomyopathy. *New Engl. J. Med.* **2017**, *376*, 61–72. [CrossRef]
45. Cadrin-Tourigny, J.; Bosman, L.P.; Nozza, A.; Wang, W.; Tadros, R.; Bhonsale, A.; Bourfiss, M.; Fortier, A.; Lie, Ø.H.; Saguner, A.M.; et al. A new prediction model for ventricular arrhythmias in arrhythmogenic right ventricular cardiomyopathy. *Eur. Hear. J.* **2019**, *40*, 1850–1858. [CrossRef] [PubMed]
46. Cadrin-Tourigny, J.; Bosman, L.P.; Wang, W.; Tadros, R.; Bhonsale, A.; Bourfiss, M.; Lie, Ø.H.; Saguner, A.M.; Svensson, A.; Andorin, A.; et al. Sudden Cardiac Death Prediction in Arrhythmogenic Right Ventricular Cardiomyo-pathy: A Multinational Collaboration. *Circ. Arrhythm. Electrophysiol.* **2021**, *14*, e008509. [CrossRef] [PubMed]
47. Van Der Voorn, S.M.; Riele, A.S.J.M.T.; Basso, C.; Calkins, H.; Remme, C.A.; Veen, T.A.B.V. Arrhythmogenic cardiomyopathy: Pathogenesis, pro-arrhythmic remodelling, and novel approaches for risk stratification and therapy. *Cardiovasc. Res.* **2020**, *116*, 1571–1584. [CrossRef]
48. Akdis, D.; Saguner, A.M.; Shah, K.; Wei, C.; Medeiros-Domingo, A.; Von Eckardstein, A.; Lüscher, T.F.; Brunckhorst, C.; Chen, H.V.; Duru, F. Sex hormones affect outcome in arrhythmogenic right ventricular cardiomyopathy/dysplasia: From a stem cell derived cardiomyocyte-based model to clinical biomarkers of disease outcome. *Eur. Hear. J.* **2017**, *38*, 1498–1508. [CrossRef] [PubMed]
49. Coats, C.J.; E Heywood, W.; Mills, K.; Elliott, P.M. Current applications of biomarkers in cardiomyopathies. *Expert Rev. Cardiovasc. Ther.* **2015**, *13*, 825–837. [CrossRef] [PubMed]
50. De Jong, S.; Van Veen, T.A.B.; De Bakker, J.M.T.; Vos, M.A.; van Rijen, H. Biomarkers of Myocardial Fibrosis. *J. Cardiovasc. Pharmacol.* **2011**, *57*, 522–535. [CrossRef]
51. De Jong, S.; Van Veen, T.A.B.; De Bakker, J.M.T.; Van Rijen, H.V.M. Monitoring cardiac fibrosis: A technical challenge. *Neth. Hear. J.* **2011**, *20*, 44–48. [CrossRef]
52. Chalikias, G.K.; Tziakas, D.N. Biomarkers of the extracellular matrix and of collagen fragments. *Clin. Chim. Acta* **2015**, *443*, 39–47. [CrossRef]
53. Spinale, F.G. Matrix Metalloproteinases. *Circ. Res.* **2002**, *90*, 520–530. [CrossRef] [PubMed]
54. Sommariva, E.; D'Alessandra, Y.; Farina, F.M.; Casella, M.; Cattaneo, F.; Catto, V.; Chiesa, M.; Stadiotti, I.; Brambilla, S.; Russo, A.D.; et al. MiR-320a as a Potential Novel Circulating Biomarker of Arrhythmogenic CardioMyopathy. *Sci. Rep.* **2017**, *7*, 1–10. [CrossRef]
55. Zhang, H.; Liu, S.; Dong, T.; Yang, J.; Xie, Y.; Wu, Y.; Kang, K.; Hu, S.; Gou, D.; Wei, Y. Profiling of differentially expressed microRNAs in arrhythmogenic right ventricular cardiomyopathy. *Sci. Rep.* **2016**, *6*, 28101. [CrossRef] [PubMed]
56. Thum, T.; Condorelli, G. Long Noncoding RNAs and MicroRNAs in Cardiovascular Pathophysiology. *Circ. Res.* **2015**, *116*, 751–762. [CrossRef]
57. Bauersachs, J. Regulation of Myocardial Fibrosis by MicroRNAs. *J. Cardiovasc. Pharmacol.* **2010**, *56*, 454–459. [CrossRef] [PubMed]

58. Thum, T.; Gross, C.; Fiedler, J.; Fischer, T.; Kissler, S.; Bussen, M.; Galuppo, P.; Just, S.; Rottbauer, W.; Frantz, S.; et al. MicroRNA-21 contributes to myocardial disease by stimulating MAP kinase signalling in fibroblasts. *Nat. Cell Biol.* **2008**, *456*, 980–984. [CrossRef] [PubMed]
59. Broch, K.; Leren, I.S.; Saberniak, J.; Ueland, T.; Edvardsen, T.; Gullestad, L.; Haugaa, K. Soluble ST2 is associated with disease severity in arrhythmogenic right ventricular cardiomyopathy. *Biomarkers* **2017**, *22*, 367–371. [CrossRef] [PubMed]
60. Hong, T.-T.; Cogswell, R.; James, C.A.; Kang, G.; Pullinger, C.R.; Malloy, M.J.; Kane, J.P.; Wojciak, J.; Calkins, H.; Scheinman, M.M.; et al. Plasma BIN1 correlates with heart failure and predicts arrhythmia in patients with arrhythmogenic right ventricular cardiomyopathy. *Hear. Rhythm.* **2012**, *9*, 961–967. [CrossRef]
61. Asimaki, A.; Protonotarios, A.; James, C.A.; Chelko, S.; Tichnell, C.; Murray, B.; Tsatsopoulou, A.; Anastasakis, A.; Riele, A.T.; Kléber, A.G.; et al. Characterizing the Molecular Pathology of Arrhythmogenic Cardiomyopathy in Patient Buccal Mucosa Cells. *Circ. Arrhythmia Electrophysiol.* **2016**, *9*, e003688. [CrossRef] [PubMed]
62. Rolf, S.; Bruns, H.-J.; Wichter, T.; Kirchhof, P.; Ribbing, M.; Wasmer, K.; Paul, M.; Breithardt, G.; Haverkamp, W.; Eckardt, L. The ajmaline challenge in Brugada syndrome: Diagnostic impact, safety, and recommended protocol. *Eur. Hear. J.* **2003**, *24*, 1104–1112. [CrossRef]
63. Peters, S. Arrhythmogenic right ventricular dysplasia-cardiomyopathy and provocable coved-type ST-segment elevation in right precordial leads: Clues from long-term follow-up. *Europace* **2008**, *10*, 816–820. [CrossRef] [PubMed]
64. Oostendorp, T.F.; Van Dessel, P.F.H.M.; Coronel, R.; Belterman, C.; Linnenbank, A.C.; Van Schie, I.H.; Van Oosterom, A.; Oosterhoff, P.; Van Dam, P.M.; De Bakker, J.M.T. Noninvasive detection of epicardial and endocardial activity of the heart. *Neth. Hear. J.* **2011**, *19*, 488–491. [CrossRef]
65. Teske, A.J.; Cox, M.G.; Riele, A.T.; De Boeck, B.W.; Doevendans, P.A.; Hauer, R.N.; Cramer, M.J. Early Detection of Regional Functional Abnormalities in Asymptomatic ARVD/C Gene Carriers. *J. Am. Soc. Echocardiogr.* **2012**, *25*, 997–1006. [CrossRef] [PubMed]
66. Haugaa, K.H.; Haland, T.F.; Leren, I.S.; Saberniak, J.; Edvardsen, T. Arrhythmogenic right ventricular cardiomyopathy, clinical manifestations, and diagnosis. *Europace* **2015**, *18*, 965–972. [CrossRef]
67. Knops, R.E.; Nordkamp, L.R.O.; Delnoy, P.-P.H.; Boersma, L.V.; Kuschyk, J.; El-Chami, M.F.; Bonnemeier, H.; Behr, E.R.; Brouwer, T.F.; Kääb, S.; et al. Subcutaneous or Transvenous Defibrillator Therapy. *N. Engl. J. Med.* **2020**, *383*, 526–536. [CrossRef]
68. Migliore, F.; Viani, S.; Bongiorni, M.G.; Zorzi, A.; Silvetti, M.S.; Francia, P.; D'Onofrio, A.; De Franceschi, P.; Sala, S.; Donzelli, S.; et al. Subcutaneous implantable cardioverter defibrillator in patients with arrhythmogenic right ventricular cardiomyopathy: Results from an Italian multicenter registry. *Int. J. Cardiol.* **2019**, *280*, 74–79. [CrossRef]
69. Link, M.S.; Laidlaw, D.; Polonsky, B.; Zareba, W.; McNitt, S.; Gear, K.; Marcus, F.; Estes, N.A.M. Ventricular Arrhythmias in the North American Multidisciplinary Study of ARVC. *J. Am. Coll. Cardiol.* **2014**, *64*, 119–125. [CrossRef]
70. Migliore, F.; Bertaglia, E.; Zorzi, A.; Corrado, D. Subcutaneous Implantable Cardioverter-Defibrillator and Arrhythmogenic Right Ventricular Cardiomyopathy. *JACC Clin. Electrophysiol.* **2017**, *3*, 785–786. [CrossRef]
71. Migliore, F.; Mattesi, G.; De Franceschi, P.; Allocca, G.; Crosato, M.; Calzolari, V.; Fantinel, M.; Ortis, B.; Facchin, D.; Daleffe, E.; et al. Multicentre experience with the second-generation subcutaneous implantable cardioverter defibrillator and the intermuscular two-incision implantation technique. *J. Cardiovasc. Electrophysiol.* **2019**, *30*, 854–864. [CrossRef]
72. Theuns, D.A.; Brouwer, T.F.; Jones, P.W.; Allavatam, V.; Donnelley, S.; Auricchio, A.; Knops, R.E.; Burke, M.C. Prospective blinded evaluation of a novel sensing methodology designed to reduce inappropriate shocks by the subcutaneous implantable cardioverter-defibrillator. *Hear. Rhythm.* **2018**, *15*, 1515–1522. [CrossRef] [PubMed]
73. Priori, S.; Blomström-Lundqvist, C.; Mazzanti, A.; Blom, N.; Borggrefe, M.; Camm, J.; Elliott, P.M.; Fitzsimons, D.; Hatala, R.; Hindricks, G.; et al. 2015 ESC Guidelines for the management of patients with ventricular arrhythmias and the prevention of sudden cardiac death. *Eur. Hear. J.* **2015**, *36*, 2793–2867. [CrossRef] [PubMed]
74. Tedford, R.J.; James, C.; Judge, D.; Tichnell, C.; Murray, B.; Bhonsale, A.; Philips, B.; Abraham, T.; Dalal, D.; Halushka, M.; et al. Cardiac Transplantation in Arrhythmogenic Right Ventricular Dysplasia/Cardiomyopathy. *J. Am. Coll. Cardiol.* **2012**, *59*, 289–290. [CrossRef] [PubMed]
75. Yancy, C.W.; Jessup, M.; Bozkurt, B.; Butler, J.; Casey, D.E., Jr.; Drazner, M.H.; Fonarow, G.C.; Geraci, S.A.; Horwich, T.; Januzzi, J.L.; et al. 2013 ACCF/AHA Guideline for the Management of Heart Failure: A report of the American College of Cardiology Foundation/American Heart Association Task Force on Practice Guidelines. *J. Am. Coll. Cardiol.* **2013**, *62*, e147–e239. [CrossRef] [PubMed]
76. Ponikowski, P.; Voors, A.A.; Anker, S.D.; Bueno, H.; Cleland, J.G.F.; Coats, A.J.S.; Falk, V.; González-Juanatey, J.R.; Harjola, V.-P.; Jankowska, E.A.; et al. 2016 ESC Guidelines for the diagnosis and treatment of acute and chronic heart failure: The Task Force for the diagnosis and treatment of acute and chronic heart failure of the European Society of Cardiology (ESC). Developed with the special contribution of the Heart Failure Association (HFA) of the ESC. *Eur. J. Heart Fail.* **2016**, *18*, 891–975. [CrossRef] [PubMed]
77. Mogensen, U.M.; Gong, J.; Jhund, P.; Shen, L.; Køber, L.; Desai, A.S.; Lefkowitz, M.P.; Packer, M.; Rouleau, J.L.; Solomon, S.D.; et al. Effect of sacubitril/valsartan on recurrent events in the Prospective comparison of ARNI with ACEI to Determine Impact on Global Mortality and morbidity in Heart Failure trial (PARADIGM-HF). *Eur. J. Hear. Fail.* **2018**, *20*, 760–768. [CrossRef]
78. Asimaki, A.; Kapoor, S.; Plovie, E.; Arndt, A.K.; Adams, E.; Liu, Z.; James, C.A.; Judge, D.; Calkins, H.; Churko, J.; et al. Identification of a New Modulator of the Intercalated Disc in a Zebrafish Model of Arrhythmogenic Cardiomyopathy. *Sci. Transl. Med.* **2014**, *6*, 240ra74. [CrossRef]

79. Chelko, S.; Asimaki, A.; Andersen, P.; Bedja, D.; Amat-Alarcon, N.; DeMazumder, D.; Jasti, R.; Macrae, C.A.; Leber, R.; Kleber, A.G.; et al. Central role for GSK3β in the pathogenesis of arrhythmogenic cardiomyopathy. *JCI Insight* **2016**, *1*, 1. [CrossRef]
80. Chelko, S.; Asimaki, A.; Lowenthal, J.; Bueno-Beti, C.; Bedja, D.; Scalco, A.; Amat-Alarcon, N.; Andersen, P.; Judge, D.P.; Tung, L.; et al. Therapeutic Modulation of the Immune Response in Arrhythmogenic Cardiomyopathy. *Circulation* **2019**, *140*, 1491–1505. [CrossRef]
81. Zhang, X.; Meng, F.; Song, J.; Zhang, L.; Wang, J.; Li, D.; Li, L.; Dong, P.; Yang, B.; Chen, Y. Pentoxifylline Ameliorates Cardiac Fibrosis, Pathological Hypertrophy, and Cardiac Dysfunction in Angiotensin II-induced Hypertensive Rats. *J. Cardiovasc. Pharmacol.* **2016**, *67*, 76–85. [CrossRef] [PubMed]
82. Szekely, Y.; Arbel, Y. A Review of Interleukin-1 in Heart Disease: Where Do We Stand Today? *Cardiol. Ther.* **2018**, *7*, 25–44. [CrossRef] [PubMed]
83. Ridker, P.M.; Everett, B.M.; Thuren, T.; MacFadyen, J.G.; Chang, W.H.; Ballantyne, C.; Fonseca, F.; Nicolau, J.; Koenig, W.; Anker, S.D.; et al. Antiinflammatory Therapy with Canakinumab for Atherosclerotic Disease. *N. Engl. J. Med.* **2017**, *377*, 1119–1131. [CrossRef] [PubMed]
84. Muchir, A.; Wu, W.; Choi, J.C.; Iwata, S.; Morrow, J.; Homma, S.; Worman, H.J. Abnormal p38 mitogen-activated protein kinase signaling in dilated cardiomyopathy caused by lamin A/C gene mutation. *Hum. Mol. Genet.* **2012**, *21*, 4325–4333. [CrossRef] [PubMed]
85. Philips, B.; Madhavan, S.; James, C.; Tichnell, C.; Murray, B.; Dalal, D.; Bhonsale, A.; Nazarian, S.; Judge, D.; Russell, S.D.; et al. Outcomes of Catheter Ablation of Ventricular Tachycardia in Arrhythmogenic Right Ventricular Dysplasia/Cardiomyopathy. *Circ. Arrhythmia Electrophysiol.* **2012**, *5*, 499–505. [CrossRef] [PubMed]
86. Garcia, F.C.; Bazan, V.; Zado, E.S.; Ren, J.-F.; Marchlinski, F. Epicardial Substrate and Outcome with Epicardial Ablation of Ventricular Tachycardia in Arrhythmogenic Right Ventricular Cardiomyopathy/Dysplasia. *Circulation* **2009**, *120*, 366–375. [CrossRef]
87. Polin, G.M.; Haqqani, H.; Tzou, W.; Hutchinson, M.; Garcia, F.C.; Callans, D.J.; Zado, E.S.; Marchlinski, F.E. Endocardial unipolar voltage mapping to identify epicardial substrate in arrhythmogenic right ventricular cardiomyopathy/dysplasia. *Hear. Rhythm.* **2011**, *8*, 76–83. [CrossRef]
88. Santangeli, P.; Tung, R.; Xue, Y.; Chung, F.-P.; Lin, Y.-J.; Di Biase, L.; Zhan, X.; Lin, C.-Y.; Wei, W.; Mohanty, S.; et al. Outcomes of Catheter Ablation in Arrhythmogenic Right Ventricular Cardiomyopathy Without Background Implantable Cardioverter Defibrillator Therapy. *JACC Clin. Electrophysiol.* **2019**, *5*, 55–65. [CrossRef]
89. Berruezo, A.; Acosta, J.; Fernández-Armenta, J.; Pedrote, A.; Barrera, A.; Arana-Rueda, E.; Bodegas, A.I.; Anguera, I.; Tercedor, L.; Penela, D.; et al. Safety, long-term outcomes and predictors of recurrence after first-line combined endoepicardial ventricular tachycardia substrate ablation in arrhythmogenic cardiomyopathy. Impact of arrhythmic substrate distribution pattern. A prospective multicentre study. *Europace* **2016**, *19*, 607–616. [CrossRef]

Journal of
Clinical Medicine

Review

Fabry Cardiomyopathy: Current Treatment and Future Options

Irfan Vardarli [1,*], Manuel Weber [2], Christoph Rischpler [2], Dagmar Führer [3], Ken Herrmann [2] and Frank Weidemann [1]

[1] Department of Medicine I, Klinikum Vest GmbH, Knappschaftskrankenhaus Recklinghausen, Academic Teaching Hospital, Ruhr-University Bochum, 45657 Recklinghausen, Germany; frank.weidemann@klinikum-vest.de
[2] Department of Nuclear Medicine, University Hospital Essen, 45147 Essen, Germany; manuel.weber@uk-essen.de (M.W.); christoph.rischpler@uk-essen.de (C.R.); ken.herrmann@uk-essen.de (K.H.)
[3] Department of Endocrinology, Diabetes and Metabolism, Clinical Chemistry—Division of Laboratory Research, Endocrine Tumor Center, WTZ/Comprehensive Cancer Center, University Hospital Essen, University of Duisburg-Essen, 45147 Essen, Germany; dagmar.fuehrer@uk-essen.de
* Correspondence: irfan.vardarli@alumni.uni-heidelberg.de; Tel.: +49-2361-563401

Abstract: Fabry disease is a multisystem X-linked lysosomal storage disorder caused by a mutation in the alpha-galactosidase A gene. Deficiency or reduced activity of alpha-galactosidase A (GLA) is leading to progressive intracellular accumulation of globotriaosylceramide (GL3) in various organs, including the heart, kidney and nerve system. Cardiac involvement is frequent and is evident as concentric left ventricular hypertrophy. Currently, the standard treatment is enzyme replacement therapy or chaperone therapy. However, early starting of therapy, before myocardial fibrosis has developed, is essential for long-term improvement of myocardial function. For future treatment options, various therapeutic approaches including gene therapy are under development. This review describes the current and potential future therapy options for Fabry cardiomyopathy.

Keywords: Fabry; cardiomyopathy; treatment; options

Citation: Vardarli, I.; Weber, M.; Rischpler, C.; Führer, D.; Herrmann, K.; Weidemann, F. Fabry Cardiomyopathy: Current Treatment and Future Options. *J. Clin. Med.* **2021**, *10*, 3026. https://doi.org/10.3390/jcm10143026

Academic Editor: Stefan Peters

Received: 10 June 2021
Accepted: 3 July 2021
Published: 7 July 2021

1. Introduction

Fabry disease (FD) is a multisystem X-linked lysosomal storage disorder caused by a mutation in the alpha-galactosidase A (GLA) gene [1]. Deficiency or reduced activity of GLA is leading to progressive accumulation of intracellular globotriaosylceramide (GL3) in various organs, including the heart, kidney and nerve system [2]. Typical manifestations include neuropathic pain, telangiectasias, anhidrosis, gastrointestinal symptoms, cornea verticillata, renal failure with unknown etiology, unexplained left ventricular (LV) hypertrophy or neurological manifestations (e.g., cryptogenic stroke) [3–8]. Regarding diagnosis of FD and Fabry cardiomyopathy, various reviews have been published [9,10].

In suspected cases, determination of GLA activity is recommended. In males, GLA activity <1% is highly suggestive for the disease of classic FD [9]. In females and in patients with late-onset mutations (e.g., N215S cardiac variant mutation) the enzyme activity may be residual or even normal; thus, in such cases, genetic testing of Fabry mutations is mandatory [11]. Basically, the additional determination of globotriaosylsphingosine (lyso-GL3) is recommended. Lyso-GL3 levels $\geq$2.7 ng/mL are associated with classical mutations [12]. For evaluation of relevant cardiac involvement, the determination of highly sensitive Troponin (hsTnT) and B-type natriuretic peptide (NT proBNP), as biomarkers, are useful [13]. In FD, hsTNT is more related to early development of cardiac fibrosis and NT proBNP to heart failure in advanced stages [14].

Although blood tests are very easy to perform, a lot of patients are diagnosed late during the disease progression. The reason for this is that symptoms can vary a lot and thus it is difficult for the clinician to assign very general symptoms to this very rare disease.

Thus, overall it takes on average 10 years from the first symptom to the correct diagnosis of FD.

In patients with FD, morbidity and poor prognosis are mainly driven by cardiomyopathy [15,16]. Currently, the standard treatment is enzyme replacement therapy or chaperone therapy [17]. However, early beginning of therapy, before myocardial fibrosis has developed, is essential for long-term improvement or stabilization of myocardial function [18]. For future treatment options, various therapeutic approaches including gene therapy are under development. This review describes the current and future therapy options for Fabry cardiomyopathy.

2. Fabry Cardiomyopathy

Left ventricular (LV) hypertrophy is the main mechanism of the Fabry cardiomyopathy. LV hypertrophy (LVH) is partly a reaction of the tissue to the GL3 deposition [10]. In addition, an increase of trophic factors, e.g., lyso-Gb3, play a role in the development of Fabry cardiomyopathy [19–26]. Furthermore, upregulation of cellular adhesion molecules in vascular endothelial cells or by oxidative stress leads to LVH [27]. Genetic aspects should also be considered. Germain et al. confirmed that p.N215S is a disease-causing Fabry mutation with severe clinical manifestations essentially limited to the heart until late adulthood, especially in males [28].

Concentric LV thickening without outflow tract obstruction [29–31], prominence of papillary muscles [30,32,33], preservation of ejection fraction and slight to mild to moderate impairment of diastolic function [15] are typical echocardiographic aspects in Fabry patients. Even in the early stages of FD, mild impairment of regional myocardial function is common, and can be assessed by strain rate or deformation imaging [16,19,29,34]. Typically, the reduction of myocardial longitudinal function starts in basal regions of posterolateral myocardium and is related to myocardial fibrosis in later stages [16]. In the end-stage cardiomyopathy, wall motion abnormalities can be observed on bidimensional echocardiography [35]. The development of replacement fibrosis, which is mostly limited to posterolateral segments of basal myocardium, is a typical morphologic sign for Fabry cardiomyopathy [19,22] and is associated with a poor prognosis [16,35]. This fibrosis can be assessed by gadolinium-contrast late enhancement (LE) magnetic resonance imaging (the gold standard for the assessment of myocardial fibrosis) or indirectly by functional deformation imaging [19,22,36,37]. Echocardiographic aspects and magnetic resonance tomography findings in various stages of Fabry cardiomyopathy were shown in Figure 1. In general, there are sufficient cardiac tools to assess early Fabry cardiomyopathy. In this context cardiac magnetic resonance tomography with T1 mapping and late enhancement imaging are very important imaging tools. Only in some patients with inconsistent diagnostic results and insufficient treatment effects cardiac biopsy might help.

Common misdiagnoses involving the heart and in particular the finding of LVH in FD are hypertensive heart disease, sarcomeric hypertrophic cardiomyopathy, cardiac amyloidosis and Friedreich cardiomyopathy. Whenever FD is suspected in hypertrophic hearts, additional questions about typical Fabry symptoms should be discussed with the patient. If the patient suffered from LVH and typical symptoms, Fabry disease is very likely and a blood test should be performed.

In case of unexplained LVH (>13 mm), FD should be suspected. In general male patients can develop LVH at the age of 20 and female patients around 10 years later. In a cohort of 100 males with unexplained LVH (≥13 mm) older than 30 years, Palecek et al. found a prevalence of 4.0% for FD. They recommend screening for FD in all men older than 30 years with unexplained LVH even in the absence of obvious extracardiac manifestations [38]. Hagège et al. investigated a cohort of 392 adult patients (278 men) with HCM defined by wall thickness ≥ 15 mm in 29 French cardiology centers. In four men (all older than 40 years; 1.5% of the cohort) the diagnosis of FD was confirmed by blood and genetic testing [39]. Nakao et al. and Sachdev et al. reported in their trials similar results [40,41].

However, other multicenter screening trials found lower prevalence of FD in patients with unexplained LVH, ranging between 0.5% and 1.5% [42,43].

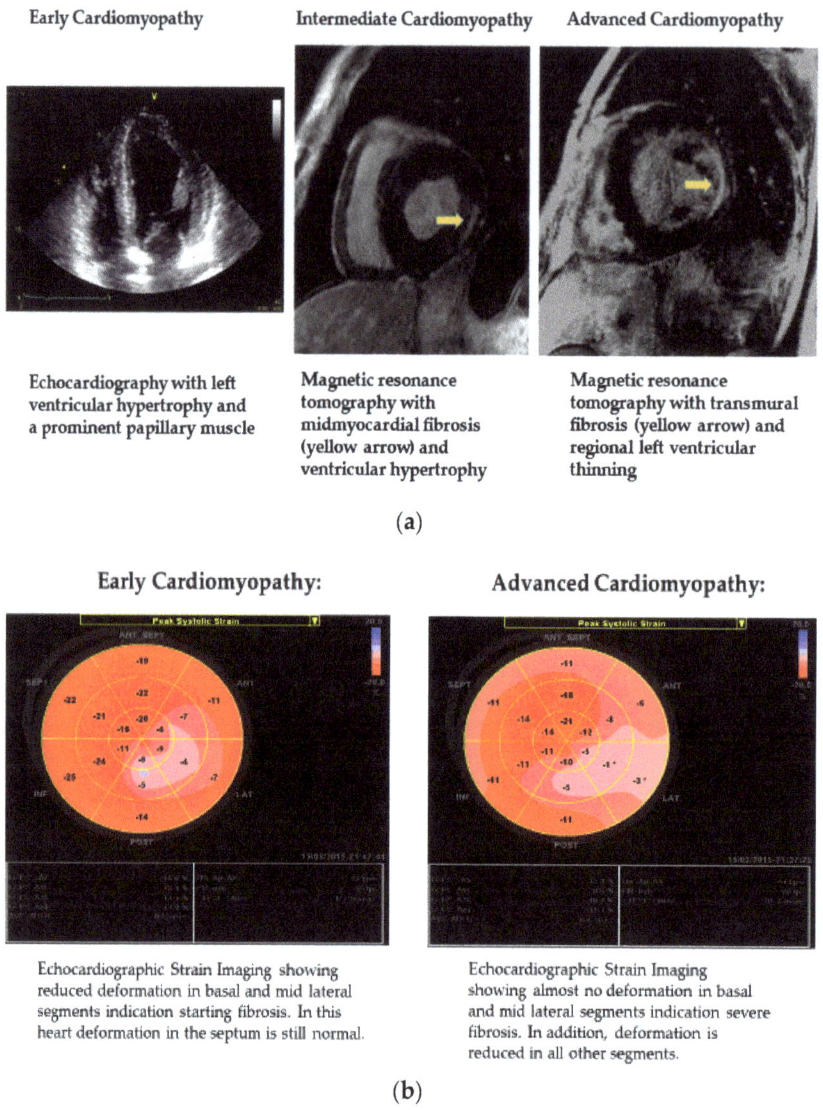

Figure 1. (**a**) Echocardiographic aspects and magnetic resonance tomography findings in various stages of Fabry cardiomyopathy. (**b**) Strain analysis in various stages of Fabry cardiomyopathy.

In all patients with a Fabry cardiomyopathy regular follow-up examinations are necessary. For cardiac test echocardiography, ECG, Holter ECG, ergometry and cardiac biomarkers should be performed. If patients are treated, all these diagnostic tests should be performed once a year. An MRI including late enhancement imaging and if possible T1 mapping should be done at least every two years [44,45].

2.1. *Treatment of Fabry Cardiomyopathy*

2.1.1. Current Treatment

Fabry cardiomyopathy, which leads to reduced life expectancy in untreated patients [46,47], can be treated with a causal therapy. The current therapy for FD (Figure 2) is enzyme replacement therapy (ERT) or in amenable mutations Chaperone therapy. ERT is administered by lifelong biweekly infusion of recombinant enzyme [48,49], which is available as agalsidase alfa (Replagal®, Shire Human Genetics Therapies AB, Stockholm, Sweden, since 2019 Takeda Pharma AG, 8152 Opfikon, Switzerland) and agalsidase beta (Fabrazyme®, Sanofi Genzyme, Cambridge, MA, USA). After enzyme replacement, microvascular GL3 depositions were cleared in the kidneys, skin and the heart of most Fabry patients [49–52]. The depletion of GL3 depositions and reduced inflammation are associated with reduced LV mass and in some patients with early stage of the disease augmentation of regional myocardial function is possible [19,29,53]. Nevertheless, the effect of ERT on life expectancy remains unclear. The timing of ERT is important, as the foremost benefit of ERT was reported in patients with less severe stage of cardiomyopathy at baseline [18,20]. Improvements of cardiomyopathy (decrease in myocardial mass, improvement of regional myocardial function and increase in exercise capacity) were observed during three years of ERT only in patients without replacement fibrosis. A reduction of LVH and stabilization of exercise capacity and LV function were found in patients with myocardial fibrosis only in one LV segment; whereas no benefit in LV function and no clear regression of LVH were seen in patients with more than one affected (myocardial fibrosis) LV segment [19]. Most patients, particularly male patients, are developing antibodies with neutralizing activity during long-term ERT [54–56]. The impact of these neutralizing antibodies on heart morphology and function remains unclear.

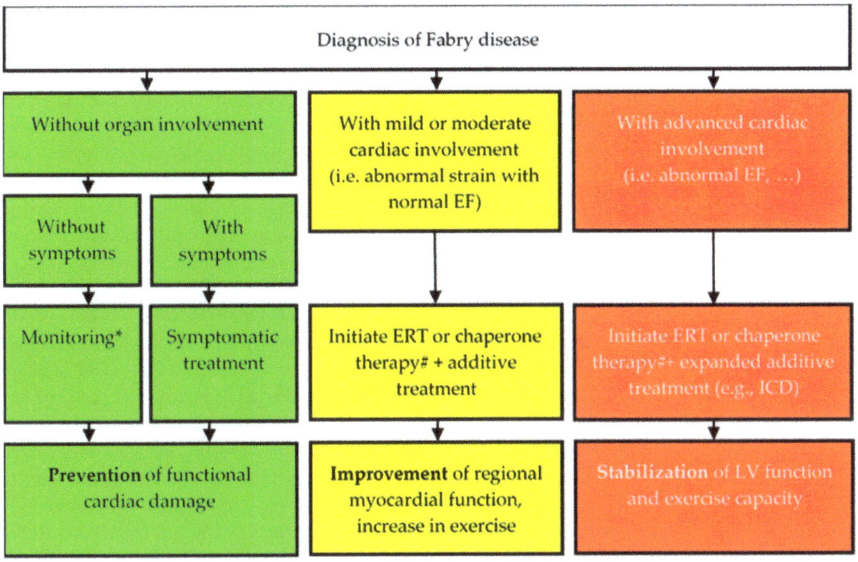

Figure 2. Current treatment algorithm for Fabry cardiomyopathy (adapted with permission from Weidemann F. et al. The Fabry cardiomyopathy: models for the cardiologist. Annu Rev Med 2011; 62: 59-67. Copyright© 2021, Marketplace™. #: only in patients with Migalastat-amenable GLA mutations possible. EF: ejection fraction, ERT: Enzyme replacement therapy, ICD: implanted cardioverter defibrillator, LV: left ventricular. * e.g., echocardiography, Holter electrocardiography (ECG). All established diagnostic tests should be performed one a year.

Chaperone therapy with Migalastat (Galafold®, Amicus Therapeutics, Cranbury, NJ, USA) with its convenient oral regimen was approved in Europe in 2016, and is an important treatment option for FD in patients with migalastat-amenable GLA mutations [17]. Germain et al. showed significant decrease in the LV mass index after ≤24 months' migalastat therapy [57]. However, as myocardial fibrosis is probably not reversible, starting treatment in early stage of the disease is crucial for improvement of prognosis [19]. Prescribing information and/or the migalastat amenability table at the website (https://www.galafoldamenabilitytable.com/hcp, accessed on 10 June 2021) should be considered for a list of amenable and non-amenable GLA mutations to migalastat. Migalastat is not recommended in patients with eGFR < 30 mL/min/1.73 m^2 [58–60].

In all patients with a cardiomyopathy additional therapy is necessary. Optimization of hypertension treatment and control of proteinuria is required. In such cases angiotensin-converting enzyme inhibitors or angiotensin receptor blockers should be preferred, with blood pressure monitoring [61,62].

Tachyarrhythmia may be treated by the use of beta-adrenergic blocking drugs, with protective effect regarding ventricular arrhythmias. Additional therapy can be applied in combination to ERT or chaperone therapy [63,64].

In case of atrial fibrillation, sinus rhythm should be restored, if possible, as brady- or tachyarrhythmia may further reduce the exercise capacity. In these patients, pulmonary vein ablation should be considered. If a restoration is not possible, frequency control should be started and therapy with oral anticoagulants is necessary [10].

In patients with bradycardia beta-adrenergic blocking drugs should be stopped and the implantation of a pacemaker should be considered [18,19]. The insertion of an implantable cardio-defibrillator should be evaluated in patients with life threatening arrhythmias, particularly in patients with end-stage cardiomyopathy [10,47].

2.1.2. Future Treatment Options/Investigational Therapies

Results from a phase 1/2 trial showed that pegunigalsidase alfa, a novel pegylated, covalently crosslinked form of alpha-GLA, may represent an advance in ERT, based on its pharmacokinetics and apparent low immunogenicity [65]. Agalsidase alfa and beta exhibit a terminal half-life ($T_{1/2\gamma}$) of ≤2 h and a maintain measurable plasma level for only <24 h [66,67]. With a $T_{1/2\gamma}$ of about 80 h, with measurable plasma levels sustained for the entire 2-week dosing interval, pegunigalsidase alfa is providing an active reservoir in the circulation to reach the target tissues [65]. Compared with agalsidase alfa or beta, patients treated with pegunigalsidase alfa developed less treatment induced antidrug antibodies (ADA) [65]. In the BALANCE trial (estimated completion date: May 2022), the BRIDGE trial (enrollment completed December 2019) and the BRIGHT trial (enrollment completed October 2020), the safety and efficacy of pegunigalsidase alpha was investigated [68]. In the BRIDGE trial, an open-label study of the safety and efficacy of pegunigalsidase alfa in patients with FD treated for at least 2 years and on a stable dose (>80%) labelled dose/kg) for at least 6 months with Replagal® (Agalsidase alfa), infusion (1 mg/kg) of the investigational medication has been administered every 2 weeks for 12 months. In the BRIGHT trial, a phase 3, open label, switch over study to assess safety, efficacy and pharmacokinetics of pegunigalsidase alfa 2 mg/kg (Bodyweight) has been administered every 4 weeks for 52 weeks in Fabry disease patients previously treated with ERT (Fabrazyme® (Agalsidase beta) or Replagal® (Agalsidase alfa)) for at least 3 years. For both studies no results have been posted yet.

Substrate reduction therapy (SRT) with Lucerastat is currently under investigation. Lucerastat, or N-butyldeoxygalactonojirimycin (Idorsia Pharmaceutical Ltd., Allschwil, Switzerland), a glucosylceramide synthase (GCS) inhibitor which prevents accumulation of Gb-3 [69] can reduce circulating levels of globotriacylceramide and other sphingolipids [70]. Venglustat (Sanofi Genzyme, Cambridge, MA, USA), another substrate reduction therapy, is currently in a phase 2 study (NCT 02489). With a high volume of distribution Lucerastat may be able to reach tissues that ERT poorly penetrates [69]. In Fabry mice it has been shown that GCS inhibitors can bring reversal of disease phenotypes which are not improved with enzyme replacement therapy [69,71,72]. The data of Welford et al. support the use for Lucerastat in Fabry patients with various genotypes, suggesting that Lucerastat could be an oral therapy suitable for all Fabry patients ignoring the primary mutation [69].

Various approaches to gene therapy are under development. Gene editing occurs ex vivo or in vivo.

With the ex vitro approach, hematopoietic stem cells are harvested from the patient. These cells receive gene editing and are then infused back into the patient for engraftment after myeloablative therapy is conducted. It has been demonstrated that CD34+ positive hematopoietic stem cells could be harvested and modified through recombinant lentivirus (LV)-mediated gene transfer of the GLA gene [73]. In the first gene therapy pilot project for FD, Khan et al. demonstrated efficient LV-mediated gene transfer into enriched Fabry patient CD34+ cells. They reported increased circulating and intracellular GLA activity, without serious safety concerns [74]. All Fabry patients (n = 5) in this pilot trial were responsive to the LV-mediated gene therapy at some level; all patients produced GLA to near normal level within one week, plasma and leukocytes demonstrates GLA activity within or above the reference range, and reductions in plasma and urine globotriaosylceramide (Gb3) and globotriaosylsphingosine (lyso-Gb3) have been demonstrated. Three patients have elected to discontinue enzyme replacement [74]. Persistent elevation of GLA activity in patients has demonstrated early safety of the protocol for this ex vivo approach, as shown also by a press release from AVROBIO [75]. However, before gene therapy can be adopted as therapeutic intervention for FD, a crucial question will be whether the current gene therapy approaches will achieve sufficient GLA activity in different tissues [75].

With the in vivo approach, a vector with gene editing is infused directly into the patient, and then cells within the patient, such as liver cells, directly undergo gene editing to express the missing protein [75]. Pre-clinical data using the liver targeted adeno-associated virus (AAV)-mediated gene transfer (ST920) has shown in alpha-gal A knockout (GLAKO) mouse model in which, after a single injection, GLA is produced by the liver and released into the bloodstream. GLA levels rise in a dose-dependent manner and have achieved levels more than 300 times those of GLA deficient mice [75]. In the first in human treatment with ST920, a recombinant AAV2/6 vector encoding the cDNA for human GAL, the safety and tolerability of ascending doses of ST920 will be elucidated (Sangamo Therapeutics, Brisbane, CA, USA). The estimated primary completion date of this phase 1/2 multicenter study (NCT04046224, ST-920-201) is December 2023 (final data collection date for primary outcome measure) [75]. The trial is currently recruiting participants in the United States. However, gene therapy might have some potential risks: unwanted immune system reactions, targeting false cells, infections induced by the virus and development of a tumor.

Another investigational approach is the administration of GLA mRNA to promote stimulated production of GLA, which is an additional unique form of therapy [76]. It has been shown that mRNA for human GLA encapsulated with lipid nanoparticles could increase GLA levels expressed in cardiac, kidney and liver tissues, resulting in enhanced globotriaosylceramide clearance [76].

3. Conclusions

Fabry cardiomyopathy, which leads to reduced life expectancy in untreated patients, can be treated with a causal therapy. However, as myocardial fibrosis is not reversible, the early starting of treatment is crucial for improvement of prognosis. New therapy concepts are under investigation in prospective studies and might help for a more efficient treatment in all stages of the cardiomyopathy.

Author Contributions: I.V., M.W., C.R., D.F., K.H. and F.W. contributed to the literature review and the preparation of the manuscript. F.W. supervised this work. All authors have read and agreed to the published version of the manuscript.

Funding: This research received no external funding.

Institutional Review Board Statement: Not applicable.

Informed Consent Statement: Not applicable.

Conflicts of Interest: Dr. Vardarli, Dr. Weber, Dr. Rischpler and Dr. Führer declare no conflicts of interest in this work. Dr. Herrmann reports personal fees from Bayer, stock options (less than 1%) from Sofie Biosciences, personal fees from SIRTEX, non-financial support from ABX, personal fees from Adacap, personal fees from Curium, personal fees from Endocyte, grants and personal fees from BTG, personal fees from IPSEN, personal fees from Siemens Healthineers, personal fees from GE Healthcare, personal fees from Amgen, personal fees from Novartis, personal fees from Y-mAbs, outside the submitted work. Dr. Weidemann has received research grants from Genzyme and Shire and speaker honoraria from Amicus, Genzyme, and Shire.

References

1. Brady, R.O.; Gal, A.E.; Bradley, R.M.; Martensson, E.; Warshaw, A.L.; Laster, L. Enzymatic defect in Fabry's disease. Ceramidetrihexosidase deficiency. *N. Engl. J. Med.* **1967**, *276*, 1163–1167. [CrossRef] [PubMed]
2. Desnick, R.J.; Brady, R.; Barranger, J.; Collins, A.J.; Germain, D.P.; Goldman, M.; Grabowski, G.; Packman, S.; Wilcox, W.R. Fabry disease, an under-recognized multisystemic disorder: Expert recommendations for diagnosis, management, and enzyme replacement therapy. *Ann. Intern. Med.* **2003**, *138*, 338–346. [CrossRef] [PubMed]
3. van der Tol, L.; Smid, B.E.; Poorthuis, B.J.; Biegstraaten, M.; Deprez, R.H.; Linthorst, G.E.; Hollak, C.E. A systematic review on screening for Fabry disease: Prevalence of individuals with genetic variants of unknown significance. *J. Med. Genet.* **2014**, *51*, 1–9. [CrossRef] [PubMed]
4. Liguori, R.; Incensi, A.; de Pasqua, S.; Mignani, R.; Fileccia, E.; Santostefano, M.; Biagini, E.; Rapezzi, C.; Palmieri, S.; Romani, I.; et al. Skin globotriaosylceramide 3 deposits are specific to Fabry disease with classical mutations and associated with small fibre neuropathy. *PLoS ONE* **2017**, *12*, e0180581. [CrossRef] [PubMed]
5. Wozniak, M.A.; Kittner, S.J.; Tuhrim, S.; Cole, J.W.; Stern, B.; Dobbins, M.; Grace, M.E.; Nazarenko, I.; Dobrovolny, R.; McDade, E.; et al. Frequency of unrecognized Fabry disease among young European-American and African-American men with first ischemic stroke. *Stroke* **2010**, *41*, 78–81. [CrossRef]
6. van der Tol, L.; Svarstad, E.; Ortiz, A.; Tondel, C.; Oliveira, J.P.; Vogt, L.; Waldek, S.; Hughes, D.A.; Lachmann, R.H.; Terryn, W.; et al. Chronic kidney disease and an uncertain diagnosis of Fabry disease: Approach to a correct diagnosis. *Mol. Genet. Metab.* **2015**, *114*, 242–247. [CrossRef] [PubMed]
7. Nagueh, S.F. Anderson-Fabry disease and other lysosomal storage disorders. *Circulation* **2014**, *130*, 1081–1090. [CrossRef] [PubMed]
8. Laney, D.A.; Peck, D.S.; Atherton, A.M.; Manwaring, L.P.; Christensen, K.M.; Shankar, S.P.; Grange, D.K.; Wilcox, W.R.; Hopkin, R.J. Fabry disease in infancy and early childhood: A systematic literature review. *Genet. Med.* **2015**, *17*, 323–330. [CrossRef]
9. Vardarli, I.; Rischpler, C.; Herrmann, K.; Weidemann, F. Diagnosis and Screening of Patients with Fabry Disease. *Ther. Clin. Risk Manag.* **2020**, *16*, 551–558. [CrossRef]
10. Weidemann, F.; Ertl, G.; Wanner, C.; Kramer, J. The Fabry cardiomyopathy—Diagnostic approach and current treatment. *Curr. Pharm. Des.* **2015**, *21*, 473–478. [CrossRef]
11. Ortiz, A.; Germain, D.P.; Desnick, R.J.; Politei, J.; Mauer, M.; Burlina, A.; Eng, C.; Hopkin, R.J.; Laney, D.; Linhart, A.; et al. Fabry disease revisited: Management and treatment recommendations for adult patients. *Mol. Genet. Metab.* **2018**, *123*, 416–427. [CrossRef]
12. Niemann, M.; Rolfs, A.; Stork, S.; Bijnens, B.; Breunig, F.; Beer, M.; Ertl, G.; Wanner, C.; Weidemann, F. Gene mutations versus clinically relevant phenotypes: Lyso-Gb3 defines Fabry disease. *Circ. Cardiovasc. Genet.* **2014**, *7*, 8–16. [CrossRef] [PubMed]
13. Weidemann, F.; Beer, M.; Kralewski, M.; Siwy, J.; Kampmann, C. Early detection of organ involvement in Fabry disease by biomarker assessment in conjunction with LGE cardiac MRI: Results from the SOPHIA study. *Mol. Genet. Metab.* **2019**, *126*, 169–182. [CrossRef]
14. Seydelmann, N.; Liu, D.; Kramer, J.; Drechsler, C.; Hu, K.; Nordbeck, P.; Schneider, A.; Stork, S.; Bijnens, B.; Ertl, G.; et al. High-Sensitivity Troponin: A Clinical Blood Biomarker for Staging Cardiomyopathy in Fabry Disease. *J. Am. Heart Assoc.* **2016**, *5*. [CrossRef]
15. Linhart, A.; Kampmann, C.; Zamorano, J.L.; Sunder-Plassmann, G.; Beck, M.; Mehta, A.; Elliott, P.M.; European FOS Investigators. Cardiac manifestations of Anderson-Fabry disease: Results from the international Fabry outcome survey. *Eur. Heart J.* **2007**, *28*, 1228–1235. [CrossRef]
16. Weidemann, F.; Breunig, F.; Beer, M.; Sandstede, J.; Stork, S.; Voelker, W.; Ertl, G.; Knoll, A.; Wanner, C.; Strotmann, J.M. The variation of morphological and functional cardiac manifestation in Fabry disease: Potential implications for the time course of the disease. *Eur. Heart J.* **2005**, *26*, 1221–1227. [CrossRef]
17. McCafferty, E.H.; Scott, L.J. Migalastat: A Review in Fabry Disease. *Drugs* **2019**, *79*, 543–554. [CrossRef]
18. Beck, M. Agalsidase alfa for the treatment of Fabry disease: New data on clinical efficacy and safety. *Expert Opin. Biol. Ther.* **2009**, *9*, 255–261. [CrossRef] [PubMed]

19. Weidemann, F.; Niemann, M.; Breunig, F.; Herrmann, S.; Beer, M.; Stork, S.; Voelker, W.; Ertl, G.; Wanner, C.; Strotmann, J. Long-term effects of enzyme replacement therapy on fabry cardiomyopathy: Evidence for a better outcome with early treatment. *Circulation* **2009**, *119*, 524–529. [CrossRef]
20. Banikazemi, M.; Bultas, J.; Waldek, S.; Wilcox, W.R.; Whitley, C.B.; McDonald, M.; Finkel, R.; Packman, S.; Bichet, D.G.; Warnock, D.G.; et al. Agalsidase-beta therapy for advanced Fabry disease: A randomized trial. *Ann. Intern. Med.* **2007**, *146*, 77–86. [CrossRef] [PubMed]
21. Aerts, J.M.; Groener, J.E.; Kuiper, S.; Donker-Koopman, W.E.; Strijland, A.; Ottenhoff, R.; van Roomen, C.; Mirzaian, M.; Wijburg, F.A.; Linthorst, G.E.; et al. Elevated globotriaosylsphingosine is a hallmark of Fabry disease. *Proc. Natl. Acad. Sci. USA* **2008**, *105*, 2812–2817. [CrossRef] [PubMed]
22. Moon, J.C.; Sachdev, B.; Elkington, A.G.; McKenna, W.J.; Mehta, A.; Pennell, D.J.; Leed, P.J.; Elliott, P.M. Gadolinium enhanced cardiovascular magnetic resonance in Anderson-Fabry disease. Evidence for a disease specific abnormality of the myocardial interstitium. *Eur. Heart J.* **2003**, *24*, 2151–2155. [CrossRef] [PubMed]
23. Sheppard, M.N.; Cane, P.; Florio, R.; Kavantzas, N.; Close, L.; Shah, J.; Lee, P.; Elliott, P. A detailed pathologic examination of heart tissue from three older patients with Anderson-Fabry disease on enzyme replacement therapy. *Cardiovasc. Pathol.* **2010**, *19*, 293–301. [CrossRef] [PubMed]
24. Elleder, M.; Bradova, V.; Smid, F.; Budesinsky, M.; Harzer, K.; Kustermann-Kuhn, B.; Ledvinova, J.; Kral, V.; Dorazilova, V. Cardiocyte storage and hypertrophy as a sole manifestation of Fabry's disease. Report on a case simulating hypertrophic non-obstructive cardiomyopathy. *Virchows Arch. A Pathol. Anat. Histopathol.* **1990**, *417*, 449–455. [CrossRef] [PubMed]
25. Elliott, P.M.; Kindler, H.; Shah, J.S.; Sachdev, B.; Rimoldi, O.E.; Thaman, R.; Tome, M.T.; McKenna, W.J.; Lee, P.; Camici, P.G. Coronary microvascular dysfunction in male patients with Anderson-Fabry disease and the effect of treatment with alpha galactosidase A. *Heart* **2006**, *92*, 357–360. [CrossRef]
26. Barbey, F.; Brakch, N.; Linhart, A.; Rosenblatt-Velin, N.; Jeanrenaud, X.; Qanadli, S.; Steinmann, B.; Burnier, M.; Palecek, T.; Bultas, J.; et al. Cardiac and vascular hypertrophy in Fabry disease: Evidence for a new mechanism independent of blood pressure and glycosphingolipid deposition. *Arterioscler. Thromb. Vasc. Biol.* **2006**, *26*, 839–844. [CrossRef]
27. Shen, J.S.; Meng, X.L.; Moore, D.F.; Quirk, J.M.; Shayman, J.A.; Schiffmann, R.; Kaneski, C.R. Globotriaosylceramide induces oxidative stress and up-regulates cell adhesion molecule expression in Fabry disease endothelial cells. *Mol. Genet. Metab.* **2008**, *95*, 163–168. [CrossRef]
28. Germain, D.P.; Brand, E.; Burlina, A.; Cecchi, F.; Garman, S.C.; Kempf, J.; Laney, D.A.; Linhart, A.; Marodi, L.; Nicholls, K.; et al. Phenotypic characteristics of the p.Asn215Ser (p.N215S) GLA mutation in male and female patients with Fabry disease: A multicenter Fabry Registry study. *Mol. Genet. Genom. Med.* **2018**, *6*, 492–503. [CrossRef]
29. Weidemann, F.; Breunig, F.; Beer, M.; Sandstede, J.; Turschner, O.; Voelker, W.; Ertl, G.; Knoll, A.; Wanner, C.; Strotmann, J.M. Improvement of cardiac function during enzyme replacement therapy in patients with Fabry disease: A prospective strain rate imaging study. *Circulation* **2003**, *108*, 1299–1301. [CrossRef]
30. Linhart, A.; Elliott, P.M. The heart in Anderson-Fabry disease and other lysosomal storage disorders. *Heart* **2007**, *93*, 528–535. [CrossRef]
31. Kampmann, C.; Baehner, F.; Whybra, C.; Martin, C.; Wiethoff, C.M.; Ries, M.; Gal, A.; Beck, M. Cardiac manifestations of Anderson-Fabry disease in heterozygous females. *J. Am. Coll. Cardiol.* **2002**, *40*, 1668–1674. [CrossRef]
32. Weidemann, F.; Wanner, C.; Breunig, F. Nomen est omen. Fabry disease. *Eur. J. Echocardiogr.* **2008**, *9*, 831–832. [CrossRef] [PubMed]
33. Weidemann, F.; Strotmann, J.M.; Niemann, M.; Herrmann, S.; Wilke, M.; Beer, M.; Voelker, W.; Ertl, G.; Emmert, A.; Wanner, C.; et al. Heart valve involvement in Fabry cardiomyopathy. *Ultrasound Med. Biol.* **2009**, *35*, 730–735. [CrossRef] [PubMed]
34. Pieroni, M.; Chimenti, C.; Ricci, R.; Sale, P.; Russo, M.A.; Frustaci, A. Early detection of Fabry cardiomyopathy by tissue Doppler imaging. *Circulation* **2003**, *107*, 1978–1984. [CrossRef] [PubMed]
35. Takenaka, T.; Teraguchi, H.; Yoshida, A.; Taguchi, S.; Ninomiya, K.; Umekita, Y.; Yoshida, H.; Horinouchi, M.; Tabata, K.; Yonezawa, S.; et al. Terminal stage cardiac findings in patients with cardiac Fabry disease: An electrocardiographic, echocardiographic, and autopsy study. *J. Cardiol.* **2008**, *51*, 50–59. [CrossRef] [PubMed]
36. Kramer, J.; Niemann, M.; Liu, D.; Hu, K.; Machann, W.; Beer, M.; Wanner, C.; Ertl, G.; Weidemann, F. Two-dimensional speckle tracking as a non-invasive tool for identification of myocardial fibrosis in Fabry disease. *Eur. Heart J.* **2013**, *34*, 1587–1596. [CrossRef]
37. Weidemann, F.; Niemann, M.; Herrmann, S.; Kung, M.; Stork, S.; Waller, C.; Beer, M.; Breunig, F.; Wanner, C.; Voelker, W.; et al. A new echocardiographic approach for the detection of non-ischaemic fibrosis in hypertrophic myocardium. *Eur. Heart J.* **2007**, *28*, 3020–3026. [CrossRef] [PubMed]
38. Palecek, T.; Honzikova, J.; Poupetova, H.; Vlaskova, H.; Kuchynka, P.; Golan, L.; Magage, S.; Linhart, A. Prevalence of Fabry disease in male patients with unexplained left ventricular hypertrophy in primary cardiology practice: Prospective Fabry cardiomyopathy screening study (FACSS). *J. Inherit. Metab. Dis.* **2014**, *37*, 455–460. [CrossRef]
39. Hagège, A.A.; Caudron, E.; Damy, T.; Roudaut, R.; Millaire, A.; Etchecopar-Chevreuil, C.; Tran, T.C.; Jabbour, F.; Boucly, C.; Prognon, P.; et al. Screening patients with hypertrophic cardiomyopathy for Fabry disease using a filter-paper test: The FOCUS study. *Heart* **2011**, *97*, 131–136. [CrossRef]

40. Nakao, S.; Takenaka, T.; Maeda, M.; Kodama, C.; Tanaka, A.; Tahara, M.; Yoshida, A.; Kuriyama, M.; Hayashibe, H.; Sakuraba, H.; et al. An atypical variant of Fabry's disease in men with left ventricular hypertrophy. *N. Engl. J. Med.* **1995**, *333*, 288–293. [CrossRef]
41. Sachdev, B.; Takenaka, T.; Teraguchi, H.; Tei, C.; Lee, P.; McKenna, W.J.; Elliott, P.M. Prevalence of Anderson-Fabry disease in male patients with late onset hypertrophic cardiomyopathy. *Circulation* **2002**, *105*, 1407–1411. [CrossRef] [PubMed]
42. Monserrat, L.; Gimeno-Blanes, J.R.; Marin, F.; Hermida-Prieto, M.; Garcia-Honrubia, A.; Perez, I.; Fernandez, X.; de Nicolas, R.; de la Morena, G.; Paya, E.; et al. Prevalence of fabry disease in a cohort of 508 unrelated patients with hypertrophic cardiomyopathy. *J. Am. Coll. Cardiol.* **2007**, *50*, 2399–2403. [CrossRef] [PubMed]
43. Elliott, P.; Baker, R.; Pasquale, F.; Quarta, G.; Ebrahim, H.; Mehta, A.B.; Hughes, D.A.; ACES study group. Prevalence of Anderson-Fabry disease in patients with hypertrophic cardiomyopathy: The European Anderson-Fabry Disease survey. *Heart* **2011**, *97*, 1957–1960. [CrossRef] [PubMed]
44. Militaru, S.; Ginghina, C.; Popescu, B.A.; Saftoiu, A.; Linhart, A.; Jurcut, R. Multimodality imaging in Fabry cardiomyopathy: From early diagnosis to therapeutic targets. *Eur. Heart J. Cardiovasc. Imaging* **2018**, *19*, 1313–1322. [CrossRef]
45. Tower-Rader, A.; Jaber, W.A. Multimodality Imaging Assessment of Fabry Disease. *Circ. Cardiovasc. Imaging* **2019**, *12*, e009013. [CrossRef]
46. Mehta, A.; Clarke, J.T.; Giugliani, R.; Elliott, P.; Linhart, A.; Beck, M.; Sunder-Plassmann, G.; FOS Investigators. Natural course of Fabry disease: Changing pattern of causes of death in FOS—Fabry Outcome Survey. *J. Med. Genet.* **2009**, *46*, 548–552. [CrossRef]
47. Waldek, S.; Patel, M.R.; Banikazemi, M.; Lemay, R.; Lee, P. Life expectancy and cause of death in males and females with Fabry disease: Findings from the Fabry Registry. *Genet. Med.* **2009**, *11*, 790–796. [CrossRef]
48. Yasuda, M.; Huston, M.W.; Pagant, S.; Gan, L.; St Martin, S.; Sproul, S.; Richards, D.; Ballaron, S.; Hettini, K.; Ledeboer, A.; et al. AAV2/6 Gene Therapy in a Murine Model of Fabry Disease Results in Supraphysiological Enzyme Activity and Effective Substrate Reduction. *Mol. Ther. Methods Clin. Dev.* **2020**, *18*, 607–619. [CrossRef]
49. Schiffmann, R.; Kopp, J.B.; Austin, H.A., 3rd; Sabnis, S.; Moore, D.F.; Weibel, T.; Balow, J.E.; Brady, R.O. Enzyme replacement therapy in Fabry disease: A randomized controlled trial. *JAMA* **2001**, *285*, 2743–2749. [CrossRef]
50. Eng, C.M.; Guffon, N.; Wilcox, W.R.; Germain, D.P.; Lee, P.; Waldek, S.; Caplan, L.; Linthorst, G.E.; Desnick, R.J.; International Collaborative Fabry Disease Study, G. Safety and efficacy of recombinant human alpha-galactosidase A replacement therapy in Fabry's disease. *N. Engl. J. Med.* **2001**, *345*, 9–16. [CrossRef] [PubMed]
51. Schaefer, R.M.; Tylki-Szymanska, A.; Hilz, M.J. Enzyme replacement therapy for Fabry disease: A systematic review of available evidence. *Drugs* **2009**, *69*, 2179–2205. [CrossRef]
52. Thurberg, B.L.; Fallon, J.T.; Mitchell, R.; Aretz, T.; Gordon, R.E.; O'Callaghan, M.W. Cardiac microvascular pathology in Fabry disease: Evaluation of endomyocardial biopsies before and after enzyme replacement therapy. *Circulation* **2009**, *119*, 2561–2567. [CrossRef] [PubMed]
53. Hughes, D.A.; Elliott, P.M.; Shah, J.; Zuckerman, J.; Coghlan, G.; Brookes, J.; Mehta, A.B. Effects of enzyme replacement therapy on the cardiomyopathy of Anderson-Fabry disease: A randomised, double-blind, placebo-controlled clinical trial of agalsidase alfa. *Heart* **2008**, *94*, 153–158. [CrossRef] [PubMed]
54. Vedder, A.C.; Breunig, F.; Donker-Koopman, W.E.; Mills, K.; Young, E.; Winchester, B.; Ten Berge, I.J.; Groener, J.E.; Aerts, J.M.; Wanner, C.; et al. Treatment of Fabry disease with different dosing regimens of agalsidase: Effects on antibody formation and GL-3. *Mol. Genet. Metab.* **2008**, *94*, 319–325. [CrossRef] [PubMed]
55. Vedder, A.C.; Linthorst, G.E.; Houge, G.; Groener, J.E.; Ormel, E.E.; Bouma, B.J.; Aerts, J.M.; Hirth, A.; Hollak, C.E. Treatment of Fabry disease: Outcome of a comparative trial with agalsidase alfa or beta at a dose of 0.2 mg/kg. *PLoS ONE* **2007**, *2*, e598. [CrossRef]
56. Benichou, B.; Goyal, S.; Sung, C.; Norfleet, A.M.; O'Brien, F. A retrospective analysis of the potential impact of IgG antibodies to agalsidase beta on efficacy during enzyme replacement therapy for Fabry disease. *Mol. Genet. Metab.* **2009**, *96*, 4–12. [CrossRef]
57. Germain, D.P.; Hughes, D.A.; Nicholls, K.; Bichet, D.G.; Giugliani, R.; Wilcox, W.R.; Feliciani, C.; Shankar, S.P.; Ezgu, F.; Amartino, H.; et al. Treatment of Fabry's Disease with the Pharmacologic Chaperone Migalastat. *N. Engl. J. Med.* **2016**, *375*, 545–555. [CrossRef]
58. Amicus Therapeutics. Galafold™ (Migalastat) Capsules, for Oral Use: US Prescribing Information. 2018. Available online: https://www.fda.gov/ (accessed on 1 February 2021).
59. European Medicines Agency. Migalastat (Galafold). EU Summary of Product Characteristics. 2018. Available online: https://www.ema.europa.eu/ (accessed on 1 February 2021).
60. Therapeutic Goods Administration. Galafold® (Migalastat): Australian Product Information. 2018. Available online: https://www.tga.gov.au/sites/defau%20lt/files/auspar-migalastat-18083%200-pi.pdf (accessed on 1 February 2021).
61. De'Oliveira, J.M.; Price, D.A.; Fisher, N.D.; Allan, D.R.; McKnight, J.A.; Williams, G.H.; Hollenberg, N.K. Autonomy of the renin system in type II diabetes mellitus: Dietary sodium and renal hemodynamic responses to ACE inhibition. *Kidney Int.* **1997**, *52*, 771–777. [CrossRef]
62. Vegter, S.; Perna, A.; Postma, M.J.; Navis, G.; Remuzzi, G.; Ruggenenti, P. Sodium intake, ACE inhibition, and progression to ESRD. *J. Am. Soc. Nephrol.* **2012**, *23*, 165–173. [CrossRef]
63. Close, L.; Elliott, P. Optimization of concomitant medication in Fabry cardiomyopathy. *Acta Paediatr.* **2007**, *96*, 81–83. [CrossRef]

64. Tahir, H.; Jackson, L.L.; Warnock, D.G. Antiproteinuric therapy and fabry nephropathy: Sustained reduction of proteinuria in patients receiving enzyme replacement therapy with agalsidase-beta. *J. Am. Soc. Nephrol.* **2007**, *18*, 2609–2617. [CrossRef] [PubMed]
65. Schiffmann, R.; Goker-Alpan, O.; Holida, M.; Giraldo, P.; Barisoni, L.; Colvin, R.B.; Jennette, C.J.; Maegawa, G.; Boyadjiev, S.A.; Gonzalez, D.; et al. Pegunigalsidase alfa, a novel PEGylated enzyme replacement therapy for Fabry disease, provides sustained plasma concentrations and favorable pharmacodynamics: A 1-year Phase 1/2 clinical trial. *J. Inherit. Metab. Dis.* **2019**, *42*, 534–544. [CrossRef]
66. Shire Human Genetic Therapies, AB. *Replagal: EPAR-Product Information*; European Medicines Agency: Stockholm, Sweden, 2016.
67. Genzyme Corporation; Fabrazyme® (Agalsidase Beta for Intravenous Infusion). *Prescribing Information*; Genzyme Corporation: Cambridge, MA, USA, 2010.
68. Pergunigalsidase Alfa (PRX-102). In *Development for the Treatment of Fabry Disease*. Available online: http://protalix.com/products/pegunigalsidase-alfa/ (accessed on 31 January 2021).
69. Welford, R.W.D.; Muhlemann, A.; Garzotti, M.; Rickert, V.; Groenen, P.M.A.; Morand, O.; Uceyler, N.; Probst, M.R. Glucosylceramide synthase inhibition with lucerastat lowers globotriaosylceramide and lysosome staining in cultured fibroblasts from Fabry patients with different mutation types. *Hum. Mol. Genet.* **2018**, *27*, 3392–3403. [CrossRef]
70. Guerard, N.; Oder, D.; Nordbeck, P.; Zwingelstein, C.; Morand, O.; Welford, R.W.D.; Dingemanse, J.; Wanner, C. Lucerastat, an Iminosugar for Substrate Reduction Therapy: Tolerability, Pharmacodynamics, and Pharmacokinetics in Patients With Fabry Disease on Enzyme Replacement. *Clin. Pharmacol. Ther.* **2018**, *103*, 703–711. [CrossRef]
71. Shen, J.S.; Arning, E.; West, M.L.; Day, T.S.; Chen, S.; Meng, X.L.; Forni, S.; McNeill, N.; Goker-Alpan, O.; Wang, X.; et al. Tetrahydrobiopterin deficiency in the pathogenesis of Fabry disease. *Hum. Mol. Genet.* **2017**, *26*, 1182–1192. [CrossRef] [PubMed]
72. Ashe, K.M.; Budman, E.; Bangari, D.S.; Siegel, C.S.; Nietupski, J.B.; Wang, B.; Desnick, R.J.; Scheule, R.K.; Leonard, J.P.; Cheng, S.H.; et al. Efficacy of Enzyme and Substrate Reduction Therapy with a Novel Antagonist of Glucosylceramide Synthase for Fabry Disease. *Mol. Med.* **2015**, *21*, 389–399. [CrossRef] [PubMed]
73. Huang, J.; Khan, A.; Au, B.C.; Barber, D.L.; Lopez-Vasquez, L.; Prokopishyn, N.L.; Boutin, M.; Rothe, M.; Rip, J.W.; Abaoui, M.; et al. Lentivector Iterations and Pre-Clinical Scale-Up/Toxicity Testing: Targeting Mobilized CD34(+) Cells for Correction of Fabry Disease. *Mol. Ther. Methods Clin. Dev.* **2017**, *5*, 241–258. [CrossRef]
74. Khan, A.; Barber, D.L.; Huang, J.; Rupar, C.A.; Rip, J.W.; Auray-Blais, C.; Boutin, M.; O'Hoski, P.; Gargulak, K.; McKillop, W.M.; et al. Lentivirus-mediated gene therapy for Fabry disease. *Nat. Commun.* **2021**, *12*, 1178. [CrossRef]
75. Felis, A.; Whitlow, M.; Kraus, A.; Warnock, D.G.; Wallace, E. Current and Investigational Therapeutics for Fabry Disease. *Kidney Int. Rep.* **2020**, *5*, 407–413. [CrossRef]
76. DeRosa, F.; Smith, L.; Shen, Y.; Huang, Y.; Pan, J.; Xie, H.; Yahalom, B.; Heartlein, M.W. Improved Efficacy in a Fabry Disease Model Using a Systemic mRNA Liver Depot System as Compared to Enzyme Replacement Therapy. *Mol. Ther.* **2019**, *27*, 878–889. [CrossRef]

Journal of
Clinical Medicine

MDPI

Review

Takotsubo Cardiomyopathy: Current Treatment

John E. Madias [1,2]

[1] Icahn School of Medicine at Mount Sinai, New York, NY 10029, USA; madiasj@nychhc.org;
Tel.: +1-(718)-334-5005; Fax: +1-(718)-334-5990
[2] Division of Cardiology, Elmhurst Hospital Center, Elmhurst, NY 11373, USA

Abstract: Management of takotsubo syndrome (TTS) is currently empirical and supportive, via extrapolation of therapeutic principles worked out for other cardiovascular pathologies. Although it has been emphasized that such non-specific therapies for TTS are consequent to its still elusive pathophysiology, one wonders whether it does not necessarily follow that the absence of knowledge of TTS' pathophysiological underpinnings should prevent us for searching, designing, or even finding, therapies efficacious for its management. Additionally, it is conceivable that therapy for TTS may be in response to pathophysiological/pathoanatomic/pathohistological consequences (e.g., "myocardial stunning/reperfusion injury"), common to both TTS and coronary artery disease, or other cardiovascular disorders). The present review outlines the whole range of management principles of TTS during its acute phase and at follow-up, including considerations pertaining to the recurrence of TTS, and commences with the idea that occasionally management of TTS should consist of mere observation along the "first do no harm" principle, while self-healing is under way. Finally, some new therapeutic hypotheses (i.e., large doses of insulin infusions in association with the employment of intravenous short- and ultrashort-acting β-blockers) are being entertained, based on previous extensive animal work and limited application in patients with neurogenic cardiomyopathy and TTS.

Keywords: takotsubo syndrome; takotsubo cardiomyopathy; therapy of takotsubo syndrome; therapy of takotsubo cardiomyopathy

Citation: Madias, J.E. Takotsubo Cardiomyopathy: Current Treatment. *J. Clin. Med.* **2021**, *10*, 3440. https://doi.org/10.3390/jcm10153440

Academic Editor: Stefan Peters

Received: 8 June 2021
Accepted: 26 July 2021
Published: 2 August 2021

1. Introduction

This review focuses exclusively on the treatment of patients with the acute phase of takotsubo syndrome (TTS), the follow-up management of this malady, and its recurrence. A disclaimer is in order in the outset regarding the term "takotsubo cardiomyopathy" since TTS is a syndrome, and not a cardiomyopathy [1], although the use of the term "takotsubo cardiomyopathy" may be excused herein, since the present review is published as part of a Special Issue of the *journal*, "Cardiomyopathies: Current Treatment and Future Options". Reference to symptoms, signs, laboratory testing, diagnostic imaging, complications, and pathophysiologic and prognostic considerations are cursorily mentioned and discussed, merely as they pertain to the different treatments of TTS, the underlying justification for their employment, the patients' response to such treatments, and side-effects arising thereof.

The pathophysiology of TTS continues to elude us [2–4]; however, it appears that an autonomic sympathetic nervous system (ASNS) seethe with resultant intense stimulation of cardiomyocytes via norepinephrine [5] and/or the cardiomyocytes' damaging effects of blood-borne catecholamines (mainly epinephrine), secreted by the adrenals [6], are instrumental to the TTS pathophenotype, a condition thus conceptualized as a "chemical myocarditis". Other plausible pathophysiologic scenarios include epicardial coronary artery spasm involving many vessels or coronary branches (i.e., some form of relatively prolonged Prinzmetal's angina) [7], coronary microvascular spasm, endothelial dysfunction, or some phenotype of coronary artery disease (CAD), any combination of the above, or in association with other mechanisms, leading to stunning/reperfusion myocardial injury, not unlike the one encountered in CAD-related ischemic injury (acute coronary syndromes [ACS], or acute myocardial infarction [AMI]) [4]. According to the latter pathophysiologic pathway, one should view with tolerance and consider the testing and/or employment of therapies designed for CAD/ACS/AMI, in the management of acute TTS [8–11].

2. Therapies as Related to the Pathophysiology of Acute TTS

It has become a cliché that we lack a specific therapy for TTS, because we have not secured a definitive pathophysiologic etiology of TTS. This may partially be a plausible assertion. If the pathophysiologic underpinnings of TTS (e.g., intense ASNS-derived cardiostimulation) which have triggered the disease are operating to the same degree, or most probably at a decreased intensity [5,6], after the patients with TTS come under our care, therapies bridling autonomic sympathetic hyperactivity may be considered appropriate (e.g., employment of β-blockers in the acute and subacute phases of TTS). Additionally, it is conceivable that, if TTS, pathophysiologically speaking, is linked to coronary vasospasm [1–3,7], nitroglycerine, organic nitrates, or calcium-blockers may be considered as appropriate therapies. Finally, if TTS is considered as a subtype of CAD or AMI [4], with underlying pathohistological features of "stunned myocardium/reperfusion injury", therapies designed for AMI, should be considered management approaches deserving evaluation [8–11].

While we are talking about our quest for unravelling the pathophysiology of, and thus providing specific therapies for TTS, we should be cognizant of the sobering fact that patients admitted with various clinical syndromes eventually diagnosed as TTS, are cared for, over many hours to sometimes days, with the provisional diagnosis(es) of CAD, AMI, or other cardiovascular or non-cardiovascular nature [12], until and even after the diagnosis of TTS has been established, following coronary angiography, showing normal coronaries or non-obstructive CAD. Accordingly, it is expected that such patients receive non-specific or empirical therapies, for many hours to days until coronary angiography discloses the absence of CAD and coronary thrombus, or the presence of non-obstructive CAD. Consequently, it may be inevitable, and not inappropriate, to treat patients with acute TTS, employing therapies for CAD, AMI, and other cardiovascular syndromes. Indeed, the commonality excessively voiced that we need special, evidence-based medicine TTS-directed randomized controlled trials (RCT) to decide on specific therapies for TTS may be impractical and perhaps not even necessary, because even at the time point of patients' hospital admission, TTS has probably been "finalized", and the condition is in its process of recovery. The above constitutes a personal opinion expressed repeatedly [6,11], may apply only to a subset of patients with TTS, and can be tangentially supported by the fact that the diagnosis of TTS is often made with considerable delay, after patients have been treated sometimes for several days as having ACS or AMI, by the rapid partial or complete recovery of the left ventricular (LV) function (sometimes within hours to 2 days), following prompt clinical presentation after the onset of the illness [13–16], or by the fact that some patients with TTS are found to have normal cardiac troponin values and/or almost normal LV function shortly after admission. Thus, therapy needs to focus on the management of established TTS pathophysiologic/pathologoanatomic/pathohistologic consequences, and complications.

3. Current Therapy of Acute TTS

What follows is a distillation of therapies practiced/proposed in the 5,534 papers, as of 31 July 2021, accessed in PubMed in response to the MeSH term "takotsubo" [17]. Many papers on TTS contain some information pertaining to its therapy [18], while some publications are focused exclusively on the management of TTS [19]. Recommendations herein are provided with the proviso that the diagnosis of TTS has been established and coronary angiography has excluded obstructive CAD, ACS, or AMI. *It may be advisable for the reader to peruse and contemplate the contents of Table 1 and Figure 1, before continuing reading of the following sections discussing individual complications.*

Table 1. Complications of TTS and corresponding recommended therapies.

Complications	Recommended Therapy (ies)
Reevaluate frequently!	**Adjust accordingly**
Asymptomatic; negative physical exam	Observe; supportive care
Angina	Nitrates; optimize volume short/ultrashort-acting β-blockers
Hypertension	Continue previous: antihypertensive regimen short/ultrashort-acting β-blockers
Tachycardia	Short/ultrashort-acting β-blockers
Hypotension	Optimize volume; D/C β-blockers; R/O LVOTO CS; phenylephrine
Bradycardia; AV blocks	D/C β-blockers; atropine pacemaker
Dyspnea; pulmonary congestion	Diuretics; oxygen
Heart failure	Diuretics; oxygen ACEi/ARB; levosimendan
Cardiogenic shock	Levosimendan; ECMO LVAD
Prolonged QTc	D/C β-blockers Pacemakers; monitoring
Atrial arrhythmias other than atrial fibrillation	β-blockers; monitoring
Atrial fibrillation	heparin; LMWH; vitamin K antagonists
PVCs/NVT	β-blockers; monitoring
Sustained VT	DC cardioversion
Ventricular fibrillation	DC-cardioversion
Ischemic stroke	Heparin; LMWH; vitamin K antagonists
Systemic or pulmonary embolism	Heparin; LMWH; vitamin K
LV thrombus	Heparin; LMWH; vitamin K antagonists
Ischemic stroke with LV thrombus	Heparin; LMWH; vitamin K antagonists; consult with Neurology
Hemorrhagic stroke with LV thrombus	Consult with Neurology and Cardiothoracic Surgery
Low LVEF with large apical akinesis/dyskinesis	Consider heparin; LMWH vitamin K antagonists
Mitral regurgitation	Optimize volume; diuretics R/O LVOTO
LVOTO	β-blockers; phenylephrine
LVOTO with CS	β-blockers cautiously vibradine; pacemaker
Left ventricular rupture	Stop anticoagulation; consult with Cardiothoracic Surgery
Right ventricular involvement	Monitor closely; diuretics
Pericarditis	Frequent ECHOs; NSAIDs consider stopping anticoagulation therapy
Torsades de pointes	Stop β-blockers; monitor QTc; pacemaker
Comorbidities	Manage as done routinely with modification as needed
Prior prescribed drugs	Continue/stop/modify as needed

Table 1. *Cont.*

Complications	Recommended Therapy (ies)
Acute kidney injury	Monitor renal function optimize volume; consider hemodialysis
Associated AMI/ACS	Manage as needed including revascularization
Associated SCAD	Manage as needed including revascularization
Cardiac arrest	Resuscitation; consideration for vest and/or ICD
Anxiety/depression	Consult with Psychiatry
Reevaluate frequently!	**Adjust accordingly!**

Abbreviations: ACEi/ARB = angiotensin-converting enzyme inhibitors/angiotensin receptor blockers; AMI/ACS = myocardial infarction/acute coronary syndromes; AV = atrioventricular; CS = cardiogenic shock; D/C = discontinue; ECHO = transthoracic echocardiogram; ECMO = extracorporeal membrane oxygenator; ICD = implanted cardioverter-defibrillator; LMWH = low-molecular-weight heparins; LV = left ventricle; LVAD = left ventricular assist device; LVEF = left ventricular ejection fraction; LVOTO = left ventricular outflow tract obstruction; NSAIDs = non-steroidal anti-inflammatory drugs; NVT = non-sustained ventricular tachycardia; PVCs = premature ventricular complexes; R/O = rule out; SCAD = spontaneous coronary artery dissection; VT = ventricular tachycardia.

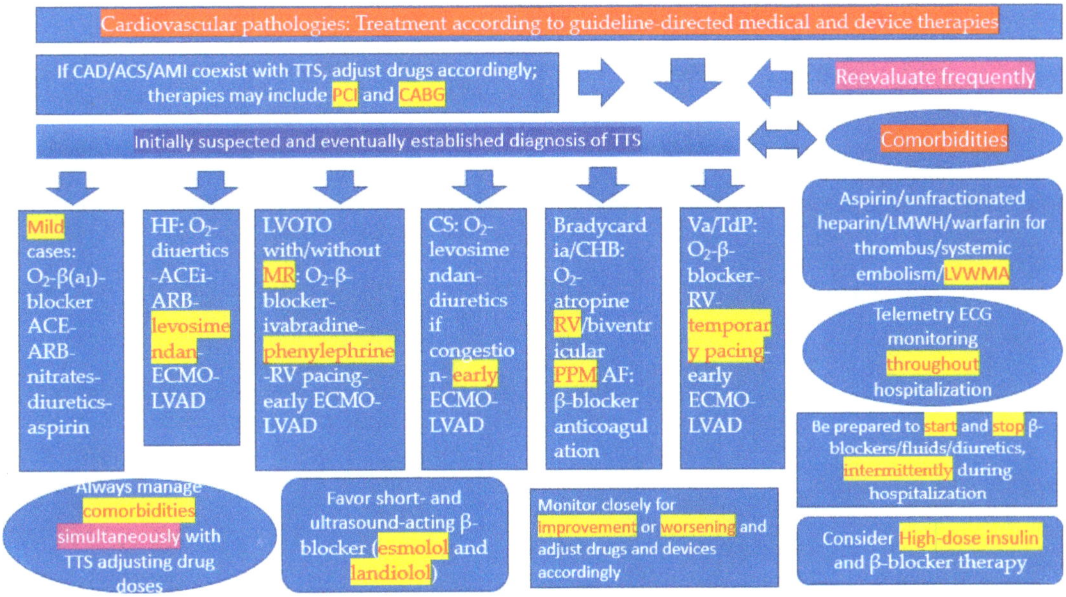

Figure 1. A graphic decisional tree of the bedside conceptualization of therapy for patients with TTS.

3.1. Asymptomatic/Normotensive/Normocardic Patients with TTS

When patients with TTS are asymptomatic with normal blood pressure (BP) and heart rate (HR), and their chest pain, dyspnea, or other symptoms or signs of disease, which brought them to seek medical attention have abated, supportive care suffices, along the lines of the Hippocratic "primum non nocere" ("first do no harm") principle [20–22]. Indeed, one should be cognizant of the possibility that pharmacological interventions in mild cases of TTS may contribute to complications, otherwise not expected had the natural course was left to evolve without any iatrogenic interference [21]. Certain drugs taken for previously present comorbidities should not be held. A short course of limited anticoagulation therapy may be needed to prevent stroke, systemic embolism, or pulmonary embolism [20–23], particularly if there is sizeable apical/midventricular akinesis/dyskinesis with apical ballooning, which predisposes to thrombus formation when coupled with the sympathetic overdrive, which induces hypercoagulability [24,25], even in asymptomatic patients and in the absence of heart failure (HF), while the patient is self-healing. In reference to prophylactic administration of anticoagulation, restraint should be exercised until one has excluded the presence of ACS or AMI via coronary angiography [21]; in the same vein, one should avoid using anticoagulants if it is suspected or shown that the underlying trigger for the TTS episode was intracerebral bleeding [21,26–28]. Continuous electrocardiographic (ECG) monitoring for emergence of arrhythmias and for QTc prolongation [29], associated with ventricular arrhythmias (VA), should be instituted and maintained throughout hospitalization, and even beyond, if left ventricular (LV) wall motion abnormalities (LVWMA), or LV thrombus, detected during hospitalization, persist at follow-up [20,30–33]. Although some physicians continue or start angiotensin-converting enzyme inhibitors/angiotensin receptor blockers (ACEi/ARB), β-blockers, diuretics and aspirin (in patients with a history of atherosclerosis or CAD), one should not forget that any therapy not proven in patients with TTS, particularly when they are asymptomatic, should be considered "quasi-experimental", tentative, and subject to close monitoring (*which applies to ALL pharmacological or other therapies administered*), continuation, or termination, depending on the response of the patients. Any treatment recommendations discussed herein emanate from general clinical reasoning consensus among experts, observational studies, and case series of patients with TTS (level of evidence C) [21,22]. Intuitively, inclusion of β-blockers may be justified, considering the nosogenic role of catecholamines in TTS; however, patients have recovered without the use of such therapy, and there is no evidence that the catecholamine-based injurious effect continues to be exerted hours or days after the inception of disease, when patients come under our care, and thus therapy with β-blockers is essential. On the other hand, precipitation of TTS by withdrawal of metoprolol in a patient has occurred [34], although that patient had LV outflow tract obstruction (LVOTO), where the β-blocker was indicated. Various cardioselective β_1-blockers (e.g., metoprolol [35], bisoprolol, esmolol [short-acting] [21,36], landiolol [ultrashort-acting]) [37–39], non-cardioselective (propranolol) [40,41] or non-cardioselective β-blockers with associated α_1-blocking effects (e.g., carvedilol or labetalol [40] have been used in patients with TTS, but no head-to-head comparisons of these drugs have been undertaken. There is also literature supporting the view that β-blockers are not beneficial in patients with TTS [42], as also shown by the reports revealing that a sizeable proportion of patients on a maintenance therapy with β-blockers have suffered TTS [43]. In general, and in reference to the employment of ACEi/ARB), β-blockers, calcium channel blockers, and aspirin, based on the literature, summarized elsewhere [20], there is no support to initiate them in asymptomatic or mildly symptomatic patients with TTS, extrapolating from the established HF management norms. Even when the above drugs are initiated on admission because of mild symptoms, there should be close monitoring to evaluate whether such therapies have not resulted in worsening in the patients. There is no other substitute than the close hemodynamic assessment of patients with TTS, particularly in the early phase of the disease (Figure 1).

The mindset in implementing therapies in patients with TTS should include the notion that the TTS phenotype may be an evolution-based protective biological algorithm to prevent death, and thus the caring physician should exercise restraint for a reflex-like implementation of pharmacology by extrapolating therapeutic modes employed in other cardiovascular pathologies [20]. Indeed, the emphasis should be on supportive care to avoid complications, while the self-restorative process to normalcy is under way.

3.2. Angina in Patients with TTS

Angina should be managed with sublingual or intravenous nitroglycerin, organic nitrates, with care not to precipitate intensification of mid-LV gradient, mediated by a reduction in systemic vascular resistance (SVR), in patients with complicated LVOTO [20]; β-blockers can also be given for angina, which may also help in alleviating LVOTO [20,35,36].

3.3. Dyspnea in Patients with TTS

Patients with TTS presenting with dyspnea should be monitored closely, regarding their hemodynamic changes and blood oxygen saturation, and insight about the extent of LV and right ventricular (RV) dysfunction, and degree of lung congestion should be sought promptly by auscultation, chest X-ray, transthoracic echocardiography (ECHO), and lung ultrasound. Diuretics, nitrates, and β-blockers, depending on the presence/absence of tachycardia, hypertension, bradycardia, hypotension, and evidence of LVOTO, may suffice. Mechanical respiratory support may be needed when pulmonary edema ensues with no response to drugs [22], and patients should be monitored for abrupt decompensation and the need for implementation of mechanical circulatory support (MCS) [22] (Section 3.13).

3.4. Hypertension and/or Tachycardia in Patients with TTS

β-blockers can be given for high BP and/or HR; short- or ultrashort-acting β-blockers should have preference, particularly during the early course of TTS, followed later by metoprolol or bisoprolol [36]. Additionally, ivabradine has been used to ameliorate sinus tachycardia [44].

3.5. Hypotension in Patients with TTS

Often patients with TTS are hypotensive on admission to the hospital, but the mechanism of this phenomenon may be an underlying decreased SVR, one of the hallmarks of TTS [20,21], mediated by downward perturbation of the sympathetic activity [45], and/or an enhanced parasympathetic activity [46], occasionally encountered in patients with TTS [5]. This can be managed by an increase in the intravenous fluid intake. Low BP should be "tolerated" providing that the cardiac output is adequate, or the organ perfusion is well maintained; however, patients receiving enhanced fluid infusions should be monitored closely (lung auscultation, blood oxygen saturation, mental state, urine volume, and the patients' subjective feeling of well-being) for adequacy of organ perfusion or emergence of pulmonary congestion. With persisting hypotension, β-blockers should not be administered, or if they have been started, they should be discontinued [19], and following adequate fluid administration, phenylephrine, an α_1-agonist should be considered in preference to positive inotropic drugs (e.g., norepinephrine) [20,21]. Additionally, continuous vigilance for present or emerging LVOTO and mitral regurgitation (MR), should be exercised via frequent application of ECHO [21].

3.6. Bradycardia and/or Atrioventricular Blocks in Patients with TTS

Sinus bradycardia or asystole are occasionally seen in patients with TTS [5], and can be managed with successive small doses of atropine. β-blockers or other drugs causing bradycardia should not be administered, or if they have been started, they should be promptly discontinued [19]. Atropine should also be used in patients with mild atrioventricular (AV) blocks, but advanced or complete heart block (CHB) should be managed with a temporary pacemaker, to be followed by permanent pacemaker (PPM) implantation decided on an individual basis [22,47–49] (Figure 2). Not all patients with TTS and CHB require PPM implantation, but some patients who have suffered TTS, triggered by CHB, certainly need to have a PPM implanted without exception [47,50]. The persistence of CHB at follow-up in patients with TTS indicates not only the need for PPM in many patients with TTS presenting or developing this complication during the acute phase of the illness, but that TTS itself most probably had been triggered by an underlying previously present AV conduction abnormality [22,48]. Remarkably, patients receiving PPM have not required further therapy for malignant VA at follow-up [51].

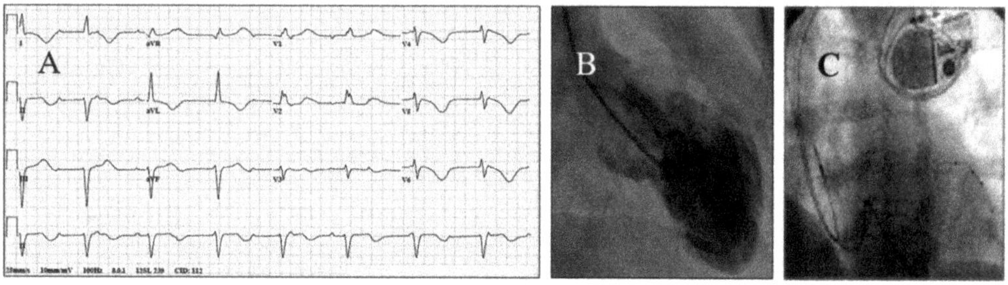

Figure 2. A patient with TTS who received a PPM for persisting CHB. A 62-year-old woman suffered TTS associated with CHB and inverted T-waves in the lateral ECG leads (**A**), for which she was initially transvenously paced, and subsequently received a PPM (biventricular) (**C**), because her CHB was persistent; ventriculography showed apical ballooning with a LVEF of 35% (**B**); an echocardiogram 15 days after the admission revealed a LVEF of 50%. CHB occasionally represents a complication of TTS, while in some cases it is the precipitant of TTS. Often, the CHB persists after the time point of normalization of LV function, and in such circumstances, there is a need for a PPM implantation. When the CHB resolves before the normalization of the LV function, a PPM may not be necessary. The CHB may be of the supra-Hisian (narrow QRS complexes) like in the present case, or of the intra-Hisian (wide QRS complexes) variety, and could precipitate VA, including TdP, mediated by the bradycardia resulting from the CHB. The present patient had a car accident due to her CHB, showed a prolonged QTc, and developed a brief episode of TdP; she was discharged with a PPM and a life vest, with an ICD not required. Reproduced and modified from Ref. [49], with the permission of the Baylor University, Medical Center.

3.7. LVEF < 30% and/or Large Apical Akinesis/Dyskinesis in Patients with TTS

Patients with a LVEF of <30% and/or marked apical akinesis/dyskinesis have worse in-hospital and follow-up prognosis [21,22], and should be closely monitored for emergence of HF, cardiogenic shock (CS), atrial arrhythmias and lethal VA, and thrombus formation [22,23]. Due to the latter, the threshold for prophylactic anticoagulation should be lower, until the LV function is markedly improved or restored to normal (Section 3.8) [21,22].

3.8. Thrombus and Prevention of Embolism in Patients with TTS

Thrombus occurs particularly in patients with a low LVEF (i.e., <30%) [21] and marked apical ballooning, and it may appear very early in the clinical course or late, 2 weeks after the inception of the illness [22,52] (Figure 3). Management of LV and/or RV, left atrial, and even left atrial appendage [53] thrombus via anticoagulation is discussed also in Section 3.1; prevention is based on early and frequent use of ECHO to detect very early development of thrombus sometimes on admission or just a few hours thereafter, or development of severe LVWMAs [20,21,23,52,54]. Unfractionated heparin, low-molecular-weight-heparin (LMWH), vitamin K antagonists, aspirin, and/or P2Y12 receptor antagonists such as clopidogrel, prasugrel, or ticagrelor, or the new oral anticoagulants can be used [20,52,54], as in other cardiovascular pathologies. Because antiplatelet agents are among the drugs which according to some "should be a part of standard treatment and initiated early" [20], this does not imply that antiplatelet drugs in isolation suffice for the management of thrombus, or severe LV dysfunction and apical ballooning, which could predispose patients with TTS to thrombus development. The bulk of the literature supports the view that heparin should be initiated in the presence of thrombus, followed by warfarin until at follow-up the thrombus has resolved, with some adding aspirin to this antithrombotic regimen [55–58]. The issue of anticoagulation should be considered broadly, encompassing its consideration for patients with TTS and severe LVWMAs and their duration without presence of intraventricular thrombus, presence of thrombus, and concern about the role of anticoagulation in causing cardiac rupture, a rare complication of TTS [20,59]. Important issues are the vigilance for the emergence of thrombus, early implementation of anticoagulation, and its maintenance for 3 to 4 or 6 months, as the resolution of the thrombus and LV dysfunction takes place.

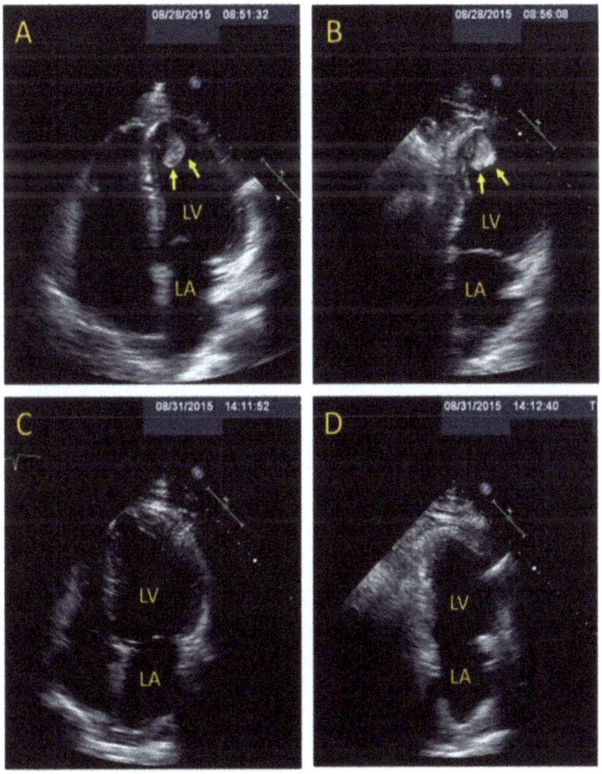

Figure 3. A patient with TTS and LV thrombus resulting in systemic embolism. A 53-year-old man suffered TTS following intense emotional stress and underwent thrombectomy for acute right superficial femoral and popliteal arterial thrombosis. Cardiac exam and troponin values were normal, and ECG showed non-specific ST-T wave changes. ECHO (4-chamber (**A**) and 2-chamber (**B**)) revealed a LV apical pedunculated and mobile thrombus measuring 2.4 × 2 cm, LV apical ballooning, and LVEF of 40% to 45%. Luminal irregularities were found at coronary angiography. A repeat ECHO 3 days after starting unfractionated heparin showed complete resolution of LV thrombus and apical akinesis (**C**,**D**). He was discharged in stable condition on warfarin for at least 3 months. LV thrombus with or without systemic embolism in TTS can occur early or late in the clinical course, and with rapid or delayed resolution. Immediate initiation of anticoagulation is warranted, and a repeat ECHO within days to 1 week is advisable to follow its course and possible early resolution. cCTS and cMRI can provide additional information. Duration of anticoagulation can be decided upon in consideration with a patient's benefit–risk ratio. Reproduced and modified from Ref. [52], with the permission of the Journal of Investigative Medicine High Impact Case Reports.

3.9. Left Ventricular Outflow Tract Obstruction in Patients with TTS

Intravenous metoprolol, esmolol, or landiolol was beneficial in patients with TTS and LVOTO via an increase in the diastolic filling time by a decrease in HR, and a decrease in contractility [21,22,35,36,39]. Consideration along with the β-blockers should be given to the use of α_1-agonist (e.g., phenylephrine) [20,21] in patients with TTS and LVOTO, in an effort to increase a possibly decreased SVR, and to increase the afterload and/or to alleviate the LVOTO. In reference to the postulated decreased SVR, mediated by an underlying altered peripheral sympathetic nerve activity in some patients with TTS [45], perhaps monitoring of sympathetic nerve input to the heart via conventional ECG electrodes [60] may evaluate for ASNS perturbations. If LVOTO is associated with CS, an intravenous infusion of short-acting β-blockers (esmolol) should be cautiously implemented, providing that there are no signs and/or symptoms of cardiac decompensation [22]. Indeed, β-blockers should be avoided in the setting of TTS with complicated LVOTO and CS [21]. Ivabradine, in place of β-blockers, has been recommended for amelioration of LVOTO, mediated by a slowing of HR [21,61]; this drug has the advantage over β-blockers that it does not negatively affect ventricular contractility. Additionally, diuretics and nitrates should be avoided since they result in intensification of LVOTO, mediated by a reduction in LV preload [21]. Instead, fluid administration to improve preload should be considered, although initiation of diuretics for associated hypoxic respiratory failure due to pulmonary edema may be required in some cases. Occasionally, LVOTO is associated with MR mediated by LVOTO-induced anterior leaflet of mitral valve systolic anterior motion (SAM) abnormality. In recalcitrant cases of LVOTO with unsatisfactory response to β-blockers and α_1-agonists, RV apical electrical pacing can be considered, extrapolating the reasoning advanced for patients with LVOTO due to obstructive cardiomyopathy [20,21,62]. Extracorporeal membrane oxygenation (ECMO) and LV assist devices (LVAD) should be considered in the management of LVOTO, and implemented relatively early, and not as the last resort when hemodynamic status has deteriorated [20]. Intra-aortic balloon pump (IABP) is contraindicated in patients with LVOTO due to its induced drop of afterload, precipitating further intensification of the intraventricular pressure gradient [20,21,51,63,64] (Figure 4), and considering the unfavorable response of patients with AMI to this modality [64].

3.10. Heart Failure in Patients with TTS

Positive inotropic agents and vasodilators should be avoided and early, instead of a delayed "heroic" treatment with MCS using venoarterial ECMO or LVAD should be considered [20,65–68]. Although close monitoring of hemodynamic consequences of pharmacological and MCS can be assessed by frequent clinical evaluation, serial noninvasive or invasive assessment of cardiac output, stroke volume, and SVR may be required in certain cases. HF may emerge in patients with TTS in association with a LV ejection fraction (LVEF) <40%, physical stressors and age >70 years [46]. ACEi/ARB, β-blockers, and diuretics are often employed, as in the management of HF resulting from other causes; however, β-blockers should not be administered, or if they have been started, they should be discontinued [19], when HF emerges or worsens, particularly in association with organ hypoperfusion. Indeed, β-blockers may be considered later, as recovery of LV dysfunction is under way, or completed [19]. Consideration of administration of a calcium sensitizer levosimendan, a non-cathecholamine inotrope, in patients with low cardiac output and HF [22,69] should be balanced with concern about the vasodilating effects of this drug, with resultant drop of the BP [20,69]. Additionally, it is reasonable to continue or start aspirin for patients with TTS and associated CAD.

3.11. Mitral Regurgitation in Patients with TTS

MR in patients with TTS is seen in association with the ballooning of midventricular and apical LV, causing leaflet tenting or tethering independent of LVOTO, or with LVOTO leading to anterior leaflet SAM abnormality. Its management should follow the principles of therapy for LVOTO (Section 3.9) and alleviation of MR with unloading vasodilators, as for other cardiovascular conditions, when MR is not associated with LVOTO. MR may be partially related to "tenting" of mitral leaflets, mechanistically associated with the LV apical-mediated and overall heart chamber enlargement, and thus may respond to all pharmacologic and LVAD-based measures [65].

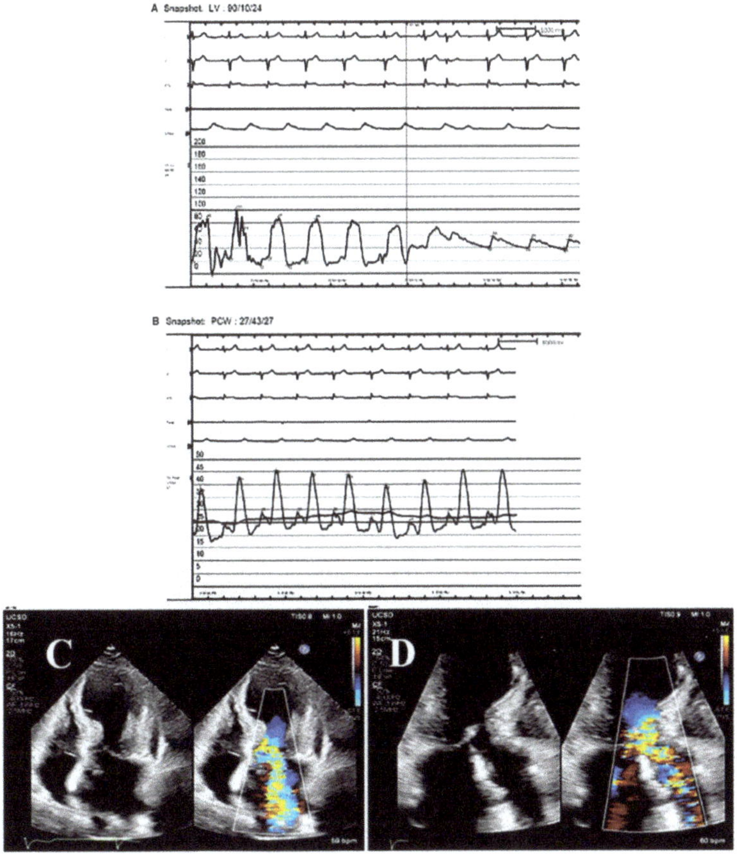

Figure 4. A patient with TTS, LVOTO, MR, and CS, responding to β-blocker and phenylephrine. A 71-year-old woman presented with chest pain, ECG lateral ST-segment elevations, and hypotension. Coronary angiography revealed no significant CAD, but a left ventriculogram showed TTS. RH catheterization revealed CS, elevated filling pressures, and V waves due to severe MR (**B**), while a dynamic LVOTO was found on LV to aorta pullback (**A**). ECHO 4-chamber view showed LVOTO and MR due to anterior mitral valve leaflet SAM (**C**), and 3-chamber view showed increase velocities across the LV outflow tract. (**D**). Worsening resulted from starting dopamine and IABP, but she improved with the initiation of phenylephrine and a low-dose β-blocker. Repeat ECHO in 3 weeks showed complete resolution of LVOTO, MR, apical akinesis, and MR. LVOTO and MR respond favorably to fluid administration to improve preload, β-blocker therapy to increase diastolic filling time, and vasopressors to raise afterload. Reproduced and modified from Ref. [64], with the permission of the European Heart Journal—Case Report.

3.12. *Right Ventricular Involvement in Patients with TTS*

RV involvement in TTS afflicts at least 1/3 of patients, is underestimated by conventional ECHO, and strain ECHO imaging is more sensitive in its detection; also, it is associated with worse in-hospital prognosis and at follow-up [70]. Such RV involvement should place physicians on the alert for other anticipated complications. Patients with RV involvement should be monitored for hypotension, RV failure, RV thrombus, and possible need for anticoagulation and fluid infusion-based resuscitation [21].

3.13. *Cardiogenic Shock in Patients with TTS*

Diagnosis of CS in patients with or without pulmonary congestion (sometimes escalated to frank pulmonary edema) and/or hypotension should be based on the presence of organ perfusion, since many patients may be hypotensive but not in CS [45]. Additionally, exclusion of LVOTO, MR, RV involvement, and cardiac rupture as the underlying mechanism of hypotension or systemic hypoperfusion and CS should be considered [21], and if found, managed accordingly (Sections 3.9, 3.11, 3.12 and 3.14). Considering the postulated role of catecholamines in the pathophysiology of TTS and precipitation of LVOTO, inotropic drugs (e.g., adrenaline, noradrenaline, dopamine, dobutamine, milrinone, and isoprenaline) to counteract hypotension and/or CS are contraindicated. Pharmacological considerations should be implemented after estimating or even objectively measuring cardiac output or index, SVR, and organ perfusion [20]. Instead the employment of levosimendan, a novel calcium sensitizer, which exerts its inotropic effect by prolonging actin–myosin interaction, leaving adrenoceptors unaffected [20,69], is recommended for patients with TTS and HF and CS [22,71], although this matter needs further assessment [72]. An additional issue to be considered, pertaining to levosimendan, is its vasodilating effect, promoting hypotension, worsening LVOTO, and further lowering the occasionally present in patients with TTS low SVR [20,69]. Additionally, the phosphodiesterase inhibitor milrinone has been considered in patients with TTS and CS [69,72]. Others absolutely disfavor the use of inotropic drugs in patients with TTT and HF or CS [20,21,65–68], a view with which this author concurs. Indeed, it may be revealing to explore carefully whether the lower mortality noted in the SWEDEHEART TTS in comparison to the InterTAK TTS cohorts in general, and in men vs. women in particular, could be traced mainly to the lower use of inotropic drugs [73], providing one performs a careful propensity score matching of many important covariates and cofounders of the 2 registries. Persisting hemodynamic instability should be managed with MCS, implementing ECMO and/or LVAD (IABP, TandemHeart, and microaxial pumps (i.e., Impella™, Abiomed, Danvers, MA)) in a bridge-to-recovery management strategy [20–22,65,68,74,75]. (Figure 5). IABP initially advocated in the management of TTS complicating CS is not anymore favored [20,51], considering its equivocal role in AMI, and particularly in patients with TTS and LVOTO where it had precipitated further hemodynamic deterioration [20,21,51]. The use of MCS, although costly, has not led to improvement in mortality, and has been linked to an increased number of patients with TTS, discharged to skilled nursing facilities [65].

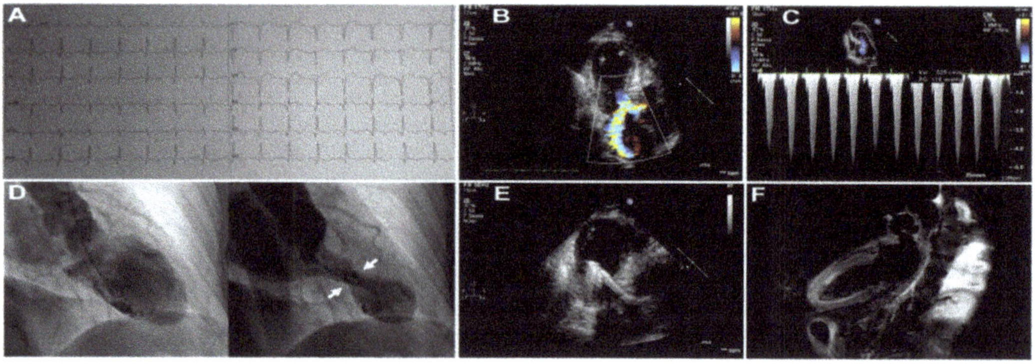

Figure 5. A patient with TTS, LVOTO, MR, and CS, treated with a percutaneous LVAD. A 71-year-old woman suffered TTS associated with CS, a LVEF of 30% (**B**,**D**), apical ballooning (**B**,**D**), LVOTO with a peak gradient of 110 mmHg (**C**), and severe MR due to anterior mitral valve leaflet SAM (**B**). An Impella 2.5 percutaneous ventricular assist device was implanted. Fluid was administered and intravenous esmolol at 50 μg/kg/min was infused. Within 4 h, LV function and lactate normalized. The LVAD was removed in 72 h, and the patient had complete recovery of her LVEF by day 30 of follow-up (**E**). The admission ECG showed ST-segment elevations in the anterolateral leads and q-waves in the inferior and anterolateral leads (**A**), and a cMRI revealed ME (**F**). MCS permits avoidance of inotropes, optimization of fluid administration, and employment of β-blockers. Reproduced and modified from Ref. [75], with the permission of the JACC: Cardiovascular Interventions.

3.14. Heart Rupture in Patients with TTS

The devastating complication of cardiac rupture in patients with TTS may be prevented by the early employment of β-blockers [43]. Considering that the mean LVEF, systolic BP, and the double product, indicative of increased oxygen demands, were higher in patients who suffered cardiac rupture as compared to those without such complication, β-blockers may be indicated in patients with this phenotype [76]. Immediate surgical repair should be attempted [76], although there is literature of patient survival with TTS and ventricular rupture managed with conservative means [77]. Patients with LV rupture and conservative management, have revealed evidence of hemorrhagic pericardial effusion, tamponade, and LV thrombus, and have been managed with pericardial drainage, or pericardial window [77].

3.15. Atrial Arrhythmias in Patients with TTS

All types of atrial arrhythmias have been observed in patients with TTS. The commonest arrhythmia encountered is sinus tachycardia, which usually responds to β-blockers. It may be prudent to start with the use of intravenous esmolol or landiolol, since these drugs can be discontinued without impunity due to their short/ultrashort-action duration, in case their use has led to worsening of HF, CS, hypotension, bradycardia, or any other complications. Additionally, ivabradine has been recommended for alleviation of sinus tachycardia in patients with TTS [61]. Atrial fibrillation (AF) a common occurrence emerging in association with an episode of TTS [78] should be managed, primarily directed at anticoagulation (Section 3.8), and slowing of heart rate, initially based on intravenous short/ultrashort-acting β-blockers, and then transitioning to long-acting β-blockers. DC-cardioversion may be considered if necessary [21]. Correction of electrolyte abnormalities is paramount in the management of atrial arrhythmias [79]. Use of calcium channel blockers for the management of AF, digitalis (particularly in the presence of LVOTO [21]), or antiarrhythmic drugs (due to their association with VA, and since some of such drugs may precipitate prolongation of QTc [80], should not be considered during the hospitalization phase of TTS.

3.16. Ventricular Arrhythmias in Patients with TTS

Patients with TTS experience VA (multiple premature ventricular contractions), ventricular tachycardias [VT] (both monomorphic and polymorphic [Torsades de Pointes] {TdP}), ventricular asystole, and pulseless electrical activity [81] (Figure 6). Vigilance for the presence of electrolyte disturbances is of paramount importance [21]. The association of VA with prolonged QTc is well established, and the need for continuous monitoring of the QTc during hospitalization has been strongly advocated [29,80]. Antiarrhythmic medications, antidepressants, or antibiotics associated with prolongation of the QTc should not be used, or promptly discontinued [22]. Treatment with β-blockers may also protect against malignant VA in patients with TTS [82], and in this setting, short-acting β-blockers should be favored [22]. Regarding the concern about the effect of β-blockers on the QTc, the issue was recently investigated, and reassuringly no prolongation of the QTc, which could have been attributed to these drugs, was noted during the first 3 days of hospitalization [83]. Sustained VA associated with CS may require MCS implementing ECMO and/or LVAD [21]. Hypokalemia should be corrected, drugs precipitating bradycardia should be avoided [19], and if such predisposing complications emerge, particularly when prolonged QTc is present, RV pacing for a protective mild increase in the underlying slow HR may be needed [78]. Episodes of TdP should be treated with DC-cardioversion shocks and magnesium sulfate [22]. An implantable cardioverter-defibrillator (ICD) should be considered if VA becomes intractable to pharmacological management [84], although it is not clear whether such action is indicated, particularly during hospitalization [21,22]. Indeed, one could resort to the use of a wearable ICD life vest in patients with recurrent VA during hospitalization, and consider implantation of an ICD based on monitoring during early follow-up, considering recovery of LV function, and while QTc is closely monitored [21,22].

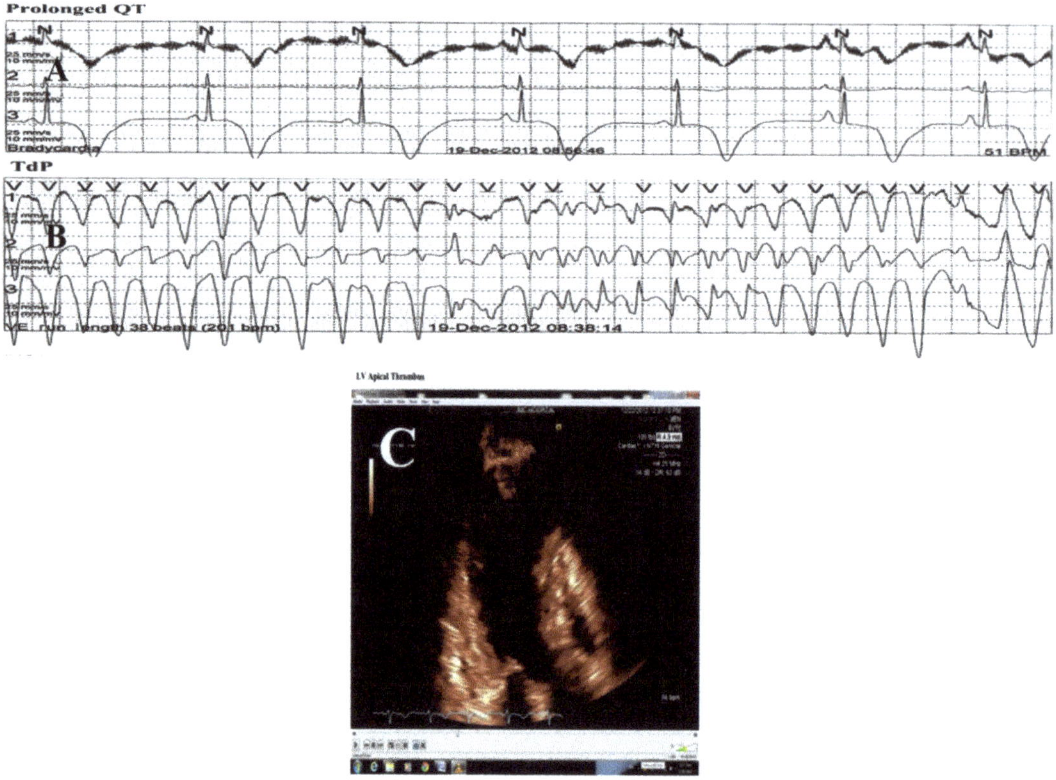

Figure 6. A patient with TTS, long QTc, and recurrent TdP and VF treated with an ICD. A 48-year-old woman with a history of postpartum depression, no CAD risk factors, and recurrent attacks of TTS of the apical variant phenotype, spanning 7 years (with the latest episode depicted herein), always precipitated by emotional stress, and resulting in chest pain, loss of consciousness, low LVEF, and sinus bradycardia (51 beats/min), inverted T-waves, long QTc (554 ms) (**A**), and repeated TdP episodes (**B**), and a LV thrombus (**C**). Coronary angiogram and LV function in between episodes were normal. She was DC-cardioverted for recurrent VF, had her β-blocker discontinued, and received magnesium, mexiletine, anticoagulation, and an ICD. LVEF normalized and the LV thrombus resolved. Reproduced and modified from Ref. [81] with the permission of the Journal of the Saudi Hear Association.

3.17. Cardiac Arrest in Patients with TTS

Although cardiac arrest precipitated by VA or asystole is encountered in patients with suspected or established TTS [22], occasionally these arrhythmias are documented in patients presenting with out-of-hospital or in-hospital cardiac arrest, and found subsequently to have TTS. Thus, an amphidromic relationship between cardiac arrest and TTS may exist; accordingly, TTS with all its consequences may emerge in patients presenting with primarily potentially lethal VA and asystole [85,86], while also VA is a frequent complication of TTS. For more on the management of patients with TTS and cardiac arrest, Section 3.16. Considering the association of AF and VA and enhanced ASNS activity, it may be of value to monitor thoracic ECG signals indicative of stellate ganglia nerve input to the heart, via currently available ECG-based technology [60].

3.18. Pericarditis in Patients with TTS

Pericarditis (acute and chronic, including Dressler's syndrome) with or without a pericardial effusion, and in association with or without cardiac tamponade has been described in patients with TTS; indeed, an amphidromic relation has been detected, in the sense that TTS may be complicated by pericarditis, and also TTS may be triggered by symptoms of pericarditis [87]. This association suggests caution in the use of thrombolytic therapy, anticoagulants, and glycoprotein IIb/IIIa inhibitors in patients with TTS and pericarditis [87]. Management is similar to idiopathic pericarditis, or pericarditis complicating other pathologies, and is based on the employment of ibuprofen or other non-steroidal anti-inflammatory drugs (NSAID), pericardiocentesis, and subxiphoid pericardial window [87].

3.19. Management of Comorbidities in Patients with Acute TTS

Management of present comorbidities in patients with TTS should continue while the patient has been admitted to the hospital and treated for TTS (Table 1 and Figure 1), providing that such therapy/ies does/do not precipitate clinical untoward responses to the patient. Accordingly, drugs for hypertension, HF, CAD, arrhythmias, diabetes, and hyperlipidemia should be continued, although doses in some of them can be modified to accommodate the new reality of TTS. Statins have been evaluated in patients with TTS, as summarized elsewhere [88], and they have not been found to exert any beneficial effects. Additionally, one should be cognizant of the occasional disease involvement of other organs (e.g., gastrointestinal tract, kidneys) precipitated by the pathophysiological processes that have triggered TTS [89]. In secondary TTS, when this disease is precipitated by physical triggers (e.g., sepsis, trauma, pulmonary insufficiency, diabetic ketoacidosis decompensation, endocrinological derangements, bleeding, surgery, anesthesia, neurologic/neurosurgical pathologies, and administration of chemotherapies), underlying precipitants should be appropriately managed, always keeping in mind that TTS is also present, and thus certain modification of provided therapies is in order. This applies primarily to the use of positive inotropes and vasodilator drugs which should not be employed in such patients with secondary TTS [22]. Instead phenylephrine for hypotension, and employment of ECMO and LVAD should be considered for severe HF and CS. In this context, detection of secondary TTS, triggered by any of the above pathologies [21], should require coronary angiography, which if it cannot be performed due to the gravity of the primary illness may lead physicians to resort to myocardial perfusion scintigraphy, or coronary computer tomography angiography (cCTA) [20] (although the latter two should not be considered equivalent to coronary angiography, which continues to be the "gold standard"); indeed, if none of the three can be performed, frequent employment of ECHO (including hand-held ECHO devices [90] in patients without a history or risk factors of CAD may be adequate for such differentiation, leaving only spontaneous coronary artery dissection as a TTS comorbidity requiring coronary arteriography [91]. Accordingly, the InterTAK group recommends cCTA as a reasonable option over coronary angiography for those with high InterTAK score and high pre-test probability for TTS; indeed, patients with low probability for TTS as per the InterTAK score, should undergo coronary angiography, while for patients with high such scores transthoracic ECHO may be considered adequate. [92]. The scenario of secondary TTS, triggered by a large array of acute medical and surgical illnesses, is exemplified by the frequent concurrent TTT and acute pathologies associated with hemodynamic instability, in patients cared for in intensive care units [93]. A great variety of pathologies triggering secondary TTS have specific management considerations, that should be taken into considerations, when one cares for such complex patient cases [21]. Indeed, a wider comorbid state has been implicated as the condition driving prognosis after TTS, particularly in connection with CS [94], prompting one to think that an intricate association of all existing comorbidities and the peculiarities of the pathophysiology of CS in TTS [20] contribute to the better recovery of LV function than seen in connection with CS in AMI, but to the worse prognosis during hospitalization and at follow-up. With this in mind, the importance of diagnosing and treating comorbidities is of great importance in this condition.

3.20. TTT Associated with CAD

Of note is that CAD and ACS, diseases that need to be differentiated from TTS, are occasionally comorbidities of TTS, and may occasionally precipitate secondarily TTS [95,96]. In such cases of concurrence of ACS and TTS, management of a coronary occlusion in a patient with AMI and TTS should be undertaken as performed routinely in accordance with issued guidelines for AMI, including the employment of percutaneous coronary interventions (PCI) [97], or even coronary artery bypass graft (CABG) surgery. In general, what is recommended is that complete revascularization be carried out particularly when myocardial ischemia/injury is due to left main coronary artery stenosis or severe multi-vessel CAD [20], along with all the preventive pharmacologic measures applied to patients with CAD and its manifestations during the acute phase of the disease and at follow-up.

4. Management of TTS in Potential Cardiac Donors

Cardiac transplantation is hampered by the scarcity of cardiac donors. This is further accentuated by the unsuitability of a proportion of donor heart grafts due to the development of secondary TTS in some of the potential cardiac donors [98]; it has been shown that heart grafts from heart donors who have suffered TTS with persisting or improving LV dysfunction have performed well without any adverse post-transplant outcomes [99]. Many of these potential heart donors with hearts revealing TTS features have suffered devastating neurological catastrophes due to head injuries or brain death from illicit drug overdoses. What is needed is to expedite the recovery of function in such heart grafts prior and after organ explantation, and during and after grafting to the hosts; these issues are currently being further investigated, and improvements need urgently to become systematized [100,101].

5. Current Follow-Up Management of Patients with TTS

Management of patients who have been discharged after an episode of TTS aims at systematic attention at follow-up with an eye for monitoring for CAD risk factors, cardiovascular and other comorbidities, and recurrence of TTS (Section 6). Early on, follow-up should evaluate whether the LVWMAs have dissipated and the LVEF has returned to normal, or to a pre-TTS status level; this can be accomplished by a repeat ECHO, or a firstly performed cardiac magnetic resonance imaging (cMRI), which in addition to the assessment of LV function can provide insights about the resolution of LV thrombus, persistence of myocardial edema (ME), and presence of myocardial fibrosis and/or scarring [102]. The outcome of atrial arrhythmias and VA, which emerged during hospitalization, or appeared after discharge, and the associated QTc prolongation in the ECG, should be of utmost concern to the physicians. During the 1st and subsequent follow-up encounters, it should be ensured that all the complications noted during the hospitalization have been resolved or require attention (e.g., persisting arrhythmias or AV blocks requiring pharmacological treatment or implantation of cardiac electronic devices (PPM and/or ICD). A combination of ACEi/ARB led to decreased 1-year mortality, although this was not the case with administration of β-blockers [42]. Anticoagulation should continue for patients who had a thrombus while they were hospitalized, or in the rare occasions that LV function has not been fully restored. The treating physicians should investigate whether the patients continue to have symptoms, and whether such persisting morbidity could be attributed to TTS or other comorbidities, or the patients have returned completely to their health status preceding their TTS episode. Indeed, current evidence showing persistent structural, functional, and myocardial metabolic dysregulation at a follow-up of 13–39 months in patients with TTS [103], should prompt us to search for specific therapies (established and new) for managing the lingering morbidity of patients who have suffered TTS.

6. Current Therapy Aimed at Preventing Recurrence of TTS

Therapy for recurrence of TTS should include regular follow-up aiming at monitoring for and managing of risk factors for CAD and other comorbidities, favoring the use of

ACEi/ARB and long-acting β-blockers (e.g., metoprolol, bisoprolol) needed for patients with comorbidities, but even for patients without such comorbidities.

However, β-blockers, ACEi/ARB, and aspirin have not prevented recurrence of TTS, its severity, or led to better survival [21,22,92,104,105], while a meta-regression study of the combined use of β-blockers and ACEi/ARB revealed a lower recurrence rate of TTC [106], a finding that requires replication. Additionally, aspirin, a frequently administered drug in patients with or suspected atherosclerosis, following discharge of patients with TTS, has not influenced favorably outcome at follow-up [107]. Endocrinological comorbidities (e.g., thyroid disorders, pheochromocytoma) should be sought after in an effort to fend off recurrence of TTS. Pheochromocytomas/paragangliomas in particular have often repeatedly been missed, and are diagnosed after recurrent episodes of TTS [108]. Considering the high rate of neurological and psychiatric comorbidities, and substance abuse in patients with TTS [42,109–111], physicians following patients with an index episode of TTS should consider systematic longitudinal management of such neurological/psychiatric pathologies, which may influence the rate of TTS recurrence. Of particular importance herein is the initiation or uptitration/downtitration of psychotropic drugs in the management of epilepsy, depression, and anxiety and the recurrence of TTS [111,112]; thus, such changes in the drug doses should be carried out in close collaboration of the patient, cardiologist, neurologist, and psychiatrist, who should also provide psychological counseling, psychotherapy, including cognitive behavioral therapy [21,22]. Currently there is no evidence that such therapeutic considerations have prevented recurrence of TTS. Additionally, expert management of chronic pulmonary pathology is recommended [22], since often decompensated chronic obstructive lung disease and asthma serve as triggers for the emergence of TTS, perhaps primed by the excessive use of bronchodilators (β_2-agonists). Since malignancies and TTS are intricately associated [113], the treating physician should look for yet undiagnosed underlying malignancy in patients with past history of TTS, particularly in the absence of obvious trigger(s) [21]; also, in patients with malignancies as a comorbidity to TTS, we should be proactive in helping our patients undergoing diagnostic procedures and pharmacological, surgical, and radiation therapies, since such exigencies are associated with recurrent TTS. Indeed, such an approach should be generalized to all patients with previous history of TTS, and patients should undergo procedures/surgeries after pretreatment over a course of a few days to weeks, with long-acting β-blockers, or as an alternative be supported with periprocedural/perioperative continuous infusions of short- or ultrashort-acting β-blockers (e.g., esmolol or landiolol). The efficacy of this hypothetical preventive approach for TTS recurrence has not been shown, but its plausible merit needs to be explored. Considering the higher propensity of women to suffer TTS, and animal models showing a preventive role of estrogens in the emergence of TTS [114], there are no clinical data supporting use of estrogens either to prevent index TTS episodes or their recurrence; however, it may be of value to reexplore the issue of a low dose estrogen supplementation for perimenopausal and postmenopausal women with the intention to prevent TTS or its recurrence [21,115].

7. Future Therapeutic Options for TTS

Considering the delays in making the diagnosis of TTS due to its similarity in clinical presentation with CAD, ACS, AMI, and HF, and the hard fact that the victims of TTS, before and after the diagnosis has been suspected and eventually established, are treated for a number of hours and often few days with therapies designed and proven beneficial for other cardiovascular pathologies, it may be unlikely that RCT could be carried out to explore for therapies which will make a difference in the management of patients with TTS. However, it is conceivable that "specific for TTS therapies" may emerge in the future, mediating an amelioration or complete reversion of pathophysiologic mechanisms, which have caused the TTS phenotype. Such therapies, may or may not be efficacious in improving the clinical course of patients with TTS, accelerating the healing process, preventing major cardiovascular and non-cardiovascular complications, and shortening the hospital stay. An impediment for a therapy that would be decisively beneficial in the management of TTS is that, even if such a therapy becomes available, it could only be implemented after the TTS is already established and the morbid pathology with its consequences is in the process of recovery. Although we do not know whether an autonomic central nervous system catecholamine storm with resultant local overstimulation of cardiomyocytes, a surge in the blood-borne catecholamine levels, spasm of the epicardial coronaries and/or coronary microcirculation, endothelial dysfunction, negative myocardial supply/demand ratio, developed LVOTO, or some other(s) not suspected as yet pathomechanism(s) are at work, what clinicians or researchers are presented with is a probably transiently dysfunctional myocardial territory, not unlike the stunned myocardium, with the features of reperfusion injury, encountered in ACS and AMI [116].

A hypothetical example of the dissociation between the pathophysiological process leading up to TTS, and a therapy designed to reverse such a nosogenic scenario can be visualized by the following: let us assume that TTS is caused by an intense relatively prolonged (more than what is encountered in Prinzmetal's angina) coronary vasospasm, affecting the epicardial coronaries and/or the coronary microcirculation, and resulting in a region with features of stunned myocardium and reperfusion injury [116]; employment of nitroglycerin, organic nitrates, or calcium blockers are not expected to exert a significant therapeutic effect leading to recovery of the myocardial region affected by the ischemic/reperfusion injury, since coronary vasospasm is not anymore exerted, or even if it is, the resultant myocardial damage has been already completed; thus even therapy along reversing the pathophysiologic trajectory resulting in TTS, does not constitute an effective management approach for established TTS.

It is conceivable that a diverse variety of pathophysiologic entities (ACS, AMI, Prinzmetal's angina, and TTS) could lead to the *same* pathophysiologic/pathoanatomic/pathohistologic outcome, i.e., that of "ischemic/reperfusion injury" [4], and thus therapies previously proposed for ACS and AMI [8,9,116], deserve a trial in patients with TTS [10,11]. Accordingly, it has been recently proposed that large doses of insulin infusions, in connection with careful monitoring to prevent hypoglycemia and hypokalemia, via concomitant infusions of dextrose and potassium supplementation, in conjunction with intravenous use of short-, or ultrashort-acting β-blockers (e.g., esmolol or landiolol) [39] (Figure 7) perhaps have beneficial therapeutic effects in patients with TTS [10,11], addressing specifically the devastating metabolic impairment (glucose and lipid pathways dysregulation, leading to decreased final glycolytic and β-oxydation metabolites and reduced availability of Krebs intermediates), noted in TTS [117,118]. This proposal is based on previous literature of animal models of stress cardiomyopathy, recently summarized [10], and limited experience in patients with neurogenic cardiomyopathy and TTS [37,38,119–122] (Figure 8). Consequently. a trial including the above therapeutic scheme deserves consideration in the management of patients with TTS. Justification of insulin employment in TTS is supported by studies using ^{18}F-FDG uptake confirming the presence of glucose metabolism disorder, similar to that observed in stunned or hibernated myocardium [123], for which insulin has been proposed [9].

An additional therapeutic parallel, tangentially supporting the consideration of insulin in the management of TTS, is the recommendation of incrementally administered high dose insulin therapy, along with intravenous calcium, in patients with drug-induced cardiac toxicity engendered by calcium blockers [124]. Additionally, since there are previous recommendations for implementation of intravenous lipid-emulsion therapy in patients with ischemic stunned myocardium/reperfusion injury [124], and calcium-blockers or β-blockers overdose [125], such therapy could be tested in animal TTS models, and if found safe and useful, be further evaluated for patients with TTS. However, we should always exercise restraint in the notion that what we view in TTS represents an adaptive protective response to the autonomic adrenergic overstimulation of the heart, and thus we should be concerned by interfering in the spontaneous self-healing process [1,20,21].

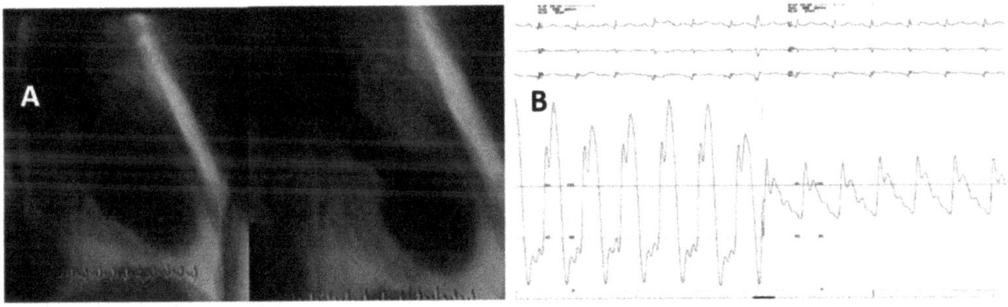

Figure 7. A patient with TTS, LVOTO, and MR treated with the ultrashort-acting β-blocker landiolol. A 72-year-old woman presented with chest pain and dyspnea triggered by emotional stress and was diagnosed with TTS and LVOTO. Her HR was 100 beats/min, BP was 96/60 mmHg. and a systolic murmur in the second right sternal border was heard. Coronary angiography did not disclose significant lesions, but LV angiography showed an apical variant TTS (**A**), MR due to anterior mitral valve leaflet SAM, with a pull-back from the LV apex to basal tract of the LV, revealing a peak gradient of 61.9 mmHg (**B**), suggestive of LVOTO. Infusion of landiolol at a dose of 4 μg/kg/min was started, which was uptitrated to 6, 8, and finally 10 μg/kg/min, under close monitoring of HR, BP, and ECHO, at which point the BP increased to 120 mmHg, the HR dropped to 50-60 beats/min, the LV gradient decreased to 20 mmHg, and the MR became mild. The dose of landiolol was decreased to 4 μg/kg/min on day 3, and the drug was terminated on day 4. Subsequently her course was uneventful and she was discharged on day 10. Reproduced and modified from Ref. [38], with the permission of Journal of General and Family Medicine.

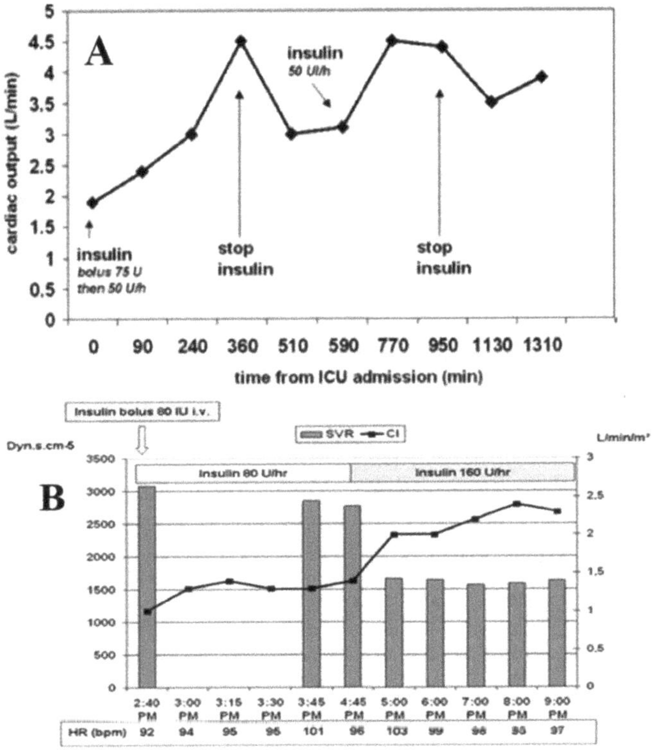

Figure 8. *Cont.*

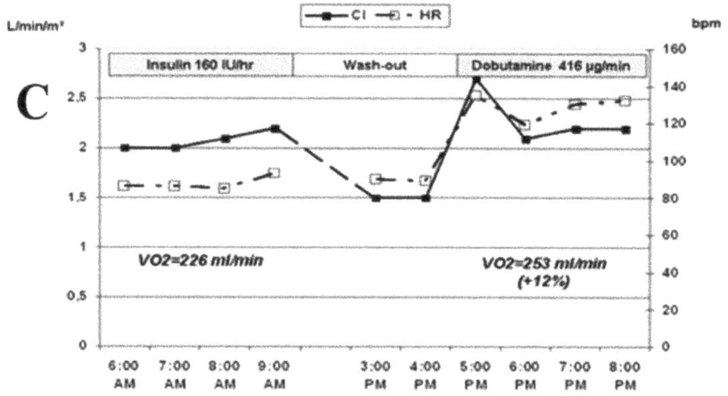

Figure 8. Hemodynamic changes in two patients with TTS treated with high doses of insulin. Effects of insulin in two patients, one with TTS after subarachnoid hemorrhage (**A**), and the other with TTS after a stroke (**B**,**C**). Vide response of cardiac output to the infusion and subsequent withdrawal of insulin (**A**). Vide response of cardiac index and SVR to 2 doses of insulin, and the stability of HR (**B**). Vide the advantages of the response of cardiac index, HR, and VO_2 to insulin versus dobutamine (**C**). Reproduced and modified from Refs. [119,121], with the permission of the Neurosurgery and BMJ Case Report.

Since experiments in a TTS rodent model with catecholamine-triggered TTS revealed that isoflurane anesthesia exerted a protective effect for development of LV dysfunction [126,127], it would be of great interest to evaluate even in a limited cohort this therapy's impact in human TTS.

Another matter of concern is the continuation of ill health at follow-up of patients with TTS with evidence of inadequate recovery of contractile function, metabolic dysfunction and systemic inflammation several months after the TTS episode [103,128,129]. What therapy should be implemented to manage these persisting problems is not currently evident. Among other well-established therapies one could consider continuation of therapy with insulin, proposed for the acute phase of TTS (vide supra), which may provide benefits to such patients. Accordingly, a time period with low doses of insulin as for diabetics with enhanced oral intake of carbohydrates and potassium to avoid hypoglycemia and/or hypokalemia, may be worth of preclinical and clinical exploration, for its effects on the post-TTS lingering morbidity.

In reference to the underlying systemic inflammation, one wonders whether a 4-pronged RCT, assigning patients to placebo, NSAID, colchicine, and corticosteroids, with an evaluation at 6 and 12 months post the episode of TTS, and assessment of symptoms, cardiopulmonary stress test, brain natriuretic peptides, C-reactive protein, ECHO strain imaging, and cMRI, may provide some answers.

A flood of articles is currently being published pertaining to the association of TTS in patients with COVID-19 admitted to intensive care units [130]. It cannot be overemphasized that a high index of suspicion needs to be imparted to all physicians that TTS may occur, and probably remains underdiagnosed, in patients with COVID-19. Concerns of the care givers should be geared towards the detection and prompt response to HF, CS, drug-induced prolongation of the QTc, and life-threatening VA in patients with COVID-19 and complicated secondary TTS [128] Finally, the heavy reliance on the frequent implementation of ECHO in patients admitted with COVID-19 cannot be overemphasized [90].

8. Prognosis of TTS

TTS, although initially thought to be an entirely benign condition, is currently felt to be a serious illness, with rates of morbidity and mortality comparable to those experienced after an AMI or other ACS [1,2,20,21]. In addition, a lingering morbidity, characterized by exercise intolerance, atypical for ischemia chest pain, exertional dyspnea, and metabolic abnormalities, persist for many months after an index episode of TTS [103]. Some patients suffer recurrence of TTS, with rare some developing multiple such episodes [131]. The early detected LV dysfunction thought initially to fully recover in a few weeks to months, based on conventional transthoracic ECHO, has been found not to be fully restored to normalcy by strain ECHO deformation studies, and some interstitial fibrosis is documented by cMRI to replace the initially observed ME [132]. In addition, patients with TTS have a high rate of cancer, neurological and psychiatric diseases [133,134], and common variety comorbidities (i.e., hypertension, diabetes), sometimes to a greater degree than patients with CAD/AMI/ACS [135], resulting to an even higher morbidity/mortality phenotypes than the latter. The issue of the prognostic role of diabetes is still unsettled, considering that a "diabetes paradox" has been identified exerting a protecting influence in the emergence of TTS, and resulting in amelioration of complications during hospitalization [136]. In general, a large array of symptoms/signs, laboratory findings, complications, comorbidities, and prognostic scores have been demonstrated, in small and large TTS patient cohorts, to be associated with worse outcome (both short-term and long term), with Table 2 providing a non-all-inclusive list of such predictors. Inconsistencies regarding prognosticators among studies, are probably related to variation in the composition of examined cohorts and/or their sizes. Finally, it appears that there are no predictors from the index episode of TTS of subsequent TTS recurrence(s) [137], and that ACE1/ARB, but not β-blockers, instituted at discharge following a TTS episode, may prevent recurrence [21,138], although this is not firmly established [42,79,88].

Table 2. Symptoms/signs, laboratory findings, complications, and comorbidities of patients with TTS, associated with worse prognosis.

Symptoms/Signs	Laboratory Findings	Complications	Comorbidities	Prognostic Scores
Tachycardia Hypotension High respiratory rate High temperature Persisting angina Dyspnea Age >70 Age <50 Male sex Physical stressors	High sensitivity troponin Hyperglycemia Hypoxia High brain natriuretic peptides Long QTc LVEF <30% High E/e′ Low LV-GLS T-wave inversion LV concentric hypertrophy Sigmoid septum ST-segment elevation Marked LVWMAs Apical variant Atypical ballooning High blood norepinephrine High tumor necrosis factor-α Myocardial edema Late recovery of LVEF High C-reactive protein High WBC count- Anemia Δnegative T-wave amplitude dispersion ΔQT dispersion; Low T3 TTS right ventricular involvement Low BMI Low eGFR cMRI-detected fibrosis Thrombolysis in myocardial infarction-2 flow cMRI late gadolinium enhancement	HF CS VA Cardiac arrest Asystole Pulseless electrical activity LV dysfunction requiring MCS Stroke Acute renal failure AF Respiratory distress needing mechanical ventilation Pulmonary edema Need for catecholamine use Need for inotropic drugs Killip class III/IV Asystole CHB MR Intraventricular thrombus	Diabetes Hypertension Neurological pathologies Psychiatric diseases Malignancies Acute pulmonary triggers Endothelial dysfunction Secondary TTS CAD Trauma Need for resuscitation eGFR Multiple noncardiac comorbidities Sepsis Admission to the ICU Peripheral artery diseas Chronic renal failure	Killip class (III and IV) on admission High GRACE score InterTAK Classification InterTAK Prognostic Score CHA2DS2-VASc risk score German and Italian Stress Cardiomyopathy (GEIST) Score

Abbreviations: AF = atrial fibrillation; BMI = body mass index; CAD = coronary artery disease; CHB = complete heart block; cMRI = cardiac magnetic resonance imaging; CS = cardiogenic shock; Δ = change; e GFR = estimated glomerular filtration rate; HF = heart failure; GLS = global longitudinal strain; ICU = Intensive Care Unit; LV = left ventricular; LVEF = left ventricular ejection fraction; LVOTO = left ventricular outflow tract obstruction; LVWMAs = left ventricular wall motion abnormalities; MCS = mechanical circulatory support; TTS = takotsubo syndrome; VA = ventricular arrhythmias; WBC = white blood cells.

9. Conclusions

The pathophysiology of TTS continues to be elusive and its management is currently based on the extrapolation of therapeutic practices proven/established for other cardiovascular diseases (CAD, AMI, HF, etc.). This may not be totally inappropriate since a secure diagnosis of TTS is made always with significant delays and thus by necessity supportive therapies in response to common symptoms and signs of cardiovascular pathology are necessary. Additionally, we should entertain the notion that whatever is the pathoetiology of TTS, the eventual emergence of stunned/reperfusion myocardial injury may call for management approaches not unique only to TTS. Due to eventual spontaneous reversibility of such pathology, frequently noted in patients with TTS, observing and monitoring asymptomatic or mildly symptomatic patients with adequate organ perfusion, while self-healing takes place may be advisable along the principle of "first do no harm". Continuation of therapies for previously present comorbidities should not be interrupted with uptitration/downtitration of drugs, as necessary. ACEi/ARB, short-acting β-blockers, anticoagulants are often implemented during hospitalization, and continued during follow-up, as needed. Earlier employment of ECMO and/or LVAD may be needed for patients in CS, and monitoring for the emergence of lethal VA, particularly associated with prolongation of the QTc interval, is imperative. Consideration should be given to favoring short- and ultrashort-acting β-blockers and implementation of large doses of insulin in the management of patients with TTS and HF or CS. Finally, the management of patients who have suffered TTS should be systematized at follow-up to include use of ACEi/ARB, reexamination of whether β-blockers prevent recurrence, employment of psychiatric evaluation and therapy, reevaluation of the inciting role of malignancy in the emergence of recurrent TTS, and management of comorbidities as they relate to recurrence of TTS.

Funding: This research received no external funding.

Institutional Review Board Statement: Not applicable.

Informed Consent Statement: Not applicable.

Data Availability Statement: Not applicable.

Conflicts of Interest: The author declares no conflict of interest.

Abbreviations

ACS	Acute Coronary Syndromes
ACEi	Angiotensin-Converting Enzyme Inhibitors
AF	Atrial Fibrillation
AMI	Acute Myocardial Infraction
ARB	Angiotensin Receptor Blockers
AV	Atrioventricular
BP	Blood Pressure
CABG	Coronary Artery Bypass Graft
CAD	Coronary Artery Disease
CHB	Complete Heart Block
cCTA	Coronary Computed Tomography Angiography
cMRI	Cardiac Magnetic Resonance Imaging
CS	Cardiogenic Shock
ECG	Electrocardiogram (phic)
ECHO	Transthoracic Echocardiography (gram)
ECMO	Extracorporeal Membrane Oxygenator
HF	Heart Failure
HR	Heart Rate
IABP	Intra-aortic Balloon Pump
ICD	Implantable Cardioverter-Defibrillator

LV	Left Ventricle (cular)
LVEF	Left ventricular Ejection Fraction
LVAD	Left Ventricular Assist Device
LVWMAs	Left Ventricular Wall Motion Abnormalities
LMWH	Low-Molecular-Wight Heparins
LVOTO	Left Ventricular Outflow Tract Obstruction
MCS	Mechanical Circulatory Supprot
ME	Myocardial Edema
MR	Mitral Regurgitation
NSAID	Non-steroidal Anti-inflammatory Drugs
PCI	Percutaneous Coronary Artery Intervention
PPM	Permanent Pacemaker
RCT	Randomized Controlled Trials
RV	Right Ventricle (cular)
SAM	Systolic Anterior Motion
SVR	Systemic Vascular Resistance
TdP	Torsades de Pointes
TTS	Takotsubo Syndrome
VA	Ventricular Arrhythmias
VT	Ventricular Tachycardia

References

1. Pelliccia, F.; Sinagra, G.; Elliott, P.; Parodi, G.; Basso, C.; Camici, P.G. Takotsubo is not a cardiomyopathy. *Int. J. Cardiol.* **2018**, *254*, 250–253. [CrossRef] [PubMed]
2. Pelliccia, F.; Kaski, J.C.; Crea, F.; Camici, P.G. Pathophysiology of takotsubo syndrome. *Circulation* **2017**, *135*, 2426–2441. [CrossRef]
3. Dias, A.; Núñez Gil, I.J.; Santoro, F.; Madias, J.E.; Pelliccia, F.; Brunetti, N.D.; Salmoirago-Blotcher, E.; Sharkey, S.W.; Eitel, I.; Akashi, Y.J.; et al. Takotsubo syndrome: State-of-the-art review by an expert panel—Part 1. *Cardiovasc. Revasc. Med.* **2019**, *20*, 70–79. [CrossRef]
4. Pelliccia, F.; Kaski, J.C.; Camici, P.G. Takotsubo syndrome's pathophysiology: Still a mystery? *Eur. Heart J.* **2019**, *40*, 1989. [CrossRef]
5. Samuels, M. The brain-heart connection. *Circulation* **2007**, *116*, 77–84. [CrossRef] [PubMed]
6. Madias, J.E. Blood norepinephrine/epinephrine/dopamine measurements in 108 patients with takotsubo syndrome from the world literature: Pathophysiological implications. *Acta Cardiol.* **2020**, *10*, 1–9, Online ahead of print. [CrossRef]
7. Madias, J.E. Pathophysiology of takotsubo syndrome: Do not forsake coronary vasospasm! *Int. J. Cardiol.* **2018**, *266*, 42. [CrossRef]
8. Sodi-Pallares, D.; Testelli, M.; Fishelder, F. Effects of an intravenous infusion of a potassium-insulin-glucose solution on the electrocardiographic signs of myocardial infarction. *Am. J. Cardiol.* **1962**, *9*, 166–181. [CrossRef]
9. Kloner, R.A.; Nesto, R.W. Glucose-insulin-potassium for acute myocardial infarction: Continuing controversy over cardioprotection. *Circulation* **2008**, *117*, 2523–2533. [CrossRef] [PubMed]
10. Madias, J.E. Insulin and takotsubo syndrome: Plausible pathophysiologic, diagnostic, prognostic, and therapeutic roles. *Acta Diabetol.* **2021**, *58*, 1–8, Online ahead of print. [CrossRef]
11. Madias, J.E. Insulin and short acting iv beta blockers: A "new" proposal for the acute management of takotsubo syndrome. *Int. J. Cardiol.* **2021**, *334*, 18–20. [CrossRef]
12. Madias, J.E. *Management of Takotsubo Syndrome in The ESC Textbook of Cardiovascular Medicine*, 3rd ed.; Camm, A.J., Luscher, T.F., Maurer, G., Serruys, P., Eds.; Oxford University Press: Oxford, UK, 2019; Chapter 30.10, pp. 1305–1306, ISBN 978-0-19-878490-6.
13. Lee, M. Time course of functional recovery in takotsubo (stress) cardiomyopathy: A serial speckle tracking echocardiography and electrocardiography study. *J. Cardiovasc Imaging.* **2020**, *28*, 50–60. [CrossRef] [PubMed]
14. Zhang, Z.; Kong, H.; Zhang, S.-Y.; Guan, T.-T. Takotsubo syndrome triggered by change in position in a patient with thoracic vertebral fracture: A case report. *Medicine* **2021**, *100*, e24088. [CrossRef] [PubMed]
15. Eitel, I.; Lücke, C.; Behrendt, F.; Sareban, M.; Gutberlet, M.; Schuler, G.; Thiele, H. Full recovery of takotsubo cardiomyopathy (apical ballooning) in two days. *Int. J. Cardiol.* **2010**, *143*, e51–e53. [CrossRef]
16. Michel, J.; Pegg, T.; Porter, D.; Fisher, N. Atypical variant stress (takotsubo) cardiomyopathy associated with gastrointestinal illness: Rapid normalisation of LV function. *N. Z. Med. J.* **2012**, *125*, 85–87. [PubMed]
17. Takotsubo Literature in PbMed. Available online: https://pubmed.ncbi.nlm.nih.gov/?term=takotsubo&sort=date (accessed on 18 July 2021).
18. Dias, A.; Núñez Gil, I.J.; Santoro, F.; Madias, J.E.; Pelliccia, F.; Brunetti, N.D., Salmoirago-Blotcher, E.; Sharkey, S.W.; Eitel, I.; Akashi, Y.J.; et al. Takotsubo syndrome: State-of-the-art review by an expert panel—Part 2. *Cardiovasc. Revasc. Med.* **2019**, *20*, 153–166. [CrossRef] [PubMed]

19. Aimo, A.; Pelliccia, F.; Panichella, G.; Vergaro, G.; Barison, A.; Passino, C.; Emdin, M.; Camici, P.G. Indications of beta-adrenoceptor blockers in Takotsubo syndrome and theoretical reasons to prefer agents with vasodilating activity. *Int. J. Cardiol.* **2021**, *333*, 45–50. [CrossRef]
20. Omerovic, E. Takotsubo syndrome-scientific basis for current treatment strategies. *Heart Fail. Clin.* **2016**, *12*, 577–586. [CrossRef]
21. Jha, S.; Zeijlon, R.; Shekka Espinosa, A.; Alkhoury, J.; Oras Omerovic, E.; Redfors, B. Clinical management in the takotsubo syndrome. *Expert Rev. Cardiovasc. Ther.* **2019**, *17*, 83–93. [CrossRef]
22. Santoro, F.; Mallardi, A.; Leopizzi, A.; Vitale, E.; Rawish, E.; Stiermaier, T.; Eitel, I.; Brunetti, N.D. Current knowledge and future challenges in takotsubo syndrome: Part 2-treatment and prognosis. *J. Clin. Med.* **2021**, *10*, 468. [CrossRef]
23. Akashi, Y.J.; Goldstein, D.S.; Barbaro, G.; Ueyama, T. Takotsubo cardiomyopathy: A new form of acute, reversible heart failure. *Circulation* **2008**, *118*, 2754–2762. [CrossRef]
24. De Gregorio, C.; Grimaldi, P.; Lentini, C. Left ventricular thrombus formation and cardioembolic complications in patients with takotsubo-like syndrome: A systematic review. *Int. J. Cardiol.* **2008**, *131*, 18–24. [CrossRef]
25. Cecchi, E.; Parodi, G.; Giglioli, C.; Passantino, S.; Bandinelli, B.; Alessandrello Liotta, A.; Bellandi, B.; Cioni, G.; Costanzo, M.; Abbate, R.; et al. Stress-induced hyperviscosity in the pathophysiology of takotsubo cardiomyopathy. *Am. J. Cardiol.* **2013**, *111*, 1523–1529. [CrossRef]
26. Fujita, K.; Fukuhara, T.; Munemasa, M.; Numba, Y.; Kuyama, H. Ampulla cardiomyopathy associated with aneurysmal subarachnoid hemorrhage: Report of 6 patients. *Surg. Neurol.* **2007**, *68*, 556–561. [CrossRef] [PubMed]
27. Oras, J.; Grivans, C.; Dalla, K.; Omerovic, E.; Rydenhag, B.; Ricksten, S.-E.; Seeman-Lodding, H. High-Sensitive troponin T and N-terminal pro B-type natriuretic peptide for early detection of stress-induced cardiomyopathy in patients with subarachnoid hemorrhage. *Neurocrit. Care* **2015**, *23*, 233–242. [CrossRef]
28. Hjalmarsson, C.; Oras, J.; Redfors, B. A case of intracerebral hemorrhage and apical ballooning: An important differential diagnosis in ST-segment elevation. *Int. J. Cardiol.* **2015**, *186*, 90–92. [CrossRef] [PubMed]
29. Madias, C.; Fitzgibbons, T.P.; Alsheikh-Ali, A.A.; Bouchard, J.L.; Kalsmith, B.; Garlitski, A.C.; Tighe, D.A.; Estes, N.A., III; Aurigemma, G.P.; Link, M.S. Acquired long QT syndrome from stress cardiomyopathy is associated with ventricular arrhythmias and torsades de pointes. *Heart Rhythm.* **2011**, *8*, 555–561. [CrossRef]
30. Bonello, L.; Com, O.; Ait-Moktar, O.; Théron, A.; Moro, P.-J.; Salem, A.; Sbragia, P.; Paganellit, F. Ventricular arrhythmias during takotsubo syndrome. *Int. J. Cardiol.* **2008**, *128*, e50–e53. [CrossRef]
31. Mahida, S.; Dalageorgou, C.; Behr, E.R. Long-QT syndrome and torsades de pointes in a patient with takotsubo cardiomyopathy: An unusual case. *Europace* **2009**, *11*, 376–378. [CrossRef] [PubMed]
32. Akashi, Y.J.; Nef, H.M.; Mollmann, H.; Ueyama, T. Stress cardiomyopathy. *Annu. Rev. Med.* **2010**, *61*, 271–286. [CrossRef]
33. Matsuoka, K.; Okubo, S.; Fujii, E.; Uchida, F.; Kasai, A.; Aoki, T.; Makino, K.; Omichi, C.; Fujimoto, N.; Ohta, S.; et al. Evaluation of the arrhythmogenecity of stress-induced "Takotsubo cardiomyopathy" from the time course of the 12-lead surface electrocardiogram. *Am. J. Cardiol.* **2003**, *92*, 230–233. [CrossRef]
34. Jefic, D.; Koul, D.; Boguszewski, A.; Martini, W. Transient left ventricular apical ballooning syndrome caused by abrupt metoprolol withdrawal. *Int. J. Cardiol.* **2008**, *131*, E35–E37. [CrossRef]
35. Migliore, F.; Bilato, C.; Isabella, G.; Iliceto, S.; Tarantini, G. Haemodynamic effects of acute intravenous metoprolol in apical ballooning syndrome with dynamic left ventricular outflow tract obstruction. *Eur. J. Heart Fail.* **2010**, *12*, 305–308. [CrossRef] [PubMed]
36. Santoro, F.; Ieva, R.; Ferraretti, A.; Fanelli, M.; Musaico, F.; Tarantino, N.; Martino, L.D.; Gennaro, L.D.; Caldarola, P.; Biase, M.D.; et al. Hemodynamic effects, safety, and feasibility of intravenous esmolol infusion during takotsubo cardiomyopathy with left ventricular outflow tract obstruction: Results from a multicenter registry. *Cardiovasc. Ther.* **2016**, *34*, 161–166. [CrossRef]
37. Chandler, B.T.; Pernu, P. Hyperinsulinaemic euglycaemic therapy use in neurogenic stunned myocardium following subarachnoid haemorrhage. *Anaesth. Intensive Care* **2018**, *46*, 575–578. [CrossRef] [PubMed]
38. Takama, T.; Fukue, M.; Sato, H.; Taniuchi, M. A case of ultrashort-acting beta-blocker landiolol hydrochloride for takotsubo syndrome with left ventricular outflow tract obstruction. *J. Gen. Fam. Med.* **2018**, *20*, 65–67. [CrossRef]
39. Krumpl, G.; Ulc, I.; Trebs, M.; Kadlecová, P.; Hodisch, J. Bolus application of landiolol and esmolol: Comparison of the pharmacokinetic and pharmacodynamic profiles in a healthy Caucasian group. *Eur. J. Clin. Pharmacol.* **2017**, *73*, 417–428. [CrossRef] [PubMed]
40. Madias, J.E. Metoprolol, propranolol, carvedilol, or labetalol for patients with Takotsubo syndrome? *Clin. Auton. Res.* **2018**, *28*, 131–132. [CrossRef] [PubMed]
41. Yoshioka, T.; Hashimoto, A.; Tsuchihashi, K.; Nagao, K.; Kyuma, M.; Ooiwa, H.; Nozawa, A.; Shimoshige, S.; Eguchi, M.; Wakabayashi, T.; et al. Clinical implications of midventricular obstruction and intravenous propranolol use in transient left ventricular apical ballooning (Tako-tsubo cardiomyopathy). *Am. Heart J.* **2008**, *155*, 526.e1–526.e7. [CrossRef]
42. Templin, C.; Ghadri, J.R.; Diekmann, J.; Napp, L.C.; Bataiosu, D.R.; Jaguszewski, M.; Cammann, V.L.; Sarcon, A.; Geyer, V.; Neumann, C.A.; et al. Clinical features and outcomes of Takotsubo (stress) cardiomyopathy. *N. Engl. J. Med.* **2015**, *373*, 929–938. [CrossRef]
43. Sharkey, S.W.; Windenburg, D.C.; Lesser, J.R.; Maron, M.S.; Hauser, R.G.; Lesser, J.N.; Haas, T.S.; Hodges, J.S.; Maron, B.J. Natural History and Expansive Clinical Profile of Stress (Tako-Tsubo) Cardiomyopathy. *J. Am. Coll. Cardiol.* **2010**, *55*, 333–341. [CrossRef] [PubMed]

44. Münzel, T.; Knorr, F.M.; Schmidt, S.; von Bardeleben, T.; Gori, E.S. Airborne disease: A case of a Takotsubo cardiomyopathy as a consequence of nighttime aircraft noise exposure. *Eur. Heart J.* **2016**, *37*, 2844. [CrossRef]
45. Schultz, T.; Shao, Y.; Redfors, B.; Sverrisdóttir, Y.B.; Råmunddal, T.; Albertsson, P.; Matejka, G.; Omerovic, E. Stress-induced cardiomyopathy in Sweden: Evidence for different ethnic predisposition and altered cardio-circulatory status. *Cardiology* **2012**, *122*, 180–186. [CrossRef]
46. Madhavan, M.; Rihal, C.S.; Lerman, A.; Prasad, A. Acute heart failure in apical ballooning syndrome (Takotsubo/stress cardiomyopathy): Clinical correlates and Mayo Clinic risk score. *J. Am. Coll. Cardiol.* **2011**, *57*, 1400–1401. [CrossRef] [PubMed]
47. Madias, J.E. Dissecting the pathophysiology of complete heart block in takotsubo syndrome. *Indian Pacing Electrophysiol. J.* **2018**, *18*, 87. [CrossRef] [PubMed]
48. Stiermaier, T.; Rommel, K.P.; Eitel, C.; Möller, C.; Graf, T.; Desch, S.; Thiele, H.; Eitel, I. Management of arrhythmias in patients with takotsubo cardiomyopathy: Is the implantation of permanent devices necessary? *Heart Rhythm.* **2016**, *13*, 1979–1986. [CrossRef]
49. Afzal, A.; Watson, J.; Choi, J.W.; Schussler, J.M.; Assar, M.D. Takotsubo cardiomyopathy in the setting of complete heart block. *Bayl. Univ. Med. Cent. Proc.* **2018**, *31*, 502–505. [CrossRef] [PubMed]
50. Benouda, L.; Roule, V.; Foucault, A.; Dahdouh, Z.; Lebon, A.; Milliez, P. Conduction disturbances in takotsubo cardiomyopathy: A cause or a consequence? *Int. J. Cardiol.* **2012**, *159*, 61–62. [CrossRef] [PubMed]
51. El-Battrawy, I.; Erath, J.W.; Lang, S.; Ansari, U.; Behnes, M.; Gietzen, T.; Zhou, X.; Borggrefe, M.; Akin, I. Takotsubo syndrome and cardiac implantable electronic device therapy. *Sci. Rep.* **2019**, *9*, 16559. [CrossRef]
52. Anabtawi, A.; Roldan, P.C.; Roldan, C.A. Takotsubo cardiomyopathy with a rapidly resolved left ventricular thrombus. *J. Investig. Med. High Impact Case Rep.* **2017**, *5*, 2324709617734238. [CrossRef]
53. Donazzan, L.; Baessato, F.; Cemin, R.; Mugnai, G.; Unterhuber, M. Atrial thrombosis during Tako-tsubo cardiomyopathy: Chance or plausible risk? *Clin. Res. Cardiol.* **2021**, *31*, 1–2, Online ahead of print. [CrossRef]
54. Herath, H.M.M.T.B.; Pahalagamage, S.P.; Lindsay, L.C.; Vinothan, S.; Withanawasam, S.; Senarathne, V.; Withana, M. Takotsubo cardiomyopathy complicated with apical thrombus formation on first day of the illness: A case report and literature review. *BMC Cardiovasc. Disord.* **2017**, *17*, 176. [CrossRef]
55. Mele, M.; Martimucci, M.; Maggi, A.; Villella, A.; Villella, M.; Langialonga, T. Cardioembolic acute myocardial infarction associated with apical ballooning: Considerations. *Int. J. Cardiol.* **2015**, *192*, 16–17. [CrossRef]
56. Samardhi, H.; Raffel, O.C.; Savage, M.; Sirisena, T.; Bett, N.; Pincus, M.; Small, A.; Walters, D.L. Takotsubo cardiomyopathy: An Australian single centre experience with medium term follow up. *Intern. Med. J.* **2012**, *42*, 35–42. [CrossRef]
57. Mrdovic, I.; Perunicic, J.; Asanin, M.; Matic, M.; Vasiljevic, Z.; Ostojic, M. Transient left ventricular apical ballooning complicated by a mural thrombus and outflow tract obstruction in a patient with pheochromocytoma. *Tex. Heart Inst. J.* **2008**, *35*, 480–482. [PubMed]
58. Azzarelli, S.; Galassi, A.R.; Amico, F.; Giacoppo, M.; Argentino, V.; Giordano, G.; Fiscella, A. Apical thrombus in a patient with takotsubo cardiomyopathy. *J. Cardiovasc. Med.* **2008**, *9*, 831–833. [CrossRef] [PubMed]
59. Mano, Y.; Baba, A.; Sukegawa, H.; Sawano, M.; Nishiyama, T.; Ohki, T. Successful conservative treatment of cardiac rupture associated with takotsubo syndrome. *Intern. Med.* **2021**, *60*, 2097–2102. [CrossRef] [PubMed]
60. Madias, J.E. A proposal for a noninvasive monitoring of sympathetic nerve activity in patients with takotsubo syndrome. *Med. Hypotheses* **2017**, *109*, 97–101. [CrossRef]
61. Madias, J.E. If channel blocker ivabradine vs. β-blockers for sinus tachycardia in patients with takotsubo syndrome. *Int. J. Cardiol.* **2016**, *223*, 877–878. [CrossRef]
62. Bui, Q.M.; Ang, L.; Phreaner, N. A case report of cardiogenic shock from takotsubo cardiomyopathy with left ventricular outflow tract obstruction: Fundamental lessons in cardiac pathophysiology. *Eur. Heart J. Case Rep.* **2021**, *5*, ytab127. [CrossRef]
63. Lyon, A.R.; Bossone, E.; Schneider, B.; Sechtem, U.; Citro, R.; Underwood, S.R.; Sheppard, M.N.; Figtree, G.; Parodi, G.; Akashi, Y.J.; et al. Current state of knowledge on Takotsubo syndrome: A position statement from the Taskforce on Takotsubo Syndrome of the Heart Failure Association of the European Society of Cardiology. *Eur. J. Heart Fail.* **2016**, *18*, 8–27. [CrossRef]
64. Thiele, H.; Zeymer, U.; Neumann, F.J.; Ferenc, M.; Olbrich, H.-G.; Hausleiter, J.; Richardt, G.; Hennersdorf, M.; Empen, K.; Fuernauet, G.; et al. Intraaortic balloon support for myocardial infarction with cardiogenic shock. *N. Engl. J. Med.* **2012**, *367*, 1287–1296. [CrossRef] [PubMed]
65. Napierkowski, S.; Banerjee, U.; Anderson, H.V.; Charitakis, K.; Madjid, M.; Smalling, R.W.; Dhoble, A. Trends and impact of the use of mechanical circulatory support for cardiogenic shock secondary to takotsubo cardiomyopathy. *Am. J. Cardiol.* **2021**, *139*, 28–33. [CrossRef]
66. Bonacchi, M.; Valente, S.; Harmelin, G.; Gensini, G.F.; Sani, G. Extracorporeal life support as ultimate strategy for refractory severe cardiogenic shock induced by Takotsubo cardiomyopathy: A new effective therapeutic option. *Artif. Organs* **2009**, *33*, 866–870. [CrossRef]
67. Bonacchi, M.; Maiani, M.; Harmelin, G.; Sani, G. Intractable cardiogenic shock in stress cardiomyopathy with left ventricular outflow tract obstruction: Is extra-corporeal life support the best treatment? *Eur. J. Heart Fail.* **2009**, *11*, 721–727. [CrossRef] [PubMed]
68. Redfors, B.; Shao, Y.; Omerovic, E. Stress-induced cardiomyopathy in a patient with chronic spinal cord transection at the level of C5: Endocrinologically mediated catecholamine toxicity. *Int. J. Cardiol.* **2012**, *159*, e61–e62. [CrossRef] [PubMed]

69. Padayachee, L. Levosimendan: The inotrope of choice in cardiogenic shock secondary to takotsubo cardiomyopathy? *Heart Lung Circ.* **2007**, *16*, S65–S70. [CrossRef]
70. Kagiyama, N.; Okura, H.; Tamada, T.; Imai, K.; Yamada, R.; Kume, T.; Hayashida, A.; Neishi, Y.; Kawamoto, T.; Yoshida, K. Impact of right ventricular involvement on the prognosis of takotsubo cardiomyopathy. *Eur. Heart J. Cardiovasc. Imaging* **2016**, *17*, 210–216. [CrossRef]
71. Ajiro, Y.; Hagiwara, N.; Katsube, Y.; Sperelakis, N.; Kasanuki, H. Levosimendan increases L-type Ca(21) current via phosphodiesterase-3 inhibition in human cardiac myocytes. *Eur. J. Pharmacol.* **2002**, *435*, 27–33. [CrossRef]
72. Santoro, F.; Ieva, R.; Ferraretti, A.; Ienco, V.; Carpagnano, G.; Lodispoto, M.; Di Biase, L.; Di Biase, M.; Brunetti, N.D. Safety and feasibility of levosimendan administration in takotsubo cardiomyopathy: A case series. *Cardiovasc. Ther.* **2013**, *31*, e133–e137. [CrossRef]
73. Redfors, B.; Omerovic, E. Takotsubo (stress) cardiomyopathy. *N. Engl. J. Med.* **2015**, *373*, 2688–2689.
74. Redfors, B.; Shao, Y.; Omerovic, E. Stress-induced cardiomyopathy in the critically ill—Why inotropes fail to improve outcome. *Int. J. Cardiol.* **2013**, *168*, 4489–4490. [CrossRef]
75. Beneduce, A.; Bertoldi, L.F.; Melillo, F.; Baldetti, L.; Spoladore, R.; Slavich, M.; Oppizzi, M.; Margonato, A.; Pappalardo, F. Mechanical circulatory with Impella percutaneous ventricular assist device as a bridge torRecovery in takotsubo syndrome complicated by cardiogenic shock and left ventricular outflow tract obstruction. *JACC Cardiovasc. Interventions* **2019**, *12*, e31–e32.
76. Kumar, S.; Kaushik, S.; Nautiyal, A.; Choudhary, S.K.; Kayastha, B.L.; Mostow, N.; Lazar, J.M. Cardiac rupture in takotsubo cardiomyopathy: A systematic review. *Clin. Cardiol.* **2011**, *34*, 672–676. [CrossRef] [PubMed]
77. Jolobe, O.M.P. Cardiac rupture with conservative treatment and survival in takotsubo cardiomyopathy. *Am. J. Emerg. Med.* **2020**, S0735–S6757. [CrossRef]
78. Pant, S.; Deshmukh, A.; Mehta, K.; Badheka, A.O.; Tuliani, T.; Patel, N.J.; Dabhadkar, K.; Prasad, A.; Paydak, H. Burden of arrhythmias in patients with takotsubo cardiomyopathy (apical ballooning syndrome). *Int. J. Cardiol.* **2013**, *170*, 64–68. [CrossRef] [PubMed]
79. Ghadri, J.R.; Wittstein, I.S.; Prasad, A.; Sharkey, S.; Dote, K.; Akashi, Y.J.; Cammann, V.L.; Crea, F.; Galiuto, L.; Desmet, W.; et al. International expert consensus document on takotsubo syndrome (Part II): Diagnostic workup, outcome, and management. *Eur. Heart J.* **2018**, *39*, 2047–2062. [CrossRef]
80. Brown, K.H.; Trohman, R.G.; Madias, C. Arrhythmias in takotsubo cardiomyopathy. *Card. Electrophysiol. Clin.* **2015**, *7*, 331–340. [CrossRef]
81. Ahmed, A.E.K.; Serafi, A.; Sunni, N.S.; Younes, H.; Hassan, W. Recurrent takotsubo with prolonged QT and torsade de pointes and left ventricular thrombus. *J. Saudi Heart Assoc.* **2017**, *29*, 44–52. [CrossRef] [PubMed]
82. Dib, C.; Prasad, A.; Friedman, P.A.; Ahmad, E.; Rihal, C.S.; Hammill, S.C.; Asirvatham, S.J. Malignant arrhythmia in apical ballooning syndrome: Risk factors and outcomes. *Indian Pacing Electrophysiol. J.* **2008**, *8*, 182–192.
83. Evison, I.; Watson, G.; Chan, C.; Bridgman, P. The effects of beta-blockers in patients with stress cardiomyopathy. *Intern. Med. J.* **2021**, *51*, 411–413. [CrossRef]
84. Chiang, C.-E. Congenital and acquired long QT syndrome. Current concepts and management. *Cardiol. Rev.* **2004**, *12*, 222–234. [CrossRef]
85. Madias, J.E. Cardiac arrest-triggered takotsubo syndrome vs. takotsubo syndrome complicated by cardiac arrest. *Int. J. Cardiol.* **2016**, *225*, 142–143. [CrossRef] [PubMed]
86. Cha, K.C.; Kim, H.I.; Kim, O.H.; Cha, Y.S.; Kim, H.; Lee, K.H.; Hwang, S.O. Echocardiographic patterns of postresuscitation myocardial dysfunction. *Resuscitation* **2018**, *124*, 90–95. [CrossRef] [PubMed]
87. Omar, H.R. Takotsubo-pericarditis association. *Am. J. Emerg. Med.* **2012**, *30*, 382–383. [CrossRef] [PubMed]
88. Santoro, F.; Ieva, R.; Musaico, F.; Ferraretti, A.; Triggiani, G.; Tarantino, N.; Di Biase, M.; Brunetti, N.D. Lack of efficacy of drug therapy in preventing takotsubo cardiomyopathy recurrence: A meta-analysis. *Clin. Cardiol.* **2014**, *37*, 434–439. [CrossRef]
89. Madias, J.E. Cardiac takotsubo syndrome in association with cerebral, renal, gastrointestinal, vascular, and perhaps total body, "takotsubo" syndrome? *J. Neurol. Sci.* **2017**, *378*, 238. [CrossRef]
90. Madias, J.E. COVID-19, POCUS, and takotsubo. *Am. J. Cardiol.* **2021**, *141*, 157. [CrossRef]
91. Y-Hassan, S. Spontaneous coronary artery dissection and takotsubo syndrome: An often overlooked association; review. *Cardiovasc. Revasc. Med.* **2018**, *19*, 717–723. [CrossRef]
92. Wischnewsky, M.B.; Candreva, A.; Bacchi, B.; Cammann, V.L.; Kato, K.; Szawan, K.A.; Gili, S.; D'Ascenzo, F.; Dichtl, W.; Citro, R.; et al. Prediction of short- and long-term mortality in takotsubo syndrome: The InterTAK prognostic score. *Eur. J. Heart Fail.* **2019**, *21*, 1469–1472. [CrossRef]
93. Oras, J.; Lundgren, J.; Redfors, B.; Brandin, D.; Omerovic, E.; Seeman-Lodding, H.; Ricksten, S.-E. Takotsubo syndrome in hemodynamically unstable patients admitted to the intensive care unit—A retrospective study. *Acta Anaesthesiol. Scand.* **2017**, *61*, 914–924. [CrossRef]
94. Limite, L.R.; Arcari, L.; Cacciotti, L.; Russo, D.; Musumeci, M.B. Cardiogenic shock in takotsubo syndrome: A clue to unravel what hides behind the curtain? *JACC Heart Fail.* **2019**, *7*, 175–176. [CrossRef] [PubMed]
95. Muksinova, M.D.; Shilova, A.S.; Gilyarov, M.Y.; Konstantinova, E.V.; Nesterov, A.P.; Udovichenko, A.E.; Svet, A.V. Takotsubo cardiomyopathy as a consequence of myocardial infarction. It is possible? *Kardiologiia* **2017**, *57*, 97–104. [CrossRef] [PubMed]

96. Redfors, B.; Ramunddal, T.; Shao, Y.; Omerovic, E. Takotsubo triggered by acute myocardial infarction: A common but overlooked syndrome? *J. Geriatr. Cardiol.* **2014**, *11*, 171–173.
97. Maeda, S.; Tamura, A.; Kawano, Y.; Naono, S.; Shinozaki, K.; Zaizen, H. Takotsubo cardiomyopathy triggered by lateral wall ST-segment elevation myocardial infarction. *J. Cardiol. Cases* **2014**, *9*, 117–120. [CrossRef] [PubMed]
98. Guglin, M. How to increase the utilization of donor hearts? *Heart Fail. Rev.* **2015**, *20*, 95–105. [CrossRef]
99. Madan, S.; Sims, D.B.; Vlismas, P.; Patel, S.R.; Saeed, O.; Murthy, S.; Forest, S.; Jakobleff, W.; Shin, J.J.; Goldstein, D.J.; et al. Cardiac transplantation using hearts with transient dysfunction: Role of takotsubo-like phenotype. *Ann. Thorac. Surg.* **2020**, *110*, 76–84. [CrossRef]
100. Madias, J.E. There should not be much doubt that neurogenic stress cardiomyopathy in cardiac is a phenotype of takotsubo syndrome. *JACC Heart Fail.* **2018**, *6*, 346–347. [CrossRef]
101. Redfors, B.; Ramunddal, T.; Oras, J.; Kristjan Karason, K.; Ricksten, S.-E.; Dellgren, G.; Omerovic, E. Successful heart transplantation from a donor with Takotsubo syndrome. *Int. J. Cardiol.* **2015**, *195*, 82–84. [CrossRef]
102. Ojha, V.; Khurana, R.; Ganga, K.P.; Kumar, S. Advanced cardiac magnetic resonance imaging in takotsubo cardiomyopathy. *Br. J. Radiol.* **2020**, *93*, 20200514. [CrossRef]
103. Scally, C.; Rudd, A.; Mezincescu, A.; Wilson, H.; Srivanasan, J.; Horgan, G.; Broadhurst, P.; Newby, D.E.; Henning, A.; Dawson, D.K. Persistent long-term structural, functional, and metabolic changes after stress-induced (takotsubo) cardiomyopathy. *Circulation* **2018**, *137*, 1039–1048. [CrossRef]
104. Palla, A.R.; Dande, A.S.; Petrini, J.; Wasserman, H.S.; Warshofsky, M.K. Pretreatment with low-dose beta-adrenergic antagonist therapy does not affect severity of Takotsubo cardiomyopathy. *Clin. Cardiol.* **2012**, *35*, 478–481. [CrossRef]
105. Isogai, T.; Matsui, H.; Tanaka, H.; Fushimi, K.; Yasunaga, H. Early β-blocker use and in-hospital mortality in patients with takotsubo cardiomyopathy. *Heart* **2016**, *102*, 1029–1035. [CrossRef]
106. Brunetti, N.D.; Santoro, F.; De Gennaro, L.; Correale, M.; Gaglione, A.; Di Biase, M.; Madias, J.E. Combined therapy with beta-blockers and ACE-inhibitors/angiotensin receptor blockers and recurrence of Takotsubo (stress) cardiomyopathy: A meta-regression study. *Int. J. Cardiol.* **2017**, *230*, 281–283. [CrossRef]
107. D'Ascenzo, F.; Gili, S.; Bertaina, M.; Iannaccone, M.; Cammann, V.L.; Di Vece, D.; Kato, K.; Saglietto, A.; Szawan, K.A.; Frangieh, A.H.; et al. Impact of aspirin on takotsubo syndrome: A propensity score-based analysis of the InterTAK Registry. *Eur. J. Heart Fail.* **2020**, *22*, 330–337. [CrossRef]
108. Y-Hassan, S.; Falhammar, H. Pheochromocytoma-and paraganglioma-triggered Takotsubo syndrome. *Endocrine* **2019**, *65*, 483–493. [CrossRef] [PubMed]
109. Compare, A.; Brugnera, A.; Spada, M.M.; Zarbo, C.; Tasca, G.A.; Sassaroli, S.; Caselli, G.; Ruggiero, G.M.; Wittstein, I. The role of emotional competence in takotsubo cardiomyopathy. *Psychosom. Med.* **2018**, *80*, 377–384. [CrossRef] [PubMed]
110. Redfors, B.; Shao, Y.; Omerovic, E. Stress-induced cardiomyopathy (takotsubo)—Broken heart and mind? *Vasc. Health Risk Manag.* **2013**, *9*, 149–154. [PubMed]
111. Schnabel, R.B.; Hasenfuß, G.; Buchmann, S.; Kahl, K.G.; Aeschbacher, S.; Osswald, S.; Angermann, C.E. Heart and brain interactions: Pathophysiology and management of cardio-psycho-neurological disorders. *Herz* **2021**, *46*, 138–149. [CrossRef]
112. Madias, J.E. Is the association of history of psychiatric disorders with takotsubo syndrome partially mediated by the underlying psychotropic drug therapy? *Int. J. Cardiol.* **2016**, *220*, 307–309. [CrossRef] [PubMed]
113. Joy, P.S.; Guddati, A.K.; Shapira, I. Outcomes of takotsubo cardiomyopathy in hospitalized cancer patients. *J. Cancer Res. Clin. Oncol.* **2018**, *144*, 1539–1545. [CrossRef] [PubMed]
114. Ueyama, T.; Ishikura, F.; Matsuda, A.; Asanuma, T.; Ueda, K.; Ichinose, M.; Kasamatsu, K.; Hano, T.; Akasaka, T.; Tsuruo, Y.; et al. Chronic estrogen supplementation following ovariectomy improves the emotional stress-induced cardiovascular responses by indirect action on the nervous system and by direct action on the heart. *Circ. J.* **2007**, *71*, 565–573. [CrossRef]
115. Madias, J.E. Estrogens for protection from an index and recurrent episodes of takotsubo syndrome? *J. Endocrinol.* in press.
116. Braunwald, E.; Kloner, R.A. The stunned myocardium: Prolonged, postischemic ventricular dysfunction. *Circulation* **1982**, *66*, 1146–1149. [CrossRef] [PubMed]
117. Godsman, N.; Kohlhaas, M.; Nickel, A.; Cheyne, L.; Marco, M.; Schweiger, L.; Hepburn, C.; Chantal Munts, C.; Welch, A.; Delibegovic, M.; et al. Metabolic alterations in a rat model of Takotsubo syndrome. *Cardiovasc. Res.* **2021**, cvab081, Online ahead of print. [CrossRef]
118. Dawson, D.K.; Neil, C.J.; Henning, A.; Cameron, D.; Jagpal, B.; Bruce, M.; Horowitz, J.; Frenneaux, M. Tako-tsubo cardiomyopathy: A heart stressed out of energy? *JACC Cardiovasc. Imaging* **2015**, *8*, 985–987. [CrossRef] [PubMed]
119. Vanderschuren, A.; Hantson, P. Hyperinsulinemic euglycemia therapy for stunned myocardium following subarachnoid hemorrhage. *J. Neurosurg.* **2009**, *110*, 64–66. [CrossRef]
120. Kenigsberg, B.B.; Barnett, C.F.; Mai, J.C.; Jason, J.; Chang, J.J. Neurogenic stunned myocardium in severe neurological injury. *Curr. Neurol. Neurosci. Rep.* **2019**, *19*, 90. [CrossRef]
121. Devos, J.; Peeters, A.; Wittebole, X.; Hantson, P. High-dose insulin therapy for neurogenic-stunned myocardium after stroke. *BMJ Case Rep.* **2012**, *2012*, bcr2012006620. [CrossRef] [PubMed]
122. Takada, T.; Jujo, K.; Ishida, I.; Hagiwara, N. Recurrent takotsubo syndrome with worsening of left ventricular outflow obstruction during hemodialysis: A case report. *Eur. Heart J. Case Rep.* **2020**, *4*, 1–6. [CrossRef]

123. Kobylecka, M.; Budnik, M.; Kochanowski, J.; Piatkowski, R.; Chojnowski, M.; Fronczewska-Wieniawska, K.; Mazurek, T.; Maczewska, J.; Peller, M.; Opolski, G.; et al. Takotsubo cardiomyopathy: FDG myocardial uptake pattern in fasting patients. Comparison of PET/CT, SPECT, and ECHO results. *J. Nucl. Cardiol.* **2018**, *25*, 1260–1270. [CrossRef] [PubMed]
124. St-Onge, M.; Anseeuw, K.; Cantrell, F.L.; Gilchrist, I.C.; Hantson, P.; Bailey, B.; Lavergne, V.; Gosselin, S.; Kerns, W., II; Laliberté, M.; et al. Experts consensus recommendations for the management of calcium channel blocker poisoning in adults. *Crit. Care Med.* **2017**, *45*, e306–e315. [CrossRef] [PubMed]
125. Doepker, B.; Healy, W.; Cortez, E.; Adkins, E.J. High-dose insulin and intravenous lipid emulsion therapy for cardiogenic shock induced by intentional calcium-channel blocker and beta-blocker overdose: A case series. *J. Emerg. Med.* **2014**, *46*, 486–490. [CrossRef] [PubMed]
126. Redfors, B.; Oras, J.; Shao, Y.; Seemann-Lodding, H.; Ricksten, S.-E.; Omerovic, E. Cardioprotective effects of isoflurane in a rat model of stress-induced cardiomyopathy (takotsubo). *Int. J. Cardiol.* **2014**, *176*, 815–821. [CrossRef]
127. Oras, J.; Redfors, B.; Ali, A.; Alkhoury, J.; Seeman-Lodding, H.; Omerovic, E.; Ricksten, S.-E. Early treatment with isoflurane attenuates left ventricular dysfunction and improves survival in experimental Takotsubo. *Acta Anaesthesiol. Scand.* **2017**, *61*, 399–407. [CrossRef]
128. Matsushita, K.; Lachmet-Thébaud, L.; Marchandot, B.; Trimaille, A.; Sato, C.; Dagrenat, C.; Greciano, S.; De Poli, F.; Leddet, P.; Peillex, M.; et al. Incomplete recovery from Takotsubo syndrome is a major determinant of cardiovascular mortality. *Circ. J.* **2021**. Online ahead of print. [CrossRef]
129. Yoneyama, K.; Akashi, Y.J. Myocardial contractile function recovery, systemic inflammation, and prognosis in takotsubo syndrome. *Circ. J.* **2021**. Online ahead of print. [CrossRef]
130. Moady, G.; Atar, S. Takotsubo syndrome during the COVID-19 pandemic, state-of -the- art review. *CJC Open* **2021**. Online ahead of print. [CrossRef]
131. Madias, J.E. Comparison of the first episode with the first recurrent episode of takotsubo syndrome in 128 patients from the world literature: Pathophysiologic connotations. *Int. J. Cardiol.* **2020**, *310*, 27–31. [CrossRef]
132. Schwarz, K.; Ahearn, T.; Srinivasan, J.; Neil, C.J.; Scally, C.; Rudd, A.; Jagpal, B.; Frenneaux, M.P.; Pislaru, C.; Horowitz, J.D.; et al. Alterations in cardiac deformation, timing of contraction and relaxation, and early myocardial fibrosis accompany the apparent recovery of acute stress-induced (takotsubo) cardiomyopathy: An end to the concept of transience. *J. Am. Soc. Echocardiogr.* **2017**, *30*, 745–755. [CrossRef]
133. Cammann, V.L.; Szawan, K.A.; Stähli, B.E.; Kato, K.; Budnik, M.; Wischnewsky, M.; Dreiding, S.; Levinson, R.A.; Di Vece, D.; Gili, S.; et al. Age-related variations in takotsubo syndrome. *J. Am. Coll. Cardiol.* **2020**, *75*, 1869–1877. [CrossRef] [PubMed]
134. Cammann, V.L.; Sarcon, A.; Ding, K.J.; Seifert, B.; Kato, K.; Di Vece, D.; Szawan, K.A.; Gili, S.; Jurisic, S.; Bacchi, B.; et al. Clinical features and outcomes of patients with malignancy and takotsubo syndrome: Observations from the International Takotsubo Registry. *J. Am. Heart Assoc.* **2019**, *8*, e010881. [CrossRef] [PubMed]
135. Stiermaier, T.; Santoro, F.; El-Battrawy, I.; Möller, C.; Graf, T.; Novo, G.; Santangelo, A.; Mariano, E.; Romeo, F.; Caldarola, P.; et al. Prevalence and prognostic impact of diabetes in takotsubo syndrome: Insights from the International, Multicenter GEIST Registry. *Diab. Care.* **2018**, *41*, 1084–1088. [CrossRef]
136. Ahuja, K.R.; Nazir, S.; Jain, V.; Isogai, T.; Saad, A.M.; Verma, B.R.; Shekhar, S.; Kumar, R.; Eltahawy, E.A.; Madias, J.E. Takotsubo syndrome: Does "diabetes paradox" exist? *Heart Lung.* **2021**, *50*, 316–322. [CrossRef] [PubMed]
137. Pelliccia, F.; Pasceri, V.; Patti, G.; Tanzilli, G.; Speciale, G.; Gaudio, C.; Camici, P.G. Long-term prognosis and outcome predictors in takotsubo syndrome: A systematic review and meta-regression study. *JACC Heart Fail.* **2019**, *7*, 143–154. [CrossRef] [PubMed]
138. Singh, K.; Carson, K.; Shah, R.; Sawhney, G.; Singh, B.; Parsaik, A.; Gilutz, H.; Usmani, Z.; Horowitz, J. Meta-analysis of clinical correlates of acute mortality in Takotsubo cardiomyopathy. *Am. J. Cardiol.* **2014**, *113*, 1420–1428. [CrossRef] [PubMed]

Journal of
Clinical Medicine

MDPI

Review

RBM20-Related Cardiomyopathy: Current Understanding and Future Options

Jan Koelemen [1,2], Michael Gotthardt [3,4,5], Lars M. Steinmetz [2,6,7] and Benjamin Meder [1,2,6,*]

1 Department of Internal Medicine III, University of Heidelberg, 69120 Heidelberg, Germany; Jan.Koelemenoglu@med.uni-heidelberg.de
2 DZHK (German Centre for Cardiovascular Research), Partner Site Heidelberg, 69120 Heidelberg, Germany; Lars.Steinmetz@stanford.edu
3 DZHK (German Centre for Cardiovascular Research), Partner Site Berlin, 10117 Berlin, Germany; gotthardt@mdc-berlin.de
4 Neuromuscular and Cardiovascular Cell Biology, Max Delbrück Center for Molecular Medicine in the Helmholtz Association, 13125 Berlin, Germany
5 Charité-Universitätsmedizin Berlin, 13353 Berlin, Germany
6 Department of Genetics and Stanford Genome Technology Center, Stanford University, Palo Alto, CA 94304, USA
7 Genome Biology Unit, European Molecular Biology Laboratory (EMBL), 69117 Heidelberg, Germany
* Correspondence: benjamin.meder@med.uni-heidelberg.de; Tel.: +49-(0)-6221-5639564; Fax: +49-(0)-6221-564645

Abstract: Splice regulators play an essential role in the transcriptomic diversity of all eukaryotic cell types and organ systems. Recent evidence suggests a contribution of splice-regulatory networks in many diseases, such as cardiomyopathies. Adaptive splice regulators, such as RNA-binding motif protein 20 (RBM20) determine the physiological mRNA landscape formation, and rare variants in the RBM20 gene explain up to 6% of genetic dilated cardiomyopathy (DCM) cases. With ample knowledge from RBM20-deficient mice, rats, swine and induced pluripotent stem cells (iPSCs), the downstream targets and quantitative effects on splicing are now well-defined and the prerequisites for corrective therapeutic approaches are set. This review article highlights some of the recent advances in the field, ranging from aspects of granule formation to 3D genome architectures underlying RBM20-related cardiomyopathy. Promising therapeutic strategies are presented and put into context with the pathophysiological characteristics of RBM20-related diseases.

Keywords: dilated cardiomyopathy; RBM20; arrhythmia; heart failure; gene therapy; alternative splicing

Citation: Koelemen, J.; Gotthardt, M.; Steinmetz, L.M.; Meder, B. RBM20-Related Cardiomyopathy: Current Understanding and Future Options. *J. Clin. Med.* **2021**, *10*, 4101. https://doi.org/10.3390/jcm10184101

Academic Editor: Stefan Peters

Received: 13 August 2021
Accepted: 8 September 2021
Published: 11 September 2021

1. RBM20 Mutations Cause Highly Penetrant Cardiomyopathies

In 2009, the first case of RBM20-associated human cardiomyopathy was described. The report mentioned two large families with autosomal dominant dilated cardiomyopathy. Clinically, they became noticeable due to young age at diagnosis, heart failure and high mortality [1]. Since then, mutations in RBM20 were recognized as an important cause of cardiomyopathy and genotype-phenotype studies suggest many patients having a progressive and complicated clinical course [1–6].

RBM20 regulates post-transcriptional splicing, particularly in sarcomeric, but also in other genes essential for myocardial homeostasis and calcium handling [1,6–8]. It is expressed in all striated muscles but highest in cardiac tissue [6]. The corresponding gene, RBM20, is located on the long arm of chromosome 10 and carries 14 exons. It encodes a 1227 amino acid protein containing two zinc finger domains, a glutamate-rich region, a leucine-rich region, an RNA-Recognition Motif (RRM)-type RNA binding domain and an arginine-/serine-rich region (RS-domain) (Figure 1) [9,10].

In patients with familial DCM, structured pedigree analysis is critical and genetic testing by sequencing of DNA commonly extracted from peripheral whole blood lymphocyte samples is recommended [11]. Pathogenic variants in RBM20 account for approximately 2–6% of the cases of familial DCM with noticeably early disease onset and clinically severe expression [2,12–14]. Figure 1 and Table 1 present reported variants with corresponding domains. Most patients carry heterozygous mutations, and the mode of inheritance is autosomal dominant [15]. Three protein regions were identified with high confidence for carrying pathogenic variants [12,15]. These are located at positions c.1601-1640 (exon 7, encoding the RRM-domain), c.1881-1920 (exon 9, encoding the highly conserved RS-domain) and c.2721-2760 (exon 11) [12,16,17]. In an international RBM20 patient registry, individuals with variants within these domains had a higher familial incidence of sudden cardiac death (SCD) and prevalence of personal history of arrhythmias than those with variants outside these hotspots or in genes such as Titin [12].

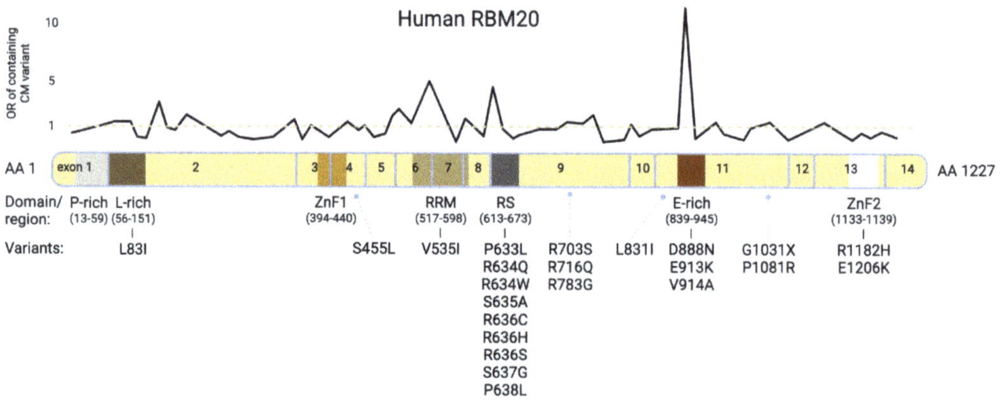

Figure 1. Modified from Parikh et al., 2019 [12]. Schematic protein structure of human RBM20 with corresponding exons. Variants shown in Table 1 are listed under the affiliated protein domains/regions. The black line chart displays the odds ratio (OR) for variant observation within the respective sections in a cardiomyopathy population vs. general population (Genome Aggregation Database [gnomAD]); underlying OR data derived from Parikh et al. [12]. Pathogenic sections predominantly concern the RS domain, the E-rich region and the RRM domain.

Table 1. RBM20 variants with corresponding exons and protein domains.

Domain	Mutation	Exon	Pathogenicity	Reference
Leu-rich-region	L83I	2	unknown	[18]
Other	S455L	4	unknown	[18]
RRM-domain	V535I	6	pathogenic	[6,16]
RS-domain	P633L	9	pathogenic	[19]
RS-domain	R634Q	9	pathogenic	[1,2,6,16]
RS-domain	R634W	9	pathogenic	[10,16]
RS-domain	S635A	9	pathogenic	[3,4,6,10]
RS-domain	R636C	9	pathogenic	[16]
RS-domain	R636H	9	pathogenic	[1,2,16,20,21]
RS-domain	R636S	9	pathogenic	[1,2,6,22]
RS-domain	S637G	9	pathogenic	[1,3,6,23]
RS-domain	P638L	9	pathogenic	[1,2,6,15,18]
Other	R703S	9	unknown	[18]
Other	R716Q	9	unknown	[6,16]
Other	R783G	9	pathogenic	[24]
Other	L831I	11	unknown	[18]
Glu-rich-region	D888N	11	unknown	[18]
Glu-rich-region	E913K	11	pathogenic	[2,25]

Table 1. *Cont.*

Domain	Mutation	Exon	Pathogenicity	Reference
Glu-rich-region	V914A	11	pathogenic	[15]
Other	G1031X *	11	pathogenic	[10,18]
Other	P1081R	11	unknown	[18]
ZnF-2	R1182H	13	unknown	[13]
ZnF-2	E1206K	13	unknown	[18]

* non-sense mutation; all others are missense mutations.

Most of the disease-causing mutations have been identified within the RS domain [1,6,9,16,26]. The RS domain generally plays an important role in pre-mRNA splicing and regulating alternative splicing by modulating the binding and assembly of the spliceosome [27–29]. In the case of RBM20, it has been shown that Serines within the Arginine–Serine–Arginine–Serine–Proline (RSRSP) stretch of the RS-Domain are physiologically phosphorylated and serve as a critical part of the nuclear localization signal (NLS) [10]. Moreover, it is believed that mutations of any residues within the RSRSP stretch, possibly accompanied by aberrant phosphorylation, may cause RBM20 mislocalization, subsequently leading to altered nuclear splicing of the target pre-mRNAs [10]. Recently, a novel angle on molecular pathophysiology of RBM20-related cardiomyopathy was established, exemplified by findings from gene-edited RBM20-p.Arg636Ser pigs [22]. It was hypothesized that the disease, beyond missplicing due to loss-of-function mutations, could also be caused by gain-of-function mutations leading to dysregulated cytoplasmic RBM20 ribonucleoprotein (RNP) granule formation [22]. Subsequently, this granule formation might mediate myocardial insufficiency, which will be further discussed below [22].

Variants outside the RS-Domain commonly do not affect splicing activity in the same way as variants within the RS-Domain [10]. However, mutations within the conserved Glutamate-rich region have been associated with disturbed alternative splicing of Titin and DCM as well [2,10,18,25,26]. It seems that they affect protein stability and hence a partial loss-of-function can occur. An altered RBM20 function was also observed in the G1031X nonsense mutation, characterized by the loss of the second zinc-finger domain [10]. Interestingly, only a homozygous son of the characterized family showed symptoms while the heterozygous mother was asymptomatic [10]. Although variants affecting the RRM-domain have not been frequently identified as causes for human RBM20-related cardiomyopathy, it has been observed that the knockout of the RRM-domain by deletion of exons 6 and 7, both in homozygous and heterozygous KO mice, affected alternative splicing of RBM20′s target genes, such as *CAMK2D* and *LDB3* [30]. Additionally, a loss of the RRM-domain and RBM20′s C-terminus led to a significant reduction of RBM20′s splicing function also in human cell culture [31].

Accurate variant calling according to current ACMG criteria is a crucial yet challenging task in rare diseases. To assist in classifying novel RBM20 variants, the corresponding location within the protein presents a suitable indicator. In this context, Gaertner et al. showed that the ratio of ryanodine receptor 2 (*RYR2*)- and titin (*TTN*)-splice variation could be also used as a tool for the classification of uncharacterized RBM20 variants if heart tissue or iPSC are available [15]. The team used qRT-PCR to measure the expression of *RYR2*-splice variants containing an additional small exon, which was previously described [8]. This quantitative expression is then put into relation with the expression of the regular *RYR2*-splice form. They were able to show that this ratio is increased in the case of pathogenic RBM20-variants [15]. As controls, they used RYR2-isoform ratios from non-failing and DCM heart samples (both negative controls), along with positive controls derived from individuals carrying the proven pathogenic RBM20-p.Pro638Leu variant. Analogous to this, they investigated the ratio of TTN-N2B to total Titin as an additional classification tool and concluded that this ratio, on the contrary, is lowered in individuals carrying pathogenic RBM20-variants [15].

2. Model Systems to Dissect the Pathophysiology and Enable Therapeutic Studies

Currently, there are several in vitro and in vivo model systems available. As the first animal model served the rat, focusing mainly on RBM20-dependent splicing regulation of *TTN* [6,32]. Left ventricular dilation and electrical abnormalities were present in these RBM20-deficient rats, showing comparatively similar pathologies as RBM20-deficient humans [1,3,6,16].

RBM20 deficiencies are also studied in established mouse models. Mouse models show advantages due to their easy handling, however, LV dysfunction primarily occurs only after stress [30]. Gene editing by targeted disruption of specific exons or CRISPR/Cas9 system has been used to create RBM20 knockout models and RBM20-mutant knockin mice mimicking human-derived mutations [3,10,30,33,34]. In mice, mutations in RBM20 are associated with signs of arrhythmia, unlike knockout models, where the reduced or eliminated expression of RBM20 resulted in a less severe phenotype, exemplified by the comparison of homozygous RBM20-p.Ser637Ala mutants with the complete knockout of RBM20 [3]. Although, in both the mutant and knockout model, splicing activity of RBM20 targets was affected, there are several examples, where the mutant leads to an altered calcium handling and subsequently to arrhythmia, while homo- and heterozygous knockouts showed regular cardiac electrical activity [3,33]. This observation suggests that not only might changes in splicing activity be the driver of this disease, but also other underlying mechanisms that likely play important roles in the pathogenesis of RBM20-related cardiomyopathy exist [3,9,19,22,33].

In genome-edited pigs, hetero- or homozygous for RBM20 alleles encoding a pathogenic human-derived RBM20-variant, it was recently discovered that RBM20 RNP granules accumulated abnormally in the sarcoplasm of the myocytes [22]. As discussed above, these findings are of greater interest and were confirmed in myocardium and reprogrammed cardiomyocytes from DCM patients carrying the same pathogenic allele [22]. In vivo, the dysregulated RNP granule aggregation was more severe in the homozygous gene-edited pigs, which lead to myocardial insufficiency and fatal circulatory failure in many of these animals [22]. Consequently, the presence of these sarcoplasmic aggregations seems to play a relevant role in the pathophysiology of RBM20-related cardiomyopathy [3,15,22]. As such, stringent observation and examination of genome-edited pigs carrying pathogenic (RBM20) variants have the potential to provide critical insights into the pathomechanism and natural course of human DCM [22]. Additionally, the pig model can also serve as a valuable large animal model for succeeding therapy studies.

The investigation of splicing defects in human heart tissue and iPSCs provides a valuable toolkit for the translation of recent in vivo and -vitro findings into a human model system [4,8,15,19,22,35–37]. Patient-specific RBM20 mutant iPSCs and isogenic gene-corrected iPSCs have been established using CRISPR/Cas9, allowing the investigation of variant-specific RBM20-dependent pathomechanisms in a controlled setting [4,19,35–37]. These sorts of models also foster larger scale therapeutic drug screenings and provide a platform to study the advantages of novel technique applications, such as nanopore sequencing, in order to further investigate the genetic background of the disease [19,36,37].

3. Trafficking of RBM20 and Aggregation Formation

Normal RBM20 synthesis and trafficking are outlined in Figure 2. Wild-type RBM20 is predominantly localized in the nucleus, being part of the spliceosome and functioning thus as a splicing cofactor. Analyses in C2C12 cells (mouse myoblast cell line) showed that RBM20 variants, such as RBM20-p.Pro638Leu or -p.Ser637Ala, lead to increased RBM20 aggregation within the cytoplasm [3,15]. Murayama et al. had shown similar results for murine p.Ser637Ala [10]. These findings from the murine models were confirmed not only in human explanted heart tissue but also in a recently published and already mentioned pig model [15,22]. Functionally, disruption of nuclear transport processes might lead to cytoplasmatic protein aggregation [38]. The mechanism responsible for this protein mislocalization is believed to be caused, for example, by aberrant phosphorylation of the RSRSP-stretch in the RS-domain [10,15]. Considering most patients are heterozygous carriers, nuclear concentrations of RBM20 remain lower, leading to functional deficiencies [15]. The described mislocalization also raises the idea that the dysregulated RNP granules could be interfering with cytoplasmic stress granules, possibly causing a detrimental cascade [3,22]. Upcoming results from currently ongoing investigations beyond nuclear splicing are eagerly awaited. The exploration and discovery of yet unidentified RBM20-partner proteins essential for its proper transportation to the nucleus and the interaction with the spliceosome and genome-foci represent additional directions of future research.

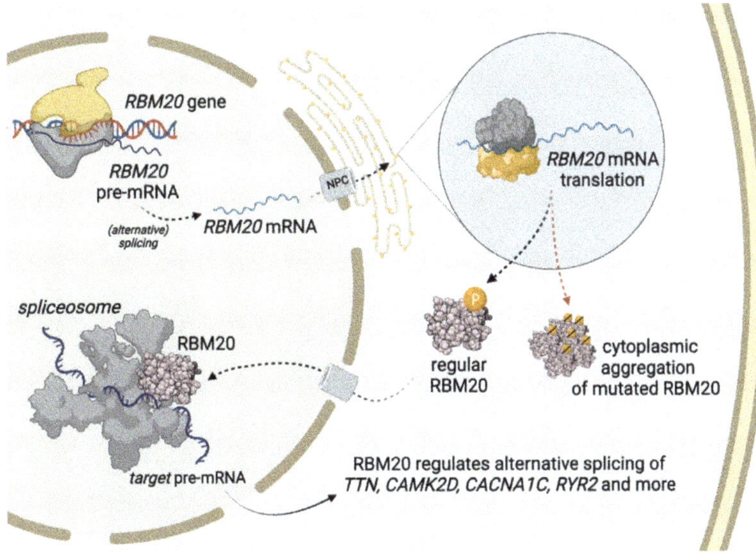

Figure 2. Modified from Schneider et al., 2019 [22]. RBM20 synthesis, trafficking and pathological cytoplasmic aggregation of RBM20-mutations. RBM20 is transcribed and its mRNA translocated through the nuclear pore complex (NPC) to the cytoplasm, where the RBM20 protein is translated. Regular RBM20 is transported back to the nucleus where it regulates alternative splicing as a part of the spliceosome. Disruption of nuclear transport processes in the presence of RBM20 mutations, however, may promote cytoplasmic protein aggregation, amongst other things by aberrant phosphorylation of the RS-Domain. This caused mislocalization may explain the altered splicing of target genes in the presence of RBM20 mutations.

Not every RBM20-variant may lead to protein mislocalization [15]. The pathogenic RBM20-p.Val914Ala variant, for instance, showed no effect on RMB20′s nuclear localization, but on downstream splicing [15]. Rare variants leading to non-sense mediated RNA decay and haploinsufficiency may result in less severe cardiomyopathy, potentially due to missing substrate for aggregates [9,10,39]. It will be interesting to investigate the resulting molecular differences in pairwise comparisons.

4. Splicing Targets and Their Function

Until now, more than 30 validated splicing targets of RBM20 have been identified with high confidence [6,8,33]. Table 2 provides an overview of these target genes with the corresponding proteins and their functions. From a pathogenetic standpoint, some of the centrally involved targets include:

Table 2. Modified from Lennermann et al., 2020 [40]. List of RBM20 target genes with corresponding protein and function.

Gene	Encoded Protein	Function	References
APTX	Aprataxin	DNA repair	[6]
CACNA1C	Calcium channel, voltage-dependent, L-type, alpha 1C sub-unit	sub-unit of the L-type calcium channel	[6]
CAMK2D	Calcium/calmodulin-dependent protein kinase II delta	Serine/threonine kinase; regulates many cardiac proteins through phosphorylation	[6,33]
CAMK2G	Calcium/calmodulin-dependent protein kinase II Gamma	Serine/threonine kinase; regulates many cardiac proteins through phosphorylation	[6]
DAB1	Disabled-1	Neuronal development	[6]
DNM3	Dynamin-3	Actin-membrane budding	[6]
DST	Dystonin	Adhesion junction plaque protein	[8]
DTNA	Dystrobrevin alpha	Part of the dystrophin-associated complex linking ECM and cytoskeleton	[6]
ENAH	Protein-enabled homolog	Actin-associated	[8]
FHOD3	Formin homology 2 domain-containing 3	Sarcomeric assembly	[6]
FNBP1	Formin-binding protein 1	Actin cytoskeleton regulation	[6]
GIT2	G protein-coupled receptor kinase interactor 2	Cytoskeletal dynamics	[6]
IMMT	Inner membrane mitochondrial protein	Part of the mitochondrial inner membrane complex	[8,37]
KALRN	Kalirin	Serine/threonine protein kinase	[6]
KCNIP2	KV channel-interacting protein 2	Sub-unit of voltage-gated potassium channel complex	[6]
LDB3	LIM domain binding 3	Sarcomeric stabilization	[6,8]
LMO7	LIM domain only protein 7	-	[8]
LRRFIP1	Leucine-rich repeat flightless-interacting protein 1	Transcriptional repressor	[8]
MECP2	Methyl CpG–binding protein 2	Transcriptional regulator; highly expressed in neuronal cells	[6]
MLIP	Muscular-enriched A-type laminin-interacting protein	Interacts with lamin A/C; potentially involved in cardiac homeostasis	[8]
MTMR1	Myotubularin-related protein 1	-	[6]
MYH7	Myosin heavy chain 7	Cardiac slow twitch myosin heavy chain beta isoform; muscle contraction	[8]
MYOM1	Myomesin-1	Sarcomeric; links titin and thick filament	[8]
NEXN	Nexilin	Actin-associated; DCM-associated	[8]
NFIA	Nuclear factor I A	Transcription factor	[6]
NPRL3	Nitrogen permease regulator-like 3	Inhibits mTORC1; necessary for cardiovascular development	[6,41]
NTRK3	Tropomyosin receptor kinase C	Neutrophin-3-receptor	[6]
OBSCN	Obscurin	Sarcomeric signaling	[8]
PDLIM3	PDZ and LIM domain protein 3	Binds alpha actinin-2; relevant for right ventricular function	[8]
PDLIM5	PDZ and LIM domain protein 5	LIM domain protein; protein-protein interaction	[6,42]
PLEKHA5	Pleckstrin homology domain-containing family A member 5	-	[6]
RALGPS1	Ral GEF with PH domain- and SH3-binding motif 1	-	[6]
RTN4	Reticulon 4	Neurite outgrowth inhibitor in the central nervous system	[8]
RYR2	Ryanodine receptor 2	Calcium receptor in the SR; allows release of Ca^{2+} into the cytosol	[8]
SEMA6D	Semaphorin 6D	Neuronal regulation	[6]
SH3KBP1	SH3 domain-containing kinase-binding protein 1	-	[6]
SLC38A10	Putative sodium-coupled neutral amino acid transporter 10	Sodium-dependent amino acid/proton antiporter	[6]
SORBS1	Sorbin and SH3 domain-containing 1	Cytoskeletal formation	[6]

Table 2. *Cont.*

Gene	Encoded Protein	Function	References
SPEN	Msx2-interacting protein	Hormone inducible transcriptional repressor	[6]
TNNT2	Cardiac troponin T	Part of the cardiac troponin complex regulating muscle contraction dependent on calcium	[8]
TPM1	Tropomyosin alpha-1 chain	Cytoskeletal; contraction	[6]
TRDN	Triadin	Forms a complex with RyR and CASQ2; calcium release from the SR	[6]
TTN	Titin	Sarcomeric spring; compliance of the heart	[6,8]
UBE2F	Ubiquitin-conjugating enzyme E2 F (putative)	-	[6]
ZNF451	E3 SUMO-protein ligase ZNF451	Protein sumoylation	[6]

4.1. *TTN*

Titin is a giant protein embedded between the Z-disk and the M-band of the sarcomere [43]. It is crucial for myocardial contraction, elasticity and a key determinant for myocardial stiffness [43,44]. A loss of function in RBM20 causes DCM, often by missplicing of *TTN* and impaired Frank–Starling mechanism [6,8,25]. One of the primary underlying molecular pathomechanisms suspected of developing RBM20-associated DCM are the newly emerging giant titin isoforms [6–8]. Regularly, RBM20 mediates exon skipping of the Titin-PEVK region; when defective, exons remain and an embryonic, large Titin isoform is produced [6,7]. This titin isoform N2BA-G leads to reduced passive tension of the cardiac sarcomere and changed cardiac energetics, consequently being involved in the pathological heart chamber dilation [17,25,45]. To find out whether mutations in RBM20 are likely functional requires molecular diagnosis. As many patients would not want to have a biopsy taken for titin isoform expression analysis, this is currently done by using titin splice reporter assays [6,31].

4.2. *RYR2*

The regulation of muscle-specific splicing of *RYR2* (Ryanodine Receptor 2) by RBM20 is well established [6–8,15]. *RYR2* encodes a calcium ion channel mainly expressed in the heart, essential for calcium homeostasis and thus for proper myocardial contraction [46,47]. Cardiomyopathy-associated RBM20 variants cause overexpression of an *RYR2*-splice variant containing an additional small exon [8]. Clinically, arrhythmias are more prevalent in RBM-associated cardiomyopathy than in most other DCM forms [5,12]. It is current thinking that myocardial remodeling and fibrosis can trigger ventricular arrhythmias, but the modification of RYR2 may also propel arrhythmic instability and thus represents an appealing therapeutic target. Results from a study focusing on *RBM20* variants responsible for arrhythmogenic cardiomyopathy proposed that affected patients should be clinically viewed similar to other arrhythmogenic cardiomyopathy or catecholaminergic polymorphic ventricular tachycardia (CPVT), which is also caused by mutations in the *RYR2* gene [12].

4.3. *CAMK2D*

The serine/threonine-specific protein kinase CaMKII-δ (Ca^{2+}/calmodulin-dependent protein kinase II) is involved in calcium homeostasis and reuptake in cardiomyocytes [48], which provides the link to RYR2 function. It was observed that mutations in RBM20 result in a CaMKII-δ isoform switch from the regular -δB and -δC isoforms to the -δA and -δ9 isoforms [33]. This alteration is responsible for an increased L-type Ca^{2+}-current with intracellular Ca^{2+}-overload and increases sarcoplasmic reticulum Ca^{2+} content in RBM20 KO cardiomyocytes, eventually promoting arrhythmogenesis [33]. It must be considered, however, that electrophysiological properties vary between rodents and humans, hence impeding the translation of findings in rodent to human-derived model systems [33]. Beyond altered Ca^{2+}-handling, Zhang et al. proposed an alternative CaMKII-based pathomechanism. The team discovered that the CaMKII-δ9 isoform may mediate cardiomyopathy by causing cardiomyocyte DNA damage and cell death due to disrupted UBE2T (Ubiquitin-conjugating enzyme E2 T)-mediated DNA repair [49].

4.4. Identification of Novel Targets

Many of RBM20′s target genes listed in Table 1 were discovered by combining data from crosslink-immunoprecipitation (CLIP-seq) with transcriptome analysis of heart tissues from wild-type and RBM20-deficient rats as well as human heart failure patients [8]. Hence, this approach remains suitable for future identifications of other involved target genes.

Recently, transcriptome analysis using long-read sequencing in the presence of RBM20 mutations has discovered novel differentially expressed RBM20-dependent transcripts. This is exemplified by the discovery of two *IMMT* (inner membrane mitochondrial protein gene) isoforms that might play a role in RBM20 cardiomyopathy [37]. These results revealed that a more widespread adoption of long-read sequencing for transcriptome analysis could identify also further differentially expressed transcripts and provide context to previously identified alternatively spliced exons [37].

4.5. Interactions between RBM20s Targets

With the help of modern technologies such as Hi-C, RNA-seq and ATAC-seq researchers can investigate genome architecture in cardiomyocytes [50]. A network of gene loci from different RBM20 targets was identified, revealing an inter-chromosomal association and interaction between each target [50].

In human embryonic stem cells (hESC), the team discovered that *TTN* pre-mRNA, the best-studied RBM20-regulated transcript in the heart, binds and accumulates RBM20 foci near its genomic locus. This RBM20 accumulation mediates spatial proximity between the *TTN* locus and other inter-chromosomal RBM20 targets like *CAMK2D* or *CACNAC1C* (Figure 3). Changes in the topological assembly of the involved targets, for example, due to experimental deletion of the *TTN* promoter in hESC significantly reduced the spatial concentration of RBM20 genome-foci [50]. This is consecutively resulting in an altered RBM20-dependent alternative splicing activity of the other targets involved [50]. These novel perceptions indicate the existence of a cardiac-specific trans-interacting chromatin domain (TID) functioning in the sense of a splicing factory [50].

4.6. Interactions with Other Splice Regulators

Interactions of RBM20 with other splice regulators have been described in the literature. It was discovered recently that in titin splicing, PTB4 (polypyrimidine tract-binding protein isoform 4) counteracts the splice repressor activity of RBM20 [31]. PTB4 and RBM20 compete for the same motive on the 5′SS downstream of the alternative *TTN* exon, consequently regulating titin isoform expression [31]. These insights into the mechanistic interactions provide a basis for the future development of RBM20 modulators which adapt titin elasticity in cardiomyopathies [31].

Most recent studies suggest that RBM20 together with PTB4 also influences the splicing pattern of *FHOD3* (formin homology 2 domain containing 3) [51,52]. *FHOD3* was identified as an RBM20 target using RNA-seq, encodes a sarcomeric protein regulating actin dynamics in cardiac tissue and is associated with HCM and DCM [6,53–56]. The teams hypothesized that both splice regulators participate in the splice site recognition by competing with the snRNP (small nuclear ribonucleic particles) spliceosomal components, which determine the targets' exon inclusion and exclusion outcome [51,52].

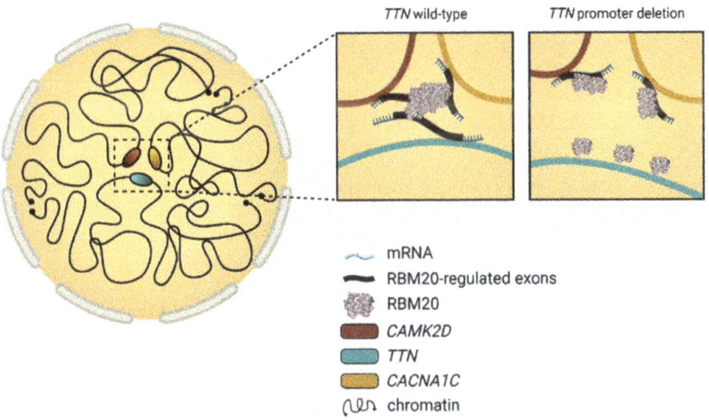

Figure 3. Modified from Bertero et al., 2019 [50]. Topological interchromosomal assembly of RBM20's target genes. Model originally proposed by Bertero et al. to regulate local chromatin organization in human cardiomyocytes. During the differentiation of cardiomyocytes, heterochromatin becomes condensed, whereas major cardiac genes such as *TTN* move from the inactive (peripheral) to the active (central) compartment of the nucleus. Transcription of *TTN* forms foci of the splicing factor RBM20, resulting in a trans-interacting chromatin domain (TID) in which other RBM20 target genes are also involved. This mechanism drives alternative splicing of the emerging transcripts and can be interrupted by alteration of *TTN* transcription [50].

5. Clinical Presentation and Risk Management

Pathogenic RBM20-variants are associated with a clinically aggressive form of DCM or left-ventricular non-compaction (LVNC; RBM20 variants are detected in ~1% of LVNC cases) [17,57,58]. In our Cardiomyopathy Center, we also observed different families with Hypertrophic Cardiomyopathy (HCM) carrying pathogenic RBM20 variants. The onset of the disease is around the mid-fourth to fifth life decade and might become apparent due to heart failure or arrhythmia [5]. Male patients generally show a more severe clinical course including significantly earlier disease onset and higher adverse event rates (heart transplantation (HTx), sudden cardiac arrest (SCA), ventricular tachycardia) [2]. In progressed stages, heart transplantation and assist devices (LVAD) are often required [1,2,5,12,13,16,18,33].

The likelihood of developing life-threatening arrhythmias is relatively high, resulting in a poor prognosis if an implanted defibrillator does not protect the patient. Of the RBM20 mutation carriers, 30% developed conduction system disorders associated with a high risk of malignant arrhythmias [5]. Data from the international RBM20 patient registry provide a valuable overview of the relative risk for RBM20 mutation carriers compared to DCM of other etiology (Table 3). Odds ratios are comparable to arrhythmogenic *LMNA*-mutation-induced DCM and significantly higher than in idiopathic or *TTNtv*-mediated DCM [12]. In the study cohort, ICD discharge and sudden cardiac arrest were observed in several mutation carriers even before the onset of left ventricular dysfunction [12]. This requires careful risk stratification in RBM20-associated cardiomyopathy and discussion of primary preventive ICD implantation.

Of patients with RBM20 cardiomyopathy, 12% receive heart transplantation due to end-stage heart failure at a remarkably young mean age of 28 years, occurring significantly earlier than in other DCM genotypes [5]. A study in a Danish population observed transplantation rates of overall 21% (34% in males) [2]. Similar results were demonstrated by Gaertner et al. in 2020, where family members carrying the pathogenic RBM20-p.Pro638Leu variant had an average event-free (HTx, LVAD or death) survival time of 28 years [15].

Table 3. Modified from Parikh et al., 2019 [12]. *RBM20*-related cardiomyopathy has a highly arrhythmogenic phenotype.

	RBM20-CM vs. DCM Odds Ratio (CI; *p*-Value)	RBM20-CM vs. *TTNtv*-CM Odds Ratio (CI; *p*-Value)	RBM20-CM vs. *LMNA*-CM Odds Ratio (CI; *p*-Value)
Evidence of sustained VA *	14.7 (6.0–36.0; $p < 0.001$)	27.3 (3.4–223.0; $p < 0.001$)	1.2 (0.6–2.4; $p = 0.65$)
Family history of SCA **	5.9 (3.1–11.2; $p < 0.001$)	6.2 (2.6–14.5; $p < 0.001$)	1.4 (0.6–2.8; $p = 0.46$)

Odds ratios for sustained ventricular arrhythmias (VA) and family history of sudden cardiac arrest (SCA) for RBM20-CM cohorts compared to DCM, titin truncating variants (*TTNtv*)-CM and Lamin A/C (*LMNA*)-CM cohorts. * Sustained VA is defined as sustained ventricular tachycardia or ventricular fibrillation on monitoring for DCM, *TTNtv* and *LMNA* and as SCA or ICD discharge for RBM20. ** SCA in RBM20 index cases only. CI = confidence interval.

6. Current Treatment Concepts in RBM20 Patients

6.1. Treatment of Heart Failure

Patients with RBM20-mediated DCM often present with systolic heart failure. Depending on the symptomatic extent of heart failure and systolic dysfunction, pharmacological treatment is carried out according to current therapeutic guidelines for acute and chronic heart failure [11,59,60]. ACE inhibitors, beta-blockers and mineralocorticoid antagonists work well in RBM20-related heart failure. The introduction of ARNI (sacubitril/valsartan) and SGLT2-inhibitors are other promising treatment options. RBM20-specific pharmacological treatments are not established.

In specialized centers worldwide, treatment with heart failure medications is advised already in the early stages of systolic dysfunction if the pathogenic mutation is known in the patient and deterioration is foreseen. These expert decisions are based on individual basis and experience and cannot be generalized at the moment.

6.2. ICD-Therapy

Current guidelines do not treat RBM20 cardiomyopathy separately from other causes of DCM. Considering available data on the risk of suffering from severe arrhythmias (Table 3), implantation of a primary prophylactic cardiac defibrillator should be discussed for individuals carrying proven pathogenic RBM20-variants [2,12]. In order to provide the same evidence that currently exists for the highly arrhythmogenic *LMNA/C* mutations [13,61–63], further studies are needed for generally recommending a primary prophylactic ICD implantation in consideration of the RBM20-mutation status.

6.3. Heart Transplantation and Assist Devices

(Temporary) support in severe heart failure can be reached by implanting a left-ventricular assist device. Heart transplantation is considered a last resort, yet indispensable due to the potentially severe clinical course of RBM20-related cardiomyopathy. As mentioned above, in a recent meta-analysis, the mean age of HTx in patients with RBM20-induced DCM was only 28 years [5]. Unlike many other genetic myopathies affecting sarcomere function, RBM20 defects mainly affect the myocardium and do not lead to skeletal myopathy [6]. This is an important aspect of considering patients for heart transplantation.

7. Future Therapeutic Options

Established generic therapies for heart failure and SCD-prevention are powerful tools to improve the prognosis of patients. However, experimental compounds or repurposing of existing drugs are attractive strategies for identifying tailored and specific RBM20-therapies. Therefore, suitable model systems are needed and stringent, and data-guided translation into the clinics is required to prevent harm by self-treatment of affected patients with experimental compounds.

7.1. RBM20 Upregulation

In 2020, Briganti et al. created an RBM20-deficient DCM model that recapitulates mRNA splicing and contractile defects of the disease using CRISPR/Cas9 in iPSC [19]. By bioinformatics screens, interesting compounds associated with RBM20 expression were identified and investigated functionally. The teams showed that the application of retinoic acid (ATRA), an active metabolite of vitamin A, upregulates RBM20 expression in murine and human-derived iPSC, partially reverting the splicing and contractile defects caused by pathogenic RBM20 variants [19]. This effect could be primarily shown in heterozygous but also in homozygous mutants, while not in the complete knockouts suggesting that the beneficial effect of ATRA remains dependent on residual RBM20 protein activity [19]. The transfer to the clinics requires functional proof in animal models and a careful clinical trial design since ATRA also has potential toxic side effects in high doses. Additionally, the RBM20-RNP-granules could be, as already mentioned, aggravated through upregulation of the RBM20-locus, potentially leading to (long-term) negative consequences.

7.2. RBM20 Downregulation

Besides the harm caused by RBM20 mutations, beneficial effects of RBM20 loss-of-function have been described as well. In heterozygous RBM20 KO-mice with an in-frame RRM deletion, a more compliant, large titin was identified, possibly leading to improved diastolic filling [30]. However, it must be considered that the impaired Frank–Starling mechanism in this scenario might outweigh the potentially beneficial effects [30].

With the development of an in vitro splice reporter assay in HEK293 cells, it was for the first time possible to screen > 34,000 small molecules for the potential treatment of diastolic dysfunction [64]. The study identified cardenolides as inhibitors of RBM20 dependent splicing, leading in the case of titin to the exclusion of PEVK exons. This again affected titin isoform expression, subsequently improving diastolic filling. These findings show that RBM20 downregulation might be helpful for future treatments of diastolic dysfunction and should be further investigated.

With the introduction of these sorts of splice reporter assays, it also remains exciting to see whether other small compounds will be identified in the future, providing novel therapeutic strategies through the regulation of RBM20 expression.

7.3. Ca^{2+}-Modulation

RBM20-dependent Ca^{2+}-homeostasis was first studied in knockdown mouse embryoid bodies [65]. Experimental data show that RBM20 loss-of-function in RBM20 KO-mice disturbed the Ca^{2+}-handling resulting in arrhythmogenic Ca^{2+}-releases/spikes from the sarcoplasmic reticulum [33]. This alteration was not only observed in homozygous but also in heterozygous mice [33]. They also discovered that the L-Type calcium channel (LTCC) activity was increased in RBM20 KO-mice, possibly due to an altered splicing of *CAMK2D* and *CACNAC1C*, likewise causing a more arrhythmogenic phenotype [33]. Wyles et al. investigated the Ca^{2+}-homeostasis in an RBM20 patient-derived iPSC model and observed improved Ca^{2+}-handling during a ß-adrenergic stress test by pretreatment with either the beta-blocker carvedilol or the L-Type-calcium-antagonist verapamil [36]. Based on the RBM20 KO-mice model, considering verapamil as a specific treatment option of arrhythmogenic dilated RBM20-cardiomyopathy was the subject of another recent study [33]. However, human data are limited and potential benefits from beta-blocker therapy would be withdrawn in this case. At the same time, calcium-antagonists have proven to be unsuccessful in the treatment of "common" heart failure.

Further evidence from current studies in iPSC and prospectively in a controlled clinical trial, is curiously awaited.

7.4. Gene Editing

As for many other genetic disorders, CRISPR/Cas9-based gene editing provides a powerful tool to investigate and possibly repair genetic abnormalities seen in RBM20 related cardiomyopathy. With the help of this technique, knockout and knockin models are already established in mouse, pig, hESC and iPSC models, and provide the basis for the identification and development of novel genetic treatment strategies [3,4,19,22,35,50].

Until now, CRISPR/Cas9-based repair approaches of pathogenic RBM20-variants are still in very early stages but represent an exciting and innovative field of research for upcoming investigations.

8. Conclusions

RBM20-related cardiomyopathy is an excellent example of how structured, collaborative clinical and experimental research can further our knowledge to a degree where clinical decision-making is considerably improved, and molecularly guided therapeutic options are emerging. With an armamentarium of potential options, the chances are high that breakthrough developments will change the course of this disease group in the near future.

Funding: This research was funded by the Leducq Foundation for funding the "Cardiac Splicing as a Therapeutic Target (CASTT)–Transatlantic Network of Excellence".

Acknowledgments: We thank the Leducq Foundation for funding the "Cardiac Splicing as a Therapeutic Target (CASTT)–Transatlantic Network of Excellence" and supporting this scientific collaboration. Our work on "RBM20-related Cardiomyopathy: Current Understanding and Future Options" is supported by the Deutsche Forschungsgemeinschaft (DFG ME 3859/4-1), the German Centre for Cardiovascular Research (DZHK), Informatics for Life (Klaus Tschira Foundation), the ERA-CVD network DETECTIN-HF and the Else-Kröner Exzellenzstipendium awarded to Benjamin Meder. All figures were created with BioRender.com.

Conflicts of Interest: L.M.S. is co-founder and shareholder of Sophia Genetics. L.M.S. has submitted a patent application on "Methods of treatment, genetic screening, and disease models for heart conditions associated with RBM20 deficiency." B.M. is involved in researching novel therapies and companion biomarkers for RBM20-related cardiomyopathies. He is a scientific advisor for therapy developments for pharmaceutical companies (Myokardia, BMS, Aavigen).

References

1. Brauch, K.M.; Karst, M.L.; Herron, K.J.; de Andrade, M.; Pellikka, P.A.; Rodeheffer, R.J.; Michels, V.V.; Olson, T.M. Mutations in Ribonucleic Acid Binding Protein Gene Cause Familial Dilated Cardiomyopathy. *J. Am. Coll. Cardiol.* **2009**, *54*, 930–941. [CrossRef]
2. Hey, T.M.; Rasmussen, T.B.; Madsen, T.; Aagaard, M.M.; Harbo, M.; Mølgaard, H.; Møller, J.E.; Eiskjær, H.; Mogensen, J. Pathogenic RBM20-Variants Are Associated With a Severe Disease Expression in Male Patients With Dilated Cardiomyopathy. *Circ. Heart Fail.* **2019**, *12*, e005700. [CrossRef] [PubMed]
3. Ihara, K.; Sasano, T.; Hiraoka, Y.; Togo-Ohno, M.; Soejima, Y.; Sawabe, M.; Tsuchiya, M.; Ogawa, H.; Furukawa, T.; Kuroyanagi, H. A missense mutation in the RSRSP stretch of Rbm20 causes dilated cardiomyopathy and atrial fibrillation in mice. *Sci. Rep.* **2020**, *10*, 17894. [CrossRef] [PubMed]
4. Streckfuss-Bömeke, K.; Tiburcy, M.; Fomin, A.; Luo, X.; Li, W.; Fischer, C.; Özcelik, C.; Perrot, A.; Sossalla, S.; Haas, J.; et al. Severe DCM phenotype of patient harboring RBM20 mutation S635A can be modeled by patient-specific induced pluripotent stem cell-derived cardiomyocytes. *J. Mol. Cell Cardiol.* **2017**, *113*, 9–21. [CrossRef]
5. Kayvanpour, E.; Sedaghat-Hamedani, F.; Amr, A.; Lai, A.; Haas, J.; Holzer, D.B.; Frese, K.S.; Keller, A.; Jensen, K.; Katus, H.A.; et al. Genotype-phenotype associations in dilated cardiomyopathy: Meta-analysis on more than 8000 individuals. *Clin. Res. Cardiol.* **2017**, *106*, 127–139. [CrossRef] [PubMed]
6. Guo, W.; Schafer, S.; Greaser, M.L.; Radke, M.H.; Liss, M.; Govindarajan, T.; Maatz, H.; Schulz, H.; Li, S.; Parrish, A.M.; et al. RBM20, a gene for hereditary cardiomyopathy, regulates titin splicing. *Nat. Med.* **2012**, *18*, 766–773. [CrossRef] [PubMed]
7. Li, S.; Guo, W.; Dewey, C.N.; Greaser, M.L. Rbm20 regulates titin alternative splicing as a splicing repressor. *Nucleic Acids Res.* **2013**, *41*, 2659–2672. [CrossRef]
8. Maatz, H.; Jens, M.; Liss, M.; Schafer, S.; Heinig, M.; Kirchner, M.; Adami, E.; Rintisch, C.; Dauksaite, V.; Radke, M.H.; et al. RNA-binding protein RBM20 represses splicing to orchestrate cardiac pre-mRNA processing. *J. Clin. Investig.* **2014**, *124*, 3419–3430. [CrossRef] [PubMed]
9. Watanabe, T.; Kimura, A.; Kuroyanagi, H. Alternative Splicing Regulator RBM20 and Cardiomyopathy. *Front. Mol. Biosci.* **2018**, *5*, 105. [CrossRef]
10. Murayama, R.; Kimura-Asami, M.; Togo-Ohno, M.; Yamasaki-Kato, Y.; Naruse, T.K.; Yamamoto, T.; Hayashi, T.; Ai, T.; Spoonamore, K.G.; Kovacs, R.J. Phosphorylation of the RSRSP stretch is critical for splicing regulation by RNA-Binding Motif Protein 20 (RBM20) through nuclear localization. *Sci. Rep.* **2018**, *8*, 8970. [CrossRef]
11. Ponikowski, P.; Voors, A.A.; Anker, S.D.; Bueno, H.; Cleland, J.G.; Coats, A.J.; Falk, V.; González-Juanatey, J.R.; Harjola, V.-P.; Jankowska, E.A. 2016 ESC Guidelines for the diagnosis and treatment of acute and chronic heart failure: The Task Force for the diagnosis and treatment of acute and chronic heart failure of the European Society of Cardiology (ESC) Developed with the special contribution of the Heart Failure Association (HFA) of the ESC. *Eur. Heart J.* **2016**, *37*, 2129–2200. [PubMed]

12. Parikh, V.N.; Caleshu, C.; Reuter, C.; Lazzeroni, L.C.; Ingles, J.; Garcia, J.; McCaleb, K.; Adesiyun, T.; Sedaghat-Hamedani, F.; Kumar, S.; et al. Regional Variation in RBM20 Causes a Highly Penetrant Arrhythmogenic Cardiomyopathy. *Circ. Heart Fail.* **2019**, *12*, e005371. [CrossRef]
13. Haas, J.; Frese, K.S.; Peil, B.; Kloos, W.; Keller, A.; Nietsch, R.; Feng, Z.; Müller, S.; Kayvanpour, E.; Vogel, B.; et al. Atlas of the clinical genetics of human dilated cardiomyopathy. *Eur. Heart J.* **2014**, *36*, 1123–1135. [CrossRef] [PubMed]
14. Kayvanpour, E.; Sedaghat-Hamedani, F.; Gi, W.T.; Tugrul, O.F.; Amr, A.; Haas, J.; Zhu, F.; Ehlermann, P.; Uhlmann, L.; Katus, H.A.; et al. Clinical and genetic insights into non-compaction: A meta-analysis and systematic review on 7598 individuals. *Clin. Res. Cardiol.* **2019**, *108*, 1297–1308. [CrossRef]
15. Gaertner, A.; Klauke, B.; Felski, E.; Kassner, A.; Brodehl, A.; Gerdes, D.; Stanasiuk, C.; Ebbinghaus, H.; Schulz, U.; Dubowy, K.O.; et al. Cardiomyopathy-associated mutations in the RS domain affect nuclear localization of RBM20. *Hum. Mutat.* **2020**, *41*, 1931–1943. [CrossRef]
16. Li, D.; Morales, A.; Gonzalez-Quintana, J.; Norton, N.; Siegfried, J.D.; Hofmeyer, M.; Hershberger, R.E. Identification of Novel Mutations in RBM20 in Patients with Dilated Cardiomyopathy. *Clin. Transl. Sci.* **2010**, *3*, 90–97. [CrossRef] [PubMed]
17. Sedaghat-Hamedani, F.; Haas, J.; Zhu, F.; Geier, C.; Kayvanpour, E.; Liss, M.; Lai, A.; Frese, K.; Pribe-Wolferts, R.; Amr, A. Clinical genetics and outcome of left ventricular non-compaction cardiomyopathy. *Eur. Heart J.* **2017**, *38*, 3449–3460. [CrossRef]
18. Refaat, M.M.; Lubitz, S.A.; Makino, S.; Islam, Z.; Frangiskakis, J.M.; Mehdi, H.; Gutmann, R.; Zhang, M.L.; Bloom, H.L.; MacRae, C.A. Genetic variation in the alternative splicing regulator RBM20 is associated with dilated cardiomyopathy. *Heart Rhythm* **2012**, *9*, 390–396. [CrossRef]
19. Briganti, F.; Sun, H.; Wei, W.; Wu, J.; Zhu, C.; Liss, M.; Karakikes, I.; Rego, S.; Cipriano, A.; Snyder, M.; et al. iPSC Modeling of RBM20-Deficient DCM Identifies Upregulation of RBM20 as a Therapeutic Strategy. *Cell Rep.* **2020**, *32*, 108117. [CrossRef]
20. Wells, Q.S.; Becker, J.R.; Su, Y.R.; Mosley, J.D.; Weeke, P.; D'Aoust, L.; Ausborn, N.L.; Ramirez, A.H.; Pfotenhauer, J.P.; Naftilan, A.J.; et al. Whole Exome Sequencing Identifies a Causal RBM20 Mutation in a Large Pedigree With Familial Dilated Cardiomyopathy. *Circ. Cardiovasc. Genet.* **2013**, *6*, 317–326. [CrossRef] [PubMed]
21. Chami, N.; Tadros, R.; Lemarbre, F.; Lo, K.S.; Beaudoin, M.; Robb, L.; Labuda, D.; Tardif, J.-C.; Racine, N.; Talajic, M.; et al. Nonsense Mutations in BAG3 are Associated With Early-Onset Dilated Cardiomyopathy in French Canadians. *Can. J. Cardiol.* **2014**, *30*, 1655–1661. [CrossRef]
22. Schneider, J.W.; Oommen, S.; Qureshi, M.Y.; Goetsch, S.C.; Pease, D.R.; Sundsbak, R.S.; Guo, W.; Sun, M.; Sun, H.; Kuroyanagi, H.; et al. Dysregulated ribonucleoprotein granules promote cardiomyopathy in RBM20 gene-edited pigs. *Nat. Med.* **2020**, *26*, 1788–1800. [CrossRef] [PubMed]
23. Millat, G.; Bouvagnet, P.; Chevalier, P.; Sebbag, L.; Dulac, A.; Dauphin, C.; Jouk, P.-S.; Delrue, M.-A.; Thambo, J.-B.; Le Metayer, P.; et al. Clinical and mutational spectrum in a cohort of 105 unrelated patients with dilated cardiomyopathy. *Eur. J. Med. Genet.* **2011**, *54*, e570–e575. [CrossRef] [PubMed]
24. Vakhrushev, Y.; Kozyreva, A.; Semenov, A.; Sokolnikova, P.; Lubimtseva, T.; Lebedev, D.; Smolina, N.; Zhuk, S.; Mitrofanova, L.; Vasichkina, E.; et al. RBM20-Associated Ventricular Arrhythmias in a Patient with Structurally Normal Heart. *Genes* **2021**, *12*, 94. [CrossRef]
25. Beqqali, A.; Bollen, I.A.; Rasmussen, T.B.; van den Hoogenhof, M.M.; van Deutekom, H.W.; Schafer, S.; Haas, J.; Meder, B.; Sørensen, K.E.; van Oort, R.J.; et al. A mutation in the glutamate-rich region of RNA-binding motif protein 20 causes dilated cardiomyopathy through missplicing of titin and impaired Frank-Starling mechanism. *Cardiovasc. Res.* **2016**, *112*, 452–463. [CrossRef] [PubMed]
26. Zahr, H.C.; Jaalouk, D.E. Exploring the Crosstalk Between LMNA and Splicing Machinery Gene Mutations in Dilated Cardiomyopathy. *Front. Genet.* **2018**, *9*, 231. [CrossRef]
27. Lin, S.; Fu, X.-D. SR proteins and related factors in alternative splicing. *Adv. Exp. Med. Biol.* **2007**, *623*, 107–122.
28. Guo, W.; Sun, M. RBM20, a potential target for treatment of cardiomyopathy via titin isoform switching. *Biophys. Rev.* **2018**, *10*, 15–25. [CrossRef]
29. Long, J.C.; Caceres, J.F. The SR protein family of splicing factors: Master regulators of gene expression. *Biochem. J.* **2009**, *417*, 15–27. [CrossRef]
30. Methawasin, M.; Hutchinson, K.R.; Lee, E.-J.; Smith III, J.E.; Saripalli, C.; Hidalgo, C.G.; Ottenheijm, C.A.; Granzier, H. Experimentally increasing titin compliance in a novel mouse model attenuates the Frank-Starling mechanism but has a beneficial effect on diastole. *Circulation* **2014**, *129*, 1924–1936. [CrossRef]
31. Dauksaite, V.; Gotthardt, M. Molecular basis of titin exon exclusion by RBM20 and the novel titin splice regulator PTB4. *Nucleic Acids Res.* **2018**, *46*, 5227–5238. [CrossRef] [PubMed]
32. Greaser, M.L.; Warren, C.M.; Esbona, K.; Guo, W.; Duan, Y.; Parrish, A.M.; Krzesinski, P.R.; Norman, H.S.; Dunning, S.; Fitzsimons, D.P.; et al. Mutation that dramatically alters rat titin isoform expression and cardiomyocyte passive tension. *J. Mol. Cell Cardiol.* **2008**, *44*, 983–991. [CrossRef] [PubMed]
33. van den Hoogenhof, M.M.G.; Beqqali, A.; Amin, A.S.; van der Made, I.; Aufiero, S.; Khan, M.A.F.; Schumacher, C.A.; Jansweijer, J.A.; van Spaendonck-Zwarts, K.Y.; Remme, C.A.; et al. RBM20 Mutations Induce an Arrhythmogenic Dilated Cardiomyopathy Related to Disturbed Calcium Handling. *Circulation* **2018**, *138*, 1330–1342. [CrossRef] [PubMed]

34. Methawasin, M.; Strom, J.G.; Slater, R.E.; Fernandez, V.; Saripalli, C.; Granzier, H. Experimentally increasing the compliance of titin through RNA binding motif-20 (RBM20) inhibition improves diastolic function in a mouse model of heart failure with preserved ejection fraction. *Circulation* **2016**, *134*, 1085–1099. [CrossRef] [PubMed]
35. Rebs, S.; Sedaghat-Hamedani, F.; Kayvanpour, E.; Meder, B.; Streckfuss-Bömeke, K. Generation of pluripotent stem cell lines and CRISPR/Cas9 modified isogenic controls from a patient with dilated cardiomyopathy harboring a RBM20 p.R634W mutation. *Stem Cell Res.* **2020**, *47*, 101901. [CrossRef]
36. Wyles, S.P.; Hrstka, S.C.; Reyes, S.; Terzic, A.; Olson, T.M.; Nelson, T.J. Pharmacological modulation of calcium homeostasis in familial dilated cardiomyopathy: An in vitro analysis from an RBM20 patient-derived iPSC model. *Clin. Transl. Sci.* **2016**, *9*, 158–167. [CrossRef]
37. Zhu, C.; Wu, J.; Sun, H.; Briganti, F.; Meder, B.; Wei, W.; Steinmetz, L.M. Single-molecule, full-length transcript isoform sequencing reveals disease-associated RNA isoforms in cardiomyocytes. *Nat. Commun.* **2021**, *12*, 4203. [CrossRef]
38. Woerner, A.C.; Frottin, F.; Hornburg, D.; Feng, L.R.; Meissner, F.; Patra, M.; Tatzelt, J.; Mann, M.; Winklhofer, K.F.; Hartl, F.U.; et al. Cytoplasmic protein aggregates interfere with nucleocytoplasmic transport of protein and RNA. *Science* **2016**, *351*, 173–176. [CrossRef]
39. Schweingruber, C.; Rufener, S.C.; Zünd, D.; Yamashita, A.; Mühlemann, O. Nonsense-mediated mRNA decay—Mechanisms of substrate mRNA recognition and degradation in mammalian cells. *Biochim. Biophys. Acta (BBA)-Gene Regul. Mech.* **2013**, *1829*, 612–623. [CrossRef]
40. Lennermann, D.; Backs, J.; van den Hoogenhof, M.M.G. New Insights in RBM20 Cardiomyopathy. *Curr. Heart Fail. Rep.* **2020**, *17*, 234–246. [CrossRef]
41. Kowalczyk, M.S.; Hughes, J.R.; Babbs, C.; Sanchez-Pulido, L.; Szumska, D.; Sharpe, J.A.; Sloane-Stanley, J.A.; Morriss-Kay, G.M.; Smoot, L.B.; Roberts, A.E. Nprl3 is required for normal development of the cardiovascular system. *Mamm. Genome* **2012**, *23*, 404–415. [CrossRef] [PubMed]
42. Ito, J.; Iijima, M.; Yoshimoto, N.; Niimi, T.; Kuroda, S.i.; Maturana, A.D. RBM 20 and RBM 24 cooperatively promote the expression of short enh splice variants. *FEBS Lett.* **2016**, *590*, 2262–2274. [CrossRef]
43. Chauveau, C.; Rowell, J.; Ferreiro, A. A Rising Titan: TTN Review and Mutation Update. *Hum. Mutat.* **2014**, *35*, 1046–1059. [CrossRef] [PubMed]
44. LeWinter, M.M.; Granzier, H.L. Cardiac titin and heart disease. *J. Cardiovasc. Pharmacol.* **2014**, *63*, 207–212. [CrossRef]
45. Deo, R.C. Alternative splicing, internal promoter, nonsense-mediated decay, or all three: Explaining the distribution of truncation variants in titin. *Circ. Cardiovasc. Genet.* **2016**, *9*, 419–425. [CrossRef]
46. Tunwell, R.E.; Wickenden, C.; Bertrand, B.M.; Shevchenko, V.I.; Walsh, M.B.; Allen, P.D.; Lai, F.A. The human cardiac muscle ryanodine receptor-calcium release channel: Identification, primary structure and topological analysis. *Biochem. J.* **1996**, *318*, 477–487. [CrossRef] [PubMed]
47. Laitinen, P.J.; Brown, K.M.; Piippo, K.; Swan, H.; Devaney, J.M.; Brahmbhatt, B.; Donarum, E.A.; Marino, M.; Tiso, N.; Viitasalo, M.; et al. Mutations of the Cardiac Ryanodine Receptor (RyR2) Gene in Familial Polymorphic Ventricular Tachycardia. *Circulation* **2001**, *103*, 485–490. [CrossRef] [PubMed]
48. Anderson, M.E. Calmodulin kinase signaling in heart: An intriguing candidate target for therapy of myocardial dysfunction and arrhythmias. *Pharmacol. Ther.* **2005**, *106*, 39–55. [CrossRef]
49. Zhang, M.; Gao, H.; Liu, D.; Zhong, X.; Shi, X.; Yu, P.; Jin, L.; Liu, Y.; Tang, Y.; Song, Y. CaMKII-δ9 promotes cardiomyopathy through disrupting UBE2T-dependent DNA repair. *Nat. Cell Biol.* **2019**, *21*, 1152–1163. [CrossRef] [PubMed]
50. Bertero, A.; Fields, P.A.; Ramani, V.; Bonora, G.; Yardimci, G.G.; Reinecke, H.; Pabon, L.; Noble, W.S.; Shendure, J.; Murry, C.E. Dynamics of genome reorganization during human cardiogenesis reveal an RBM20-dependent splicing factory. *Nat. Commun.* **2019**, *10*, 1538. [CrossRef]
51. Fochi, S.; Lorenzi, P.; Galasso, M.; Stefani, C.; Trabetti, E.; Zipeto, D.; Romanelli, M.G. The Emerging Role of the RBM20 and PTBP1 Ribonucleoproteins in Heart Development and Cardiovascular Diseases. *Genes* **2020**, *11*, 402. [CrossRef]
52. Lorenzi, P.; Sangalli, A.; Fochi, S.; Dal Molin, A.; Malerba, G.; Zipeto, D.; Romanelli, M.G. RNA-binding proteins RBM20 and PTBP1 regulate the alternative splicing of FHOD3. *Int. J. Biochem. Cell Biol.* **2019**, *106*, 74–83. [CrossRef] [PubMed]
53. Taniguchi, K.; Takeya, R.; Suetsugu, S.; Kan-o, M.; Narusawa, M.; Shiose, A.; Tominaga, R.; Sumimoto, H. Mammalian formin fhod3 regulates actin assembly and sarcomere organization in striated muscles. *J. Biol. Chem.* **2009**, *284*, 29873–29881. [CrossRef] [PubMed]
54. Arimura, T.; Takeya, R.; Ishikawa, T.; Yamano, T.; Matsuo, A.; Tatsumi, T.; Nomura, T.; Sumimoto, H.; Kimura, A. Dilated cardiomyopathy-associated FHOD3 variant impairs the ability to induce activation of transcription factor serum response factor. *Circ. J.* **2013**, *77*, 2990–2996. [CrossRef]
55. Wooten, E.C.; Hebl, V.B.; Wolf, M.J.; Greytak, S.R.; Orr, N.M.; Draper, I.; Calvino, J.E.; Kapur, N.K.; Maron, M.S.; Kullo, I.J. Formin homology 2 domain containing 3 variants associated with hypertrophic cardiomyopathy. *Circ. Cardiovasc. Genet.* **2013**, *6*, 10–18. [CrossRef]
56. Ushijima, T.; Fujimoto, N.; Matsuyama, S.; Kan-o, M.; Kiyonari, H.; Shioi, G.; Kage, Y.; Yamasaki, S.; Takeya, R.; Sumimoto, H. The actin-organizing formin protein Fhod3 is required for postnatal development and functional maintenance of the adult heart in mice. *J. Biol. Chem.* **2018**, *293*, 148–162. [CrossRef] [PubMed]

57. van Waning, J.I.; Caliskan, K.; Hoedemaekers, Y.M.; van Spaendonck-Zwarts, K.Y.; Baas, A.F.; Boekholdt, S.M.; van Melle, J.P.; Teske, A.J.; Asselbergs, F.W.; Backx, A.P. Genetics, clinical features, and long-term outcome of noncompaction cardiomyopathy. *J. Am. Coll. Cardiol.* **2018**, *71*, 711–722. [CrossRef]
58. Miszalski-Jamka, K.; Jefferies, J.L.; Mazur, W.; Głowacki, J.; Hu, J.; Lazar, M.; Gibbs, R.A.; Liczko, J.; Kłyś, J.; Venner, E. Novel genetic triggers and genotype–phenotype correlations in patients with left ventricular noncompaction. *Circ. Cardiovasc. Genet.* **2017**, *10*, e001763. [CrossRef] [PubMed]
59. Yancy, C.W.; Jessup, M.; Bozkurt, B.; Butler, J.; Casey, D.E.; Colvin, M.M.; Drazner, M.H.; Filippatos, G.S.; Fonarow, G.C.; Givertz, M.M.; et al. 2017 ACC/AHA/HFSA Focused Update of the 2013 ACCF/AHA Guideline for the Management of Heart Failure. *J. Am. Coll. Cardiol.* **2017**, *70*, 776–803. [CrossRef] [PubMed]
60. Yancy, C.W.; Jessup, M.; Bozkurt, B.; Butler, J.; Casey, D.E.; Drazner, M.H.; Fonarow, G.C.; Geraci, S.A.; Horwich, T.; Januzzi, J.L.; et al. 2013 ACCF/AHA Guideline for the Management of Heart Failure. *J. Am. Coll. Cardiol.* **2013**, *62*, e147–e239. [CrossRef] [PubMed]
61. Malhotra, R.; Mason, P.K. Lamin A/C deficiency as a cause of familial dilated cardiomyopathy. *Curr. Opin. Cardiol.* **2009**, *24*, 203–208. [CrossRef]
62. Anselme, F.; Moubarak, G.; Savouré, A.; Godin, B.; Borz, B.; Drouin-Garraud, V.; Gay, A. Implantable cardioverter-defibrillators in lamin A/C mutation carriers with cardiac conduction disorders. *Heart Rhythm* **2013**, *10*, 1492–1498. [CrossRef] [PubMed]
63. Hasselberg, N.E.; Haland, T.F.; Saberniak, J.; Brekke, P.H.; Berge, K.E.; Leren, T.P.; Edvardsen, T.; Haugaa, K.H. Lamin A/C cardiomyopathy: Young onset, high penetrance, and frequent need for heart transplantation. *Eur. Heart J.* **2017**, *39*, 853–860. [CrossRef] [PubMed]
64. Liss, M.; Radke, M.H.; Eckhard, J.; Neuenschwander, M.; Dauksaite, V.; von Kries, J.P.; Gotthardt, M. Drug discovery with an RBM20 dependent titin splice reporter identifies cardenolides as lead structures to improve cardiac filling. *PLoS ONE* **2018**, *13*, e0198492. [CrossRef] [PubMed]
65. Beraldi, R.; Li, X.; Martinez Fernandez, A.; Reyes, S.; Secreto, F.; Terzic, A.; Olson, T.M.; Nelson, T.J. Rbm20-deficient cardiogenesis reveals early disruption of RNA processing and sarcomere remodeling establishing a developmental etiology for dilated cardiomyopathy. *Hum. Mol. Genet.* **2014**, *23*, 3779–3791. [CrossRef] [PubMed]

Journal of
Clinical Medicine

MDPI

Review

Genetic Insights into Primary Restrictive Cardiomyopathy

Andreas Brodehl [1,*] and Brenda Gerull [2,*]

1 Erich and Hanna Klessmann Institute, Heart and Diabetes Center NRW, University Hospital of the Ruhr-University Bochum, Georgstrasse 11, 32545 Bad Oeynhausen, Germany
2 Comprehensive Heart Failure Center (CHFC), Department of Medicine I, University Clinic Würzburg, Am Schwarzenberg 15, 97078 Würzburg, Germany
* Correspondence: abrodehl@hdz-nrw.de (A.B.); gerull_b@ukw.de (B.G.); Tel.: +49-(0)-5731-973530 (A.B.); +49-(0)-931-20146457 (B.G.)

Abstract: Restrictive cardiomyopathy is a rare cardiac disease causing severe diastolic dysfunction, ventricular stiffness and dilated atria. In consequence, it induces heart failure often with preserved ejection fraction and is associated with a high mortality. Since it is a poor clinical prognosis, patients with restrictive cardiomyopathy frequently require heart transplantation. Genetic as well as non-genetic factors contribute to restrictive cardiomyopathy and a significant portion of cases are of unknown etiology. However, the genetic forms of restrictive cardiomyopathy and the involved molecular pathomechanisms are only partially understood. In this review, we summarize the current knowledge about primary genetic restrictive cardiomyopathy and describe its genetic landscape, which might be of interest for geneticists as well as for cardiologists.

Keywords: restrictive cardiomyopathy; cardiomyopathy; cardiovascular genetics; desmin; troponin; filamin-C

Citation: Brodehl, A.; Gerull, B. Genetic Insights into Primary Restrictive Cardiomyopathy. *J. Clin. Med.* **2022**, *11*, 2094. https://doi.org/10.3390/jcm11082094

Academic Editor: Stefan Peters

Received: 14 March 2022
Accepted: 6 April 2022
Published: 8 April 2022

1. Introduction

In clinical practice, cardiomyopathies are divided according to structural and functional criteria into different classes [1,2]. Classification according to their etiology revealed a non-negligible percentage of genetic cases for all structural cardiomyopathies [3]. In comparison to hypertrophic cardiomyopathy (HCM) with an estimated prevalence of 1:500 [4], the prevalence of restrictive cardiomyopathy (RCM) is currently unknown [5]. However, because of the rarity of primary RCM, its genetic background is poorly defined compared with other cardiomyopathies. Beside primary RCM, it can manifest as a part of systemic diseases such as amyloidosis [6], which can also be genetically caused, for example, by mutations in the *TTR* (transthyretin) gene [7]. In addition, RCM can also be part of different syndromic diseases, e.g., Alström syndrome (MIM, #203800) [8] or Myhre syndrome (MIM, #139210) [9]. In this review, we will focus on the genetic etiology of primary RCM and will summarize the current knowledge of the RCM-associated genes.

2. Clinical Description

RCM is characterized by severely enlarged atria, normal-sized ventricles, with increased myocardial stiffness leading to impaired ventricular filling and diastolic dysfunction (Figure 1). Systolic function and ventricular wall thicknesses are often normal. Patients present with symptoms of left and/or right ventricular heart failure with preserved ejection fraction (HFpEF), atrial fibrillation, ventricular arrhythmias and frequently conduction disorders [10]. The overall prognosis is poor and the 5-year survival rate of adult patients with a confirmed genetic cause was 56% [11]. Specific therapies of non-infiltrative genetic forms do not exist. Non-specific therapies include fluid and sodium restrictions and medical treatment of heart failure with reduction of volume overload as well as anticoagulation and antiarrhythmic therapy. Very often heart transplantation (HTx) is the only option for long-term survival [12].

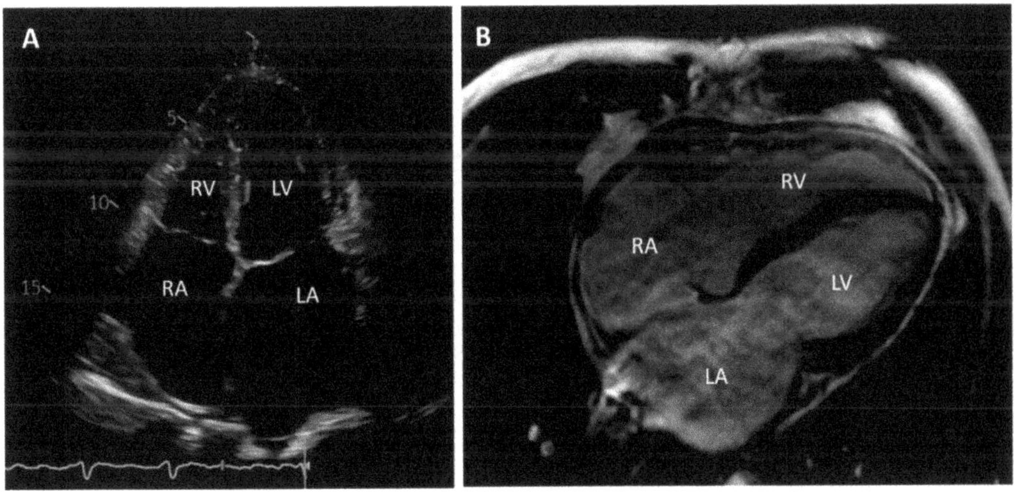

Figure 1. (**A**) Apical four chamber view during systole of an echocardiogram (**B**) and four chamber view of cardiac magnetic resonance image of a 50-year-old patient carrying a pathogenic *FLNC* mutation. Note the enlarged atria, normal ventricular sizes and wall thicknesses. RA = right atrium; RV = right ventricle; LA = left atrium; LV = left ventricle.

3. Genetic Landscape of Restrictive Cardiomyopathy

Currently, pathogenic mutations in 19 different genes have been identified in patients with RCM (Table 1 and Figure 2A). Since RCM is a rare cardiomyopathy with an unknown prevalence [13], the genetic landscape is not completely discovered. At present, for several of the known RCM genes, only a single family or even a single index patient has been reported. All known RCM genes are localized on autosomes (Figure 2B) and in most cases, the mutations are inherited in an autosomal dominant mode or appear as de novo mutations. However, there are also some examples for a recessive inheritance pattern [14]. The majority of RCM genes encode for sarcomere, cytoskeleton or Z-disc proteins, e.g., the cardiac troponins, desmin or filamin-C (Figure 2A). Remarkably, there is a significant genetic overlap with other cardiomyopathies especially with HCM and to some extent with dilated cardiomyopathy (DCM), left-ventricular non-compaction cardiomyopathy (LVNC) or arrhythmogenic cardiomyopathy (ACM) (Figure 3). Currently, it is unknown why mutations in the same gene cause different cardiomyopathies. However, additional genetic modifiers as well as diverse environmental factors can be suggested to be contributing to these phenotypical differences. Sometimes, different phenotypes including RCM are even present within the same family [15,16].

Remarkably, there is also a genetic overlap between RCM and myofibrillar myopathy (MFM, MIM, #601419). MFM is a group of genetic muscle diseases characterized by myofibrillar disorganization and abnormal intra-sarcoplasmic protein aggregates [17]. It can affect the skeletal and/or cardiac muscle. Mutations in seven genes cause MFM (*DES* [18], *CRYAB* [19], *FLNC* [20], *LMNA* [21], *BAG3* [22], *TTN* [23,24], *MYL2* [25]) as well as RCM (Table 1). The genetic overlap between both diseases (Figure 3) might indicate a detrimental involvement of pathological cardiac protein aggregates [26].

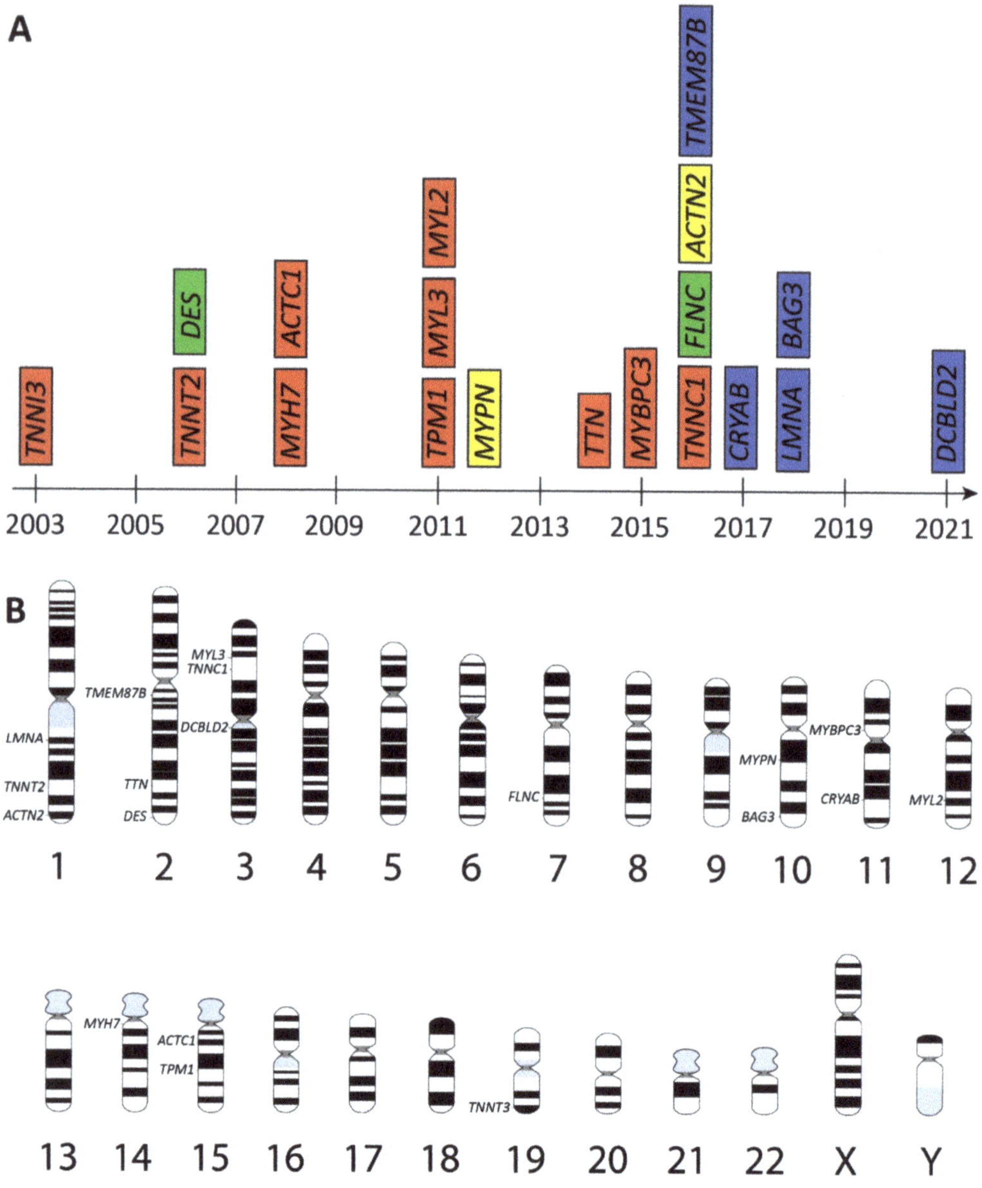

Figure 2. Overview of RCM genes. (**A**) Genes associated with restrictive cardiomyopathy (RCM) according to the year of discovery. Different subcellular localizations are color-coded (red = sarcomere; green = cytoskeleton; yellow = Z-disc and blue = others). (**B**) Chromosomal location of RCM-associated genes. Schematic idiograms were licensed from shutterstock.de.

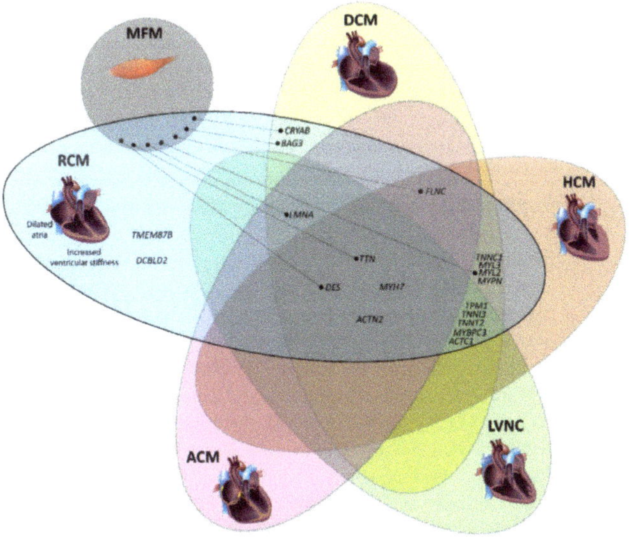

Figure 3. Venn diagram showing the genetic overlap of restrictive cardiomyopathy (RCM) with other cardiomyopathies. ACM = arrhythmogenic cardiomyopathy; DCM = dilated cardiomyopathy; HCM = hypertrophic cardiomyopathy; LVNC = left ventricular non-compaction cardiomyopathy; and MFM = myofibrillar myopathy. Gene names according to the HUGO Gene Nomenclature Committee, HGNC (https://www.genenames.org/ (accessed on 13 March 2022)). Sub-images of the DCM or HCM heart were licensed from shutterstock.de.

Table 1. Overview about RCM-associated genes and proteins.

Gene	Cytogenetic Location	Encoded Protein	Subcellular Protein Localization	First Description	References
TNNI3	19q13.42	cardiac troponin I	Sarcomere	2003	[27]
TNNT2	1q32.1	cardiac troponin T	Sarcomere	2006	[28]
DES	2q35	desmin	Intermediate filament	2006	[29]
ACTC1	15q14	cardiac actin	Sarcomere	2008	[30]
MYH7	14q11.2	β myosin heavy chain	Sarcomere	2008	[31]
TPM1	15q22.2	tropomyosin 1	Sarcomere	2011	[32]
MYL3	3p21.31	essential myosin light chain 3	Sarcomere	2011	[32]
MYL2	12q24.11	cardiac regulatory myosin light chain	Sarcomere	2011	[32]
MYPN	10q21.3	myopalladin	Sarcomere, Z-disc	2012	[33]
TTN	2q31.2	titin	Sarcomere	2014	[34]
MYBPC3	11p11.2	cardiac myosin binding protein C	Sarcomere	2015	[35]
TNNC1	3p21.1	cardiac troponin C	Sarcomere	2016	[36]
FLNC	7q32.1	filamin C	Intercalated disc, Z-disc, sarcolemma	2016	[37]
TMEM87B	2q13	transmembrane protein 87 B	Membrane	2016	[38]
ACTN2	1q43	α actinin 2	Z-disc	2016	[39]
CRYAB	11q23.1	αB crystallin	IF associated protein, intercalated disc, Z-disc	2017	[40] [1]
LMNA	1q22	lamin A/C	Nuclear lamina	2018	[41]
BAG3	10q26.11	bcl2 associated athanogene 3	Cytosol	2018	[42]
DCBLD2	3q12.1	discoidin cub and lccl domain containing protein 2	Membrane	2021	[43] [2]

[1] RCM-associated with skeletal myopathy. [2] RCM-associated with atrial fibrillation, tachycardia, developmental delay and dysmorphic features.

3.1. Mutations in Genes Encoding for Sarcomere Proteins

The majority of known RCM-associated mutations are found in ten genes encoding for sarcomere proteins (Figure 2A). These mutations affect the thin and thick filaments as well as titin filaments.

3.1.1. Cardiac Troponins (TNNI3, TNNT2, TNNC1) and Alpha-Tropomyosin (TPM1)

The cardiac troponin complex is composed of three subunits controlling the position of tropomyosin, essential for the regulation of striated muscle contraction and located along the sarcomere thin filament [44]. Disruption of regulatory function due to mutations leads to cardiac dysfunction and cardiomyopathy. Since the early 1990s, cardiac troponins are known as disease genes for HCM [45], however, they expand their disease spectrum to all genetic forms of cardiomyopathies including RCM.

The gene encoding the cardiac isoform of troponin I (TNNI3) is the main target gene for RCM within the thin filaments and the sarcomeres. Almost all mutations are located in the regulatory C-terminal region interacting with actin and the N-terminal domain of TNNC1 (Table 2 and Figure 4). A high proportion of de novo mutations in infants and children with a poor outcome are described. Few mutations are solely reported to cause an RCM phenotype, but most of them are also found in patients with HCM. Studies on skinned fibers by Gomes et al. suggest that TNNI3 mutations increase Ca^{2+} sensitivity of force development and decrease the ability of TNNI3 to inhibit actomyosin ATPase activity, leading to impaired relaxation properties and diastolic dysfunction [46]. Additionally, it has been shown that mutant alleles, such as p.L144Q, p.R145W and p.R170W, incorporate into the thin filaments to a lower extent compared to wildtype affecting the structural stability of the filaments [47,48]. Overall, it appears that similar mutations can cause a hypertrophic, dilated or restrictive phenotype assuming that genetic modifiers or other environmental factors influence the age of onset and phenotypic expression. A transgenic mouse model (cTNI-193His) corresponding to the human p.R192H mutation mimics the RCM phenotype in mice and suggests that impaired relaxation resulting from Ca^{2+} hypersensitivity [49] and diastolic dysfunction occurring in a dose-dependent manner and indicating that the dosage of mutant protein may be important for the severity of impaired diastole [50].

In contrast to TNNI3, a restrictive phenotype appears to be less common in the two other troponin genes. Mutations in TNNT2 are mainly reported in rare cases where other cardiomyopathy phenotypes also occur in the same family. Furthermore, two compound heterozygous mutations in the cardiac TNNC1 evolved in a restrictive phenotype in two infants (Table 2) [36]. Kawai et al. developed a knock-in mouse model (TnC-A8V), which mimics the human phenotype of enlarged atria, hyper contractility and diastolic dysfunction. The authors suggest perturbed cross-bridge kinetics by myosin rod hypophosphorylation as a potential novel mechanism [51].

Alpha tropomyosin (encoded by TPM1) is a long, double-stranded, helical coiled-coil protein that is wrapped about the long axis of the actin backbone (Figure 4, red structure) and serves to block the active site on actin, thereby inhibiting actin and myosin from binding under resting conditions. TPM1 and the troponin complex constitute the Ca^{2+}-sensitive switch that regulates the contraction of cardiac muscle fibers. Several missense mutations have been described causing either HCM or DCM [52]. Recently, Dorsch et al. reported a 6-year-old child with severe RCM carrying two TPM1 variants in compound heterozygous state requiring HTx, whereas family members with one of the two variants expressed an HCM-like phenotype [16]. In summary, the one case indicates that TPM1 is a very rare disease gene and the RCM phenotype may only occur in compound heterozygosity.

Table 2. Overview about known RCM-associated thin filament mutations.

Mutation	Age of Onset and Clinical Features	Family History	MAF [1]	Comments	References
			TNNI3		
p.D127Y	infant, HF, VAD	de novo	-	contractile dysfunctions and effects on thin filament structure	[53]
p.L144Q	adult, HF	unknown	-		[27]
p.L144H	young adults, HF	familial	-		[54]
p.R145W	children and adults, HF	familial, autosomal dominant	3/280226	variant also associated with HCM; Dutch founder mutation; segregation in several families	[27,39,55]
p.R145Q	children	familial, far relative HCM	-	associated with HCM	[55]
p.S150P	child, SCD	familial	-	one Chinese family with several affected members	[56]
c.549+2delT	infant, died at age 2	de novo	-	predicts splicing defect and truncation	[55]
p.D168fsX176	child, HF, died at age 28y	de novo	-	protein reduction	[57]
p.R170G	child, HF	de novo	-		[47]
p.R170W	infant	de novo	-	variant also associated with HCM	[47,58]
p.R170Q	child, HF	de novo	-	variant also associated with HCM	[30,54]
p.A171T	adult, HF, AF	unknown	-		[27]
p.E177fsX209	child	de novo	-		[30]
p.K178E	6y, HF	de novo	-		[27]
p.K178del	child	de novo	-		[55]
p.D190H	mainly adults, HF, SCD	familial	-	named in ClinVar as p.D190G	[27]
p.R192C	child	familial	-	carries also mosaicism of p.R145Q; associated also with HCM in far relative	[55]
p.R192H	children, young adult, HF	de novo	-	independent reports of de novo mutations; variants also associated with HCM	[27,59,60]
p.K193E	adults, AF, SCD	familial	-	cousin developed HCM	[61]
p.I195fs	young adult, HF, HTx	de novo	-	dominant-negative effect	[62]
p.D196H	three adults, HF, HTx	familial, homozygous	-	heterozygous carrier asymptomatic	[63]
p.R204H	children, HF, HTx, VSD in one case	de novo	-	independent reports of de novo mutations	[59,64,65]
			TNNT2		
p.I89N	two adult cases within one family	familial	0.00002	mixed phenotype with HCM and DCM	[66]
p.R104C	children, young adult, HF	familial	-	mixed phenotype with HCM in the family	[67]
p.E69del	infant, HF, VAD	de novo	-		[28]

Table 2. *Cont.*

Mutation	Age of Onset and Clinical Features	Family History	MAF [1]	Comments	References
p.E146K	child	familial	0.00003	variant also associated with other CMPs	[30]
			TNNC1		
p.A8V; p.D145E	two infants died	familial, compound heterozygous	0.00001 0.0001	HCM which evolved into RCM	[36]
			TPM1		
p.E62Q; p.M281T	child	familial, compound heterozygous	- 0.00001	each single variant leads to a HCM like phenotype	[16]
			ACTC1		
p.D313H	child	familial	-	father was diagnosed with DCM	[30]

[1] MAF = Minor allele frequency according to Genome Aggregation Database (February 2022), https://gnomad.broadinstitute.org (accessed on 13 March 2022). AF = atrial fibrillation, CMPs = cardiomyopathies, DCM = dilated cardiomyopathy, HCM = hypertrophic cardiomyopathy, HF = heart failure, HTx = heart transplantation, RCM = restrictive cardiomyopathy, SCD = sudden cardiac death, VAD = ventricular assist device, VSD = ventricular septal defect.

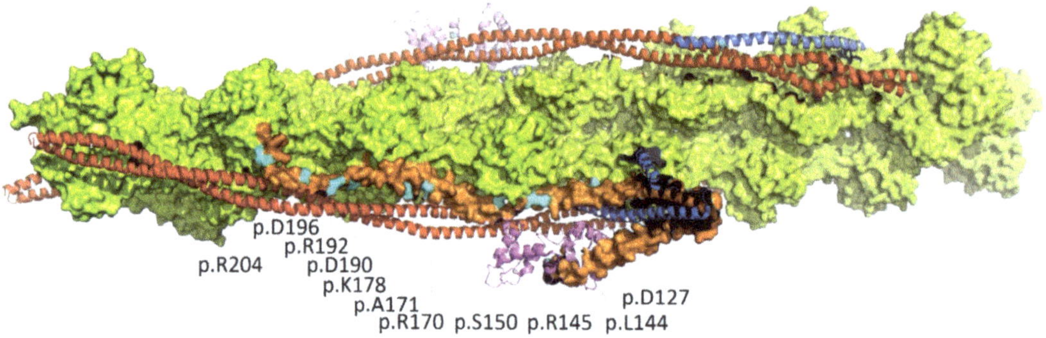

Figure 4. Schematic molecular structure of the thin filaments in the Ca^{2+} free state [68] (https://www.rcsb.org/structure/6KN7 (accessed on 13 March 2022)). Actin is shown in light green, tropomyosin is shown in red, cardiac troponin T is shown in blue, troponin C is shown in violet and troponin I is shown in orange. The localizations of the RCM-associated *TNNI3* missense mutations are shown in cyan. The majority of RCM-associated *TNNI3* missense mutations are localized in the C-terminal part of troponin-I.

3.1.2. Cardiac Actin (ACTC1)

Human cardiac α-actin, encoded by ACTC1, is one of the six human actin isoforms. Using fluorescence in situ hybridization technique Ueyama et al. showed that ACTC1 is localized on chromosome 15q14 [69]. Cardiac α-actin is highly conserved between different species and skeletal and cardiac α-actin are co-expressed in cardiomyocytes [70]. As a monomer, actin has a globular structure (G-actin) and polymerize into filaments (F-actin). Actin is the major structural component of the thin filaments (Figure 4, green structure) and is eminent for the contraction cycle and force generation of cardiomyocytes [71].

Kaski et al. described for the first time an RCM causing mutation in ACTC1 (p.D313H) [30]. The father developed DCM and the sister of the index patient showed a mixed RCM/DCM phenotype, but no genetic sequence analysis was performed for both [30]. Functional analysis was not performed in this study. However, ACTC1-p.D313H is localized in the tropomyosin binding region which supports its functional impact. In addition, ACTC1 mutations can cause DCM [72], HCM [73], LVNC [74] and septal defects [75] (Figure 3).

3.1.3. Myosin Heavy and Light Chains (MYH7, MYL2 and MYL3)

The thick filaments of the cardiac and skeletal sarcomere are mainly formed by myosin. Human cardiac myosin is a hexameric protein complex consisting of β myosin heavy chains (encoded my MYH7), two essential light chains (encoded by MYL3) and two regular myosin light chains (encoded by MYL2) [76–78]. Myosin proteins consist of a head, neck and tail domain. The head domains interact with the thin filaments and contain the N-terminal globular motor domains [79] performing the power stroke during contraction [80]. The neck region is bound by the myosin light chains [81] and the tail domains build a coiled-coil [82].

In all three myosin genes, mutations have been found in RCM patients (Table 3). For the first time, Karam et al. described in 2008 a de novo mutation in the MYH7 gene (p.P838L) in an infantile patient with RCM [31]. Several further pathogenic MYH7 mutations have been described for RCM (Table 3). The majority of these mutations are missense mutations. Beside RCM, MYH7 mutations are particularly causative for HCM [83] and to a less extent for DCM [84], LVNC [74] and ACM [85].

In 2011, Caleshu et al. reported a female RCM patient carrying MYL2-p.G57E and in addition MYL3-p.E143K^{hom} [32]. The described index patient carrying these myosin light chain variants do not present a family history of cardiomyopathies [32], which might be caused by a recessive inheritance. The mutation MYL3-p.E143K^{hom} was also identified before in the homozygous state in HCM patients [86]. Transgenic mice with the cardiac expression of human MYL3-p.E143K developed an increased ventricular stiffness, cardiac interstitial fibrosis and showed ultrastructural defects of the sarcomeres leading to a restrictive phenotype [87]. *MYL2* and *MYL3* mutations also cause HCM [88,89] and DCM [90] (Figure 3).

Table 3. Overview about known RCM-associated myosin mutations (*MYH7, MYL2, MYL3*).

Mutation	Age of Onset and Clinical Features	Family History	MAF [1]	Comments	References
		MYH7			
p.Y386C	infant, coronary artery bridging	unknown	-		[91]
p.R721K	adult, AF,	familial	-	in combination with *ABCC9*-p.R1186Q	[92]
p.G768R	adult, AF, death at age 42	unknown	-		[39]
	infant, HTx	unknown	-		[93]
p.R783H	adult, AVB, death at age 54	familial	0.00002	son has HCM	[39]
p.P838L	infant	de novo	-		[31]
p.L840M	child	unknown	-	in combination with *MYBPC3*-p.P147L	[39]
p.R870C	two adults, AF	familial	0.00002	myofibrillar disarray, cardiomyocyte necrosis, abnormal nuclei morphology	[94]
p.I909M	adult, AVB, AF, death at age 56	unknown	-		[39]
p.T1188CfsX22	adult, in combination with LVH	de novo	-		[95]
		MYL2			
p.G57E	adult	absent	0.000004	in combination with *MYL3*-p.E143K^{hom}	[32]
		MYL3			
MYL3-p.E143K^{hom}	adult	absent	0.00001	in combination with *MYL2*-p.G57E	[32]

[1] MAF = Minor allele frequency according to Genome Aggregation Database (February 2022), https://gnomad.broadinstitute.org (accessed on 13 March 2022). AF = atrial fibrillation, AVB = atrioventricular block, HCM = hypertrophic cardiomyopathy, HTx = heart transplantation, LVH = left ventricular hypertrophy, VUS = variant of unknown significance.

3.1.4. Cardiac Myosin Binding Protein C (MYBPC3)

Another main disease gene for HCM and to a minor extent DCM and LVNC is the gene encoding the cardiac myosin binding protein C (MYBPC3). One study by Wu et al. showed that one de novo variant, previously also associated with HCM (p.E334K) and one truncation variant p.Q463X might cause RCM as part of the phenotypic spectrum [35].

3.1.5. Titin (TTN)

Titin is the largest known human protein and represents the third filament system in cardiac and skeletal muscle [96]. Its primary role is maintaining sarcomere organization, generation of passive tension during muscle stretching and modulating contraction. The major cardiac phenotype caused by TTN mutations is DCM, however so far almost exclusively truncation variants are proven to be causative accounting for 30% of affected individuals with DCM [97,98]. Recently, multiple pathogenic mechanisms have been suggested including haploinsufficiency, truncated titin polypeptides as well as post-translational modifications of titin [99,100]. The role of missense variants is poorly understood, but at least for DCM their relevance as causative remains questionable; they may have a modifying effect [101]. Rarely, other cardiac phenotypes such as HCM, RCM and ACM have been suggested to be associated with TTN variants. In particular a de novo missense mutation, p.Y7621C, located in the A/I junction of titin has been shown to segregate in a family with five affected members aged 12–35 years with typical features of a restrictive physiology suggesting that other missense mutations may also relevant for RCM in particular if they appear de novo [34].

3.2. *Mutations in Genes Encoding Non-Saromere Proteins*

Although the majority of RCM-associated mutations has been found in genes encoding for different sarcomere proteins (Figure 2A), mutations in non-sarcomeric genes are also relevant. Several different mutations have been reported, for example in the DES and FLNC genes.

3.2.1. Desmin (DES)

The DES gene encodes the cytoplasmic muscle specific intermediate filament protein desmin. Intermediate filaments connect different cell organelles such as the cardiac desmosomes, costameres, Z-discs, mitochondria and the cell nuclei [102,103]. Cardiac desmosomes are cell–cell junctions localized at the intercalated disc mediating the cell–cell adhesion of the cardiomyocytes [104]. Desmin filaments are coupled to the desmosomes via the cytolinker protein, desmoplakin [105]. Costameres are multi-protein complexes localized at the sarcolemma and connect the extracellular matrix with the myofibrils [106]. The intermediate filaments are connected via different cytolinker proteins, e.g., plectin with the Z-bands and the costameres [107]. Due to its central role in the cardiac intermediate filament system and its connections with several multi-protein complexes or cell organelles, desmin is highly relevant for the structural integrity of the cardiomyocytes. DES-deficient mice developed severe cardiomyopathy in combination with skeletal myopathy characterized by fragile myofibrils, severe cardiac fibrosis, cardiomyocyte necrosis and abnormal calcium deposits [108,109]. DES mutations in humans are associated with different skeletal and cardiac myopathies [110–114]. In 2006, Hager and colleagues described for the first time a patient with RCM carrying the mutation DES-p.E245D. Later, it was recognized that this mutation causes a splicing defect leading to an in-frame skipping of exon-3 causing a deletion of 32 amino acids within the rod domain [115,116]. Several other pathogenic RCM-associated DES mutations have been reported [14,117–122] (Figure 5 and Table 4).

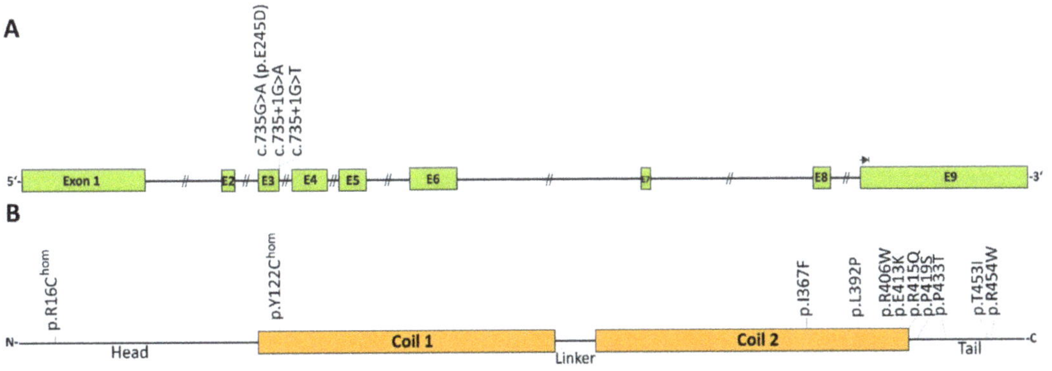

Figure 5. Schematic overview of RCM associated DES mutations. (**A**) Schematic overview about the DES gene consisting of nine exons (NM_001927.4). Three splice site mutations have been identified in RCM patients at the donor splice site of exon 3. (**B**) Schematic domain organization of desmin and the localization of the known RCM-associated DES missense mutations.

Most of the DES mutations are missense or small in-frame deletion mutations leading to a detrimental effect on the filament assembly process [123,124]. The desmin monomer consists of a central α-helical rod domain flanked by non-helical head and tail domains [125]. Two desmin monomers form coiled–coil dimers driven by the annealing of a hydrophobic seam [126]. These dimers form anti parallel tetramers [127]. Eight tetramers anneal into unit-length filaments (ULFs) which have a size of about 60 nm [128]. ULFs are the essential building blocks of intermediate filaments and hybridize longitudinally into regular intermediate filaments [125,129]. As intermediate filaments do not have a polar orientation, they can fuse end-to-end [130–132]. DES mutations can disturb the filament assembly at different steps [123,124].

Table 4. Overview about known RCM-associated *DES* mutations.

Mutation	Age of Onset and Clinical Features	Family History	MAF [1]	Comments	References
c.735+1G>A	adult, SM	de novo	-	induces a splice defect, skipping of exon-3	[133]
c.735+1G>T	adults, SM	two patients	-	induces a splice defect, skipping of exon-3	[119]
p.R16C	adult, AVB, HTx	one patient	0.000006570	homozygous	[134]
p.Y122H	adult, AVB	one patient	-	homozygous	[14]
c.735G>C (p.E245D)	adults, AF	several family members, only index patient was genotyped	-	induces a splice defect, skipping of exon-3	[116]
p.I367F	adults, AVB, SM	several family members	-	index patient diagnosed with HCM [135]	[15,135]
p.L392P	adult, AVB, SM	one patient	-		[135]
p.R406W	adults, AVB	three affected members	-	a different index patient presented ACM in combination with SM [112]	[117,134]
p.E413K	adults, AVB, AF, SCD	four affected members	-		[136,137]
p.R415Q	adult, AF	several family members	-	different phenotypes, unclear if a splice defect is caused (last bp of exon-6)	[15]
p.P419S	adults, AVB, SM	two patients	-		[135]
p.P433T	adult, AVB, SM	one patient	-		[120]
p.T453I	adult, AVB	de novo	-		[134]
p.R454W	adults, AVB, SM	two patients	-		[112]

[1] MAF = Minor allele frequency according to Genome Aggregation Database, https://gnomad.broadinstitute.org/ (accessed on 13 March 2022). ACM = arrhythmogenic cardiomyopathy, AF = atrial fibrillation, AVB = atrioventricular block, HCM = hypertrophic cardiomyopathy, HTx = heart transplantation, SCD = sudden cardiac death, SM = skeletal myopathy.

3.2.2. Myopalladin (MYPN)

Myopalladin belongs beside myotillin (MYOT) and palladin (PALLD) to the actin-binding and immunoglobulin-containing proteins within the Z-disc [138,139]. It contains five immunoglobulin (Ig) domains and a proline-rich motif [138]. In 2012, Purevjav et al. described a MYPN nonsense mutation (p.Q529X) in two affected siblings with RCM [33]. Beside RCM, MYPN mutations are also found in patients with DCM [140], HCM [141] and nemaline myopathy (MIM, #617336) [142].

3.2.3. α-Actinin-2 (ACTN2)

The ACTN2 gene was mapped to chromosome 1q43 [143] and consists of 21 exons [144]. α-Actinin-2 is the main structural component of the Z-discs in striated muscles [145] and belongs to the spectrin protein family [146]. The typical structural element of this protein family are the spectrin-like repeats [147], which are formed by three α-helices forming a left-handed supercoil [148]. α-Actinin-2 forms anti parallel dimers and consists of an N-terminal actin binding domain, a central ROD domain and a calmodulin-like domain (CAMD) (Figure 6) [149].

In 2016, Kostareva et al. screened a cohort of 24 unrelated RCM patients using a broad cardiomyopathy next generation sequencing (NGS) panel and identified, among others, the likely pathogenic mutation ACTN2-p.N175Y (Table 1) [39]. Besides RCM, pathogenic mutations in ACTN2 are associated with DCM [150], HCM [151], LVNC [152] or ACM [153] indicating a broad spectrum of cardiac phenotypes associated with those mutations (Figure 3). In addition, ACTN2 mutations can also cause skeletal myopathies [154].

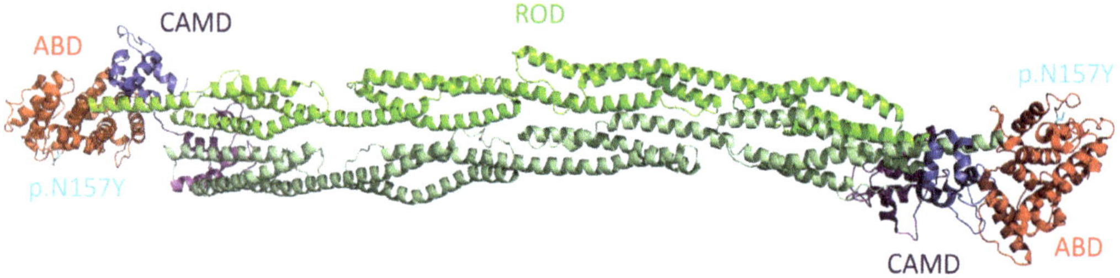

Figure 6. Structural overview of the anti parallel α-actinin-2 dimer (https://www.rcsb.org/structure/4D1E) (accessed on 13 March 2022) [149]. The N-terminal. Actin-binding domains are shown in red. Four spectrin-like repeats build the central cylindrical rod domain (green). A C-terminal calmodulin-like domain is built by two EF hand motifs (purple and blue). The position of the RCM-associated mutation ACTN2-p.N157Y within the actin-binding domain is shown in cyan.

3.2.4. Filamin-C (FLNC)

Originally, mutations in FLNC were identified in patients with MFM (MIM, #609524) [155] or distal myopathy (MIM, #614065) [156]. The FLNC gene consists of 48 exons and is mapped on human chromosome 7q32 [157]. It encodes filamin-C, which is a cytolinker protein. Filamin-C contains an N-terminal actin-binding domain and 24 immunoglobulin-(Ig) domains, which are separated by two hinge regions (Figure 7) [158]. The dimerization of filamin-C is mediated by a protein–protein interaction of its 24th Ig-domains [159]. In cardiomyocytes, filamin-C is localized at the intercalated discs, the sarcolemma and the Z-discs [158,160]. Several binding partners including titin [161,162], integrin β1A and myotilin [163] as well as actin and sarcoglycans [164] have been reported. For a detailed overview see [158].

Valdés-Mas et al. identified in 2014, by whole-exome sequencing several FLNC mutations in patients with HCM [165]. Of note, FLNC mutations can likewise cause DCM [166], ACM [167] or non-compaction cardiomyopathy [168]. RCM-associated FLNC mutations were described in two families for the first time in 2016 [37]. Since then, several other

FLNC missense mutations have been identified in RCM patients (Table 5 and Figure 7). Whereas DCM-associated FLNC truncation mutations are presumably leading to haploinsufficiency [169], an abnormal aggregation leading in consequence to sarcomeric disarray has been demonstrated for some missense mutations [37,165,170]. Several (zebra)fish and mouse models for FLNC have been generated revealing different muscle and heart defects [166,171–178]. Of note, even in Drosophila melanogaster loss of the filamin ortholog 'Cheerio' causes Z-disc and sarcomere defects [162]. Recently, two iPSC lines from donors with RCM carrying FLNC missense mutations have been generated, but their characterization is ongoing [179,180]. Tucker et al. inserted the mutation FLNC-p.V2297M using genome editing by 'Clustered Regularly Interspaced Short Palindromic Repeats' (CRISPR)-Cas9 into a human embryonic stem cell line (hESC). The fractional shortening was decreased in hESC-derived cardiomyocytes [181].

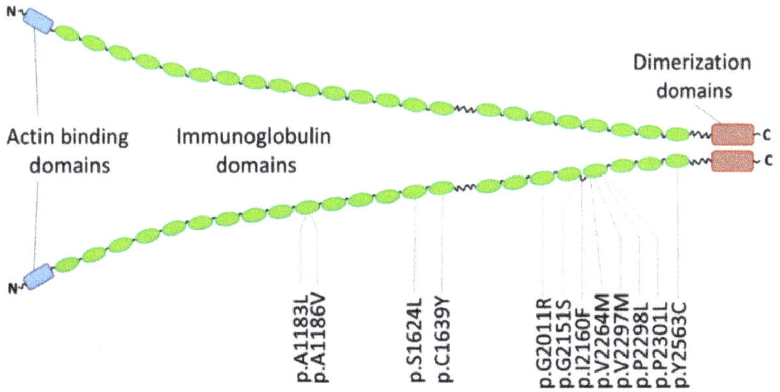

Figure 7. Schematic overview about the domain organization of filamin-C and the localization of the known RCM-associated FLNC missense mutations.

Table 5. Overview about the known RCM-associated *FLNC* mutations.

Mutation	Clinical Features	Family History	MAF [1]	Comments	References
p.A1183L	RCM and congenital myopathy	one patient	-		[176]
p.A1186V	RCM and congenital myopathy	three unrelated index patients	-	de novo	[176]
	RCM	one patient	-	de novo, early onset	[182]
p.S1624L	RCM	four affected family members	0.00003		[37]
p.C1639Y	RCM	one patient	-	de novo, early onset	[182]
p.G2011R	RCM	one patient	-	iPSC model	[180]
p.G2151S	RCM	two patients	-	in addition *PTPN11*-p.Q510R	[183]
p.I2160F	RCM	three affected family members	-		[37]
p.V2264M	RCM, SM	one patient	-	iPSC model	[179]
p.V2297M	RCM, AF	five affected family members	0.000004		[181]
p.P2298L	RCM	eight patients (four genotyped)	-		[184]
p.P2301L	RCM, AF, muscular weakness	one patient	-	de novo	[183]
p.Y2563C	RCM	two monozygotic twins	-	de novo	[184]

[1] MAF = Minor allele frequency according to Genome Aggregation Database (January 2022), https://gnomad.broadinstitute.org/(accessed on 13 March 2022). AF = atrial fibrillation, RCM = restrictive cardiomyopathy, SM = skeletal myopathy.

3.2.5. Lamin A/C (LMNA)

Lamin A/C belongs to the intermediate filament protein family (type V) [125] and forms the nuclear lamina [185]. The nuclear lamina is a molecular meshwork, which is important for the structural integrity of the nuclei and regulates the chromatin organization [186].

Recently, Paller et al. found a 1 bp deletion in exon 5 of the LMNA gene (c.835delG, p.E279RfsX201) in a RCM patient who developed additionally skeletal muscle weakness and atrial fibrillation [41]. Histology analysis revealed hypertrophy and cardiac fibrosis in the explanted myocardial tissue [41]. Beside RCM, LMNA mutations cause DCM [187], ACM [188], LVNC [189], Emery–Dreifuss muscular dystrophy (MIM, #181350) [190], familial lipodystrophy (MIM #151660) [191] and Hutchinson–Gilford progeria syndrome (HGPS, MIM #176670) [192]. The nuclear envelope and the connected nuclear lamina of cardiomyocytes are sensitive structures where mutations affect several other proteins, e.g., TMEM43 may cause different cardiomyopathies [193].

3.2.6. Transmembrane Protein 87B (TMEM87B)

TMEM87B encodes a multi-pass transmembrane protein, which is involved in endosome to Golgi apparatus retrograde transport [194].

Yu et al. described the hemizygous missense mutation TMEM87B-p.N456D in combination with a 1.7 Mb microdeletion on the second allele in a patient who developed RCM in combination with an atrial septal defect, craniofacial abnormalities, dysmorphic features, microcephaly and skeletal dysplasia [38]. Using anti sense morpholino injections, it has been shown by Russel et al. that TMEM87B knockdown causes cardiac hypoplasia and cardiac defects in zebrafish embryos [195].

3.2.7. αB-Crystallin (CRYAB)

CRYAB (or HSPB5) encodes αB-crystallin, which belongs to the small heat shock protein (sHSP) family [196]. Several sHSPs are expressed in the human heart. Originally, αB-crystallin was discovered as a major component of the vertebrate eye lenses [197]. However, it is also highly expressed in the heart and in the skeletal muscle [198,199]. In 1998, Vicart et al. identified in a French family with MFM in combination with HCM and cataract the pathogenic missense mutation CRYAB-p.R120G (Figure 8). Of note, this mutation causes, comparable to DES mutation, an abnormal aggregation of desmin and αB-crystallin in skeletal and cardiac myocytes [19]. Interestingly, Sacconi et al. described the same triad of clinical symptoms in a family carrying a different CRYAB mutation [200]. CRYAB mutations can also cause isolated cataract without cardiac involvement [201] or vice versa isolated DCM without cataract [202]. Recently, the CRYAB mutation p.D109G has been described in a small German family with RCM in combination with SM [40]. Interestingly, R120 and D109 form two ion bridges stabilizing the dimerization of αB-crystallin (Figure 8). The αB-crystallin dimers form large oligomers [203] which have an ATP-independent chaperone-like activity [204]. In addition, αB-crystallin binds also to different cytoskeletal and sarcomere proteins, e.g., titin [205].

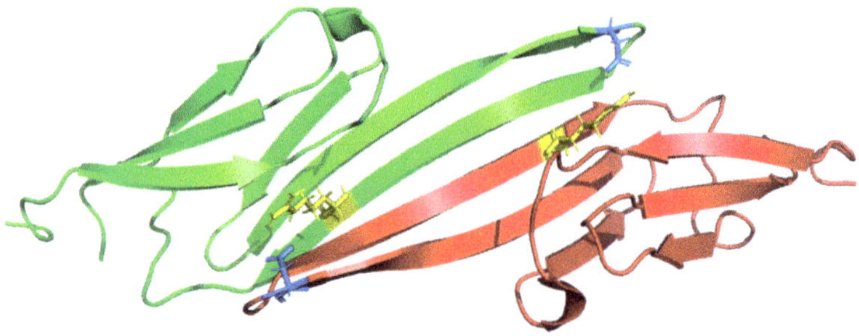

Figure 8. Molecular structure of the αB-crystallin domain determined by nuclear magnetic resonance (NMR) spectroscopy (https://www.rcsb.org/structure/2KLR) (accessed on 13 March 2022) [206]. Two ion bridges are formed between aspartate p.D109 (blue) and arginine p.R120 (yellow) mediating its dimerization. Of note, the mutation CRYAB-p.D109G is associated with RCM in combination with skeletal myopathy [40] and -p.R120G causes MFM in combination with HCM and cataract [19,207].

3.2.8. Bcl2 Associated Athanogene 3 (BAG3)

The BAG3 gene consists of four exons and encodes Bcl2 associated athanogene 3 [208]. BAG3 is a co-chaperone binding to the ATPase domain of heat shock protein Hsc70/Hsp70 and regulating its chaperone function [209]. BAG3 is structurally organized in an N-terminal tryptophan-tryptophan (WW) domain, two IPV domains, two 14-3-3 binding motifs, a proline-rich region and a C-terminal BAG domain [210,211]. The protein–protein interaction of BAG3 with Hsc70/Hsp70 is mediated by its BAG domain [212]. BAG3 acts as an ATP exchange factor stabilizing the ATPase domain of Hsc70/Hsp70 without bound ATP [213]. Since the multi-domain organization of BAG3, numerous other binding partners have been described. For example, BAG3 binds to several members of the sHSP family including αB-Crystallin [214–218]. Briefly summarized, BAG3 has a central and important role in protein quality control and chaperone-assisted selective autophagy [219].

Several pathogenic mutations in BAG3 have been described in patients with DCM [220] or with MFM [221]. In addition, BAG3 mutations are found in patients with RCM in combination with MFM [42]. Recently, Kimura et al. generated a transgenic mouse model with an overexpression of BAG3-p.P209L conjugated with green fluorescent protein. These mice develop RCM and severe cardiac fibrosis. At the cellular level, disorganization of the Z-disc and abnormal protein aggregation were present [222]. In contrast, the knock-in mouse model carrying the equivalent murine mutation Bag3-p.P215L does not develop a cardiac phenotype [223].

3.2.9. Discoidin Cub and Lccl Domain Containing Protein-2 (DCBLD2)

Recently, Alhamoudi et al. described the homozygous nonsense mutation DCBLD2-p.W27X in a 5-year-old Arabic patient with severe RCM, tachycardia, atrial fibrillation, dysmorphic features and developmental delay. Functional analyses using primary dermal fibroblast from the mutation carrier indicated reduced cell proliferation and altered amounts of calcium and reactive oxygen species in comparison to normal fibroblasts [43]. DCBLD2 encodes a ubiquitously expressed type-I transmembrane protein [224,225]. It is involved in vascular smooth muscle cell proliferation [226], vascular endothelial growth factor (VEGF) signaling [227] and epithelial–mesenchymal transition [228]. However, the exact molecular functions of DCBLD2 contributing to RCM and other cardiomyopathies are currently unknown and deserve increased research attention in the future.

4. Summary and Outlook

Currently, mutations in over 19 different disease-causing genes have been discovered in patients with primary RCM. However, the genetic landscape of RCM is overlapping with the genetic background of other cardiomyopathies. Genes encoding for sarcomere proteins such as cardiac troponin-I are the major RCM genes. However, more recently, the prevalence of mutations in specific non-sarcomeric genes such as *DES* or *FLNC* has increased; broad NGS gene panels or whole exome sequencing should be considered if a genetic etiology is suspected. This might be also beneficial, since the genetic landscape of RCM remains incomplete. Therefore, multi-center studies enrolling larger patient cohorts are needed to provide a robust overview about the genetic etiology of RCM. In addition, these studies might reveal the age of onset associated with specific genotypes.

As no sufficient treatment for RCM is currently available, there is a highly unmet medical need for the development of more precise genetic or molecular therapies. However, there is hope on the horizon with novel therapies targeting the sarcomere. In particular, for the obstructive form of HCM the allosteric inhibitor of the cardiac specific myosin adenosine triphosphatase (MYK-461) has shown symptomatic improvement in a phase 3 trial and may also be applicable for patients with RCM and sarcomeric mutations leading to an excessive cross bridging with actin [229]. The opposite setting, small molecules, such as omecamtiv mecarbil and danicamtiv, increasing contractility may be effective in particular in patients with sarcomere mutations and DCM [230].

Another exciting strategy can be seen in genome editing using CRISPR-Cas9 [231] or RNA editing using Cas7-11 [232] in combination with adequate cardiomyocyte specific delivery vectors, e.g., adeno-associated viruses [233,234], will help to reach this goal in the future. Recently, CRISPR-Cas9 has been used for example for correcting DCM associated truncating *TTN* mutations [235] and deserves interest in the context of RCM in the future.

Author Contributions: Conceptualization, A.B. and B.G.; writing—original draft preparation, A.B. and B.G.; writing—review and editing, A.B. and B.G.; visualization, A.B. and B.G.; funding acquisition, A.B. and B.G. All authors have read and agreed to the published version of the manuscript.

Funding: We acknowledge support by the DFG Open Access Publication Funds of the Ruhr-University Bochum (funding number: 5678). Funding to B.G. was also provided by the German Research Foundation (project number: 453989101).

Institutional Review Board Statement: Not applicable.

Informed Consent Statement: Not applicable.

Conflicts of Interest: The authors declare no conflict of interest. The funders had no role in the design of the study; in the collection, analyses, or interpretation of data; in the writing of the manuscript, or in the decision to publish the results.

References

1. McKenna, W.J.; Maron, B.J.; Thiene, G. Classification, epidemiology, and global burden of cardiomyopathies. *Circ. Res.* **2017**, *121*, 722–730. [CrossRef] [PubMed]
2. White, P.; Myers, M. The classification of cardiac diagnosis. *JAMA* **1921**, *77*, 1414–1415.
3. Gerull, B.; Klaassen, S.; Brodehl, A. The genetic landscape of cardiomyopathies. In *Genetic Causes of Cardiac Disease*; Erdmann, J., Moretti, A., Eds.; Springer: Cham, Switzerland, 2019; pp. 45–91.
4. Butzner, M.; Leslie, D.L.; Cuffee, Y.; Hollenbeak, C.S.; Sciamanna, C.; Abraham, T. Stable rates of obstructive hypertrophic cardiomyopathy in a contemporary era. *Front. Cardiovasc. Med.* **2021**, *8*, 765876. [CrossRef]
5. Elliott, P.; Andersson, B.; Arbustini, E.; Bilinska, Z.; Cecchi, F.; Charron, P.; Dubourg, O.; Kuhl, U.; Maisch, B.; McKenna, W.J.; et al. Classification of the cardiomyopathies: A position statement from the european society of cardiology working group on myocardial and pericardial diseases. *Eur. Heart J.* **2008**, *29*, 270–276. [CrossRef] [PubMed]
6. Cuddy, S.A.M.; Falk, R.H. Amyloidosis as a systemic disease in context. *Can. J. Cardiol.* **2020**, *36*, 396–407. [CrossRef] [PubMed]
7. Ruberg, F.L.; Grogan, M.; Hanna, M.; Kelly, J.W.; Maurer, M.S. Transthyretin amyloid cardiomyopathy: JACC state-of-the-art review. *J. Am. Coll. Cardiol.* **2019**, *73*, 2872–2891. [CrossRef] [PubMed]
8. Paisey, R.B.; Steeds, R.; Barrett, T.; Williams, D.; Geberhiwot, T.; Gunay-Aygun, M. Alstrom syndrome. In *GeneReviews((R))*; Adam, M.P., Ardinger, H.H., Pagon, R.A., Wallace, S.E., Bean, L.J.H., Gripp, K.W., Mirzaa, G.M., Amemiya, A., Eds.; University of Washington: Seattle, DC, USA, 1993.
9. Starr, L.J.; Lindor, N.M.; Lin, A.E. Myhre syndrome. In *GeneReviews((R))*; Adam, M.P., Ardinger, H.H., Pagon, R.A., Wallace, S.E., Bean, L.J.H., Gripp, K.W., Mirzaa, G.M., Amemiya, A., Eds.; University of Washington: Seattle, DC, USA, 1993.
10. Seferovic, P.M.; Polovina, M.; Bauersachs, J.; Arad, M.; Gal, T.B.; Lund, L.H.; Felix, S.B.; Arbustini, E.; Caforio, A.L.P.; Farmakis, D.; et al. Heart failure in cardiomyopathies: A position paper from the heart failure association of the european society of cardiology. *Eur. J. Heart Fail.* **2019**, *21*, 553–576. [CrossRef]
11. Kubo, T.; Gimeno, J.R.; Bahl, A.; Steffensen, U.; Steffensen, M.; Osman, E.; Thaman, R.; Mogensen, J.; Elliott, P.M.; Doi, Y.; et al. Prevalence, clinical significance, and genetic basis of hypertrophic cardiomyopathy with restrictive phenotype. *J. Am. Coll. Cardiol.* **2007**, *49*, 2419–2426. [CrossRef]
12. DePasquale, E.C.; Nasir, K.; Jacoby, D.L. Outcomes of adults with restrictive cardiomyopathy after heart transplantation. *J. Heart Lung Transplant.* **2012**, *31*, 1269–1275. [CrossRef]
13. Muchtar, E.; Blauwet, L.A.; Gertz, M.A. Restrictive cardiomyopathy: Genetics, pathogenesis, clinical manifestations, diagnosis, and therapy. *Circ. Res.* **2017**, *121*, 819–837. [CrossRef]
14. Brodehl, A.; Pour Hakimi, S.A.; Stanasiuk, C.; Ratnavadivel, S.; Hendig, D.; Gaertner, A.; Gerull, B.; Gummert, J.; Paluszkiewicz, L.; Milting, H. Restrictive cardiomyopathy is caused by a novel homozygous desmin (DES) mutation p.Y122H leading to a severe filament assembly defect. *Genes* **2019**, *10*, 918. [CrossRef] [PubMed]
15. Ripoll-Vera, T.; Zorio, E.; Gamez, J.M.; Molina, P.; Govea, N.; Cremer, D. Phenotypic patterns of cardiomyopathy caused by mutations in the desmin gene. A clinical and genetic study in two inherited heart disease units. *Rev. Esp. Cardiol.* **2015**, *68*, 1027–1029. [CrossRef] [PubMed]
16. Dorsch, L.M.; Kuster, D.W.D.; Jongbloed, J.D.H.; Boven, L.G.; van Spaendonck-Zwarts, K.Y.; Suurmeijer, A.J.H.; Vink, A.; du Marchie Sarvaas, G.J.; van den Berg, M.P.; van der Velden, J.; et al. The effect of tropomyosin variants on cardiomyocyte function and structure that underlie different clinical cardiomyopathy phenotypes. *Int. J. Cardiol.* **2021**, *323*, 251–258. [CrossRef] [PubMed]

17. Fichna, J.P.; Maruszak, A.; Zekanowski, C. Myofibrillar myopathy in the genomic context. *J. Appl. Genet.* **2018**, *59*, 431–439. [CrossRef]
18. Munoz-Marmol, A.M.; Strasser, G.; Isamat, M.; Coulombe, P.A.; Yang, Y.; Roca, X.; Vela, E.; Mate, J.L.; Coll, J.; Fernandez-Figueras, M.T.; et al. A dysfunctional desmin mutation in a patient with severe generalized myopathy. *Proc. Natl. Acad. Sci. USA* **1998**, *95*, 11312–11317. [CrossRef]
19. Vicart, P.; Caron, A.; Guicheney, P.; Li, Z.; Prevost, M.C.; Faure, A.; Chateau, D.; Chapon, F.; Tome, F.; Dupret, J.M.; et al. A missense mutation in the αB-crystallin chaperone gene causes a desmin-related myopathy. *Nat. Genet.* **1998**, *20*, 92–95. [CrossRef]
20. Kley, R.A.; Hellenbroich, Y.; van der Ven, P.F.; Furst, D.O.; Huebner, A.; Bruchertseifer, V.; Peters, S.A.; Heyer, C.M.; Kirschner, J.; Schroder, R.; et al. Clinical and morphological phenotype of the filamin myopathy: A study of 31 German patients. *Brain* **2007**, *130 Pt 12*, 3250–3264. [CrossRef]
21. Dhawan, P.S.; Liewluck, T.; Knapik, J.; Milone, M. Myofibrillar myopathy due to dominant LMNA mutations: A report of 2 cases. *Muscle Nerve* **2018**, *57*, E124–E126. [CrossRef]
22. Odgerel, Z.; Sarkozy, A.; Lee, H.S.; McKenna, C.; Rankin, J.; Straub, V.; Lochmuller, H.; Paola, F.; D'Amico, A.; Bertini, E.; et al. Inheritance patterns and phenotypic features of myofibrillar myopathy associated with a BAG3 mutation. *Neuromuscul. Disord.* **2010**, *20*, 438–442. [CrossRef]
23. Pfeffer, G.; Barresi, R.; Wilson, I.J.; Hardy, S.A.; Griffin, H.; Hudson, J.; Elliott, H.R.; Ramesh, A.V.; Radunovic, A.; Winer, J.B.; et al. Titin founder mutation is a common cause of myofibrillar myopathy with early respiratory failure. *J. Neurol. Neurosurg. Psychiatry* **2014**, *85*, 331–338. [CrossRef]
24. Izumi, R.; Niihori, T.; Aoki, Y.; Suzuki, N.; Kato, M.; Warita, H.; Takahashi, T.; Tateyama, M.; Nagashima, T.; Funayama, R.; et al. Exome sequencing identifies a novel TTN mutation in a family with hereditary myopathy with early respiratory failure. *J. Hum. Genet.* **2013**, *58*, 259–266. [CrossRef] [PubMed]
25. Weterman, M.A.; Barth, P.G.; van Spaendonck-Zwarts, K.Y.; Aronica, E.; Poll-The, B.T.; Brouwer, O.F.; van Tintelen, J.P.; Qahar, Z.; Bradley, E.J.; de Wissel, M.; et al. Recessive MYL2 mutations cause infantile type I muscle fibre disease and cardiomyopathy. *Brain* **2013**, *136 Pt 1*, 282–293. [CrossRef]
26. Cimiotti, D.; Budde, H.; Hassoun, R.; Jaquet, K. Genetic restrictive cardiomyopathy: Causes and consequences—An integrative approach. *Int. J. Mol. Sci.* **2021**, *22*, 558. [CrossRef]
27. Mogensen, J.; Kubo, T.; Duque, M.; Uribe, W.; Shaw, A.; Murphy, R.; Gimeno, J.R.; Elliott, P.; McKenna, W.J. Idiopathic restrictive cardiomyopathy is part of the clinical expression of cardiac troponin I mutations. *J. Clin. Investig.* **2003**, *111*, 209–216. [CrossRef]
28. Peddy, S.B.; Vricella, L.A.; Crosson, J.E.; Oswald, G.L.; Cohn, R.D.; Cameron, D.E.; Valle, D.; Loeys, B.L. Infantile restrictive cardiomyopathy resulting from a mutation in the cardiac troponin T gene. *Pediatrics* **2006**, *117*, 1830–1833. [CrossRef] [PubMed]
29. Hager, S.; Mahrholdt, H.; Goldfarb, L.G.; Goebel, H.H.; Sechtem, U. Images in cardiovascular medicine. Giant right atrium in the setting of desmin-related restrictive cardiomyopathy. *Circulation* **2006**, *113*, e53–e55. [CrossRef] [PubMed]
30. Kaski, J.P.; Syrris, P.; Burch, M.; Tome-Esteban, M.T.; Fenton, M.; Christiansen, M.; Andersen, P.S.; Sebire, N.; Ashworth, M.; Deanfield, J.E.; et al. Idiopathic restrictive cardiomyopathy in children is caused by mutations in cardiac sarcomere protein genes. *Heart* **2008**, *94*, 1478–1484. [CrossRef]
31. Karam, S.; Raboisson, M.J.; Ducreux, C.; Chalabreysse, L.; Millat, G.; Bozio, A.; Bouvagnet, P. A de novo mutation of the beta cardiac myosin heavy chain gene in an infantile restrictive cardiomyopathy. *Congenit. Heart Dis.* **2008**, *3*, 138–143. [CrossRef]
32. Caleshu, C.; Sakhuja, R.; Nussbaum, R.L.; Schiller, N.B.; Ursell, P.C.; Eng, C.; De Marco, T.; McGlothlin, D.; Burchard, E.G.; Rame, J.E. Furthering the link between the sarcomere and primary cardiomyopathies: Restrictive cardiomyopathy associated with multiple mutations in genes previously associated with hypertrophic or dilated cardiomyopathy. *Am. J. Med. Genet. Part A* **2011**, *155*, 2229–2235. [CrossRef]
33. Purevjav, E.; Arimura, T.; Augustin, S.; Huby, A.C.; Takagi, K.; Nunoda, S.; Kearney, D.L.; Taylor, M.D.; Terasaki, F.; Bos, J.M.; et al. Molecular basis for clinical heterogeneity in inherited cardiomyopathies due to myopalladin mutations. *Hum. Mol. Genet.* **2012**, *21*, 2039–2053. [CrossRef]
34. Peled, Y.; Gramlich, M.; Yoskovitz, G.; Feinberg, M.S.; Afek, A.; Polak-Charcon, S.; Pras, E.; Sela, B.A.; Konen, E.; Weissbrod, O.; et al. Titin mutation in familial restrictive cardiomyopathy. *Int. J. Cardiol.* **2014**, *171*, 24–30. [CrossRef] [PubMed]
35. Wu, W.; Lu, C.X.; Wang, Y.N.; Liu, F.; Chen, W.; Liu, Y.T.; Han, Y.C.; Cao, J.; Zhang, S.Y.; Zhang, X. Novel phenotype-genotype correlations of restrictive cardiomyopathy with myosin-binding protein C (MYBPC3) gene mutations tested by next-generation sequencing. *J. Am. Heart Assoc.* **2015**, *4*, e001879. [CrossRef] [PubMed]
36. Ploski, R.; Rydzanicz, M.; Ksiazczyk, T.M.; Franaszczyk, M.; Pollak, A.; Kosinska, J.; Michalak, E.; Stawinski, P.; Ziolkowska, L.; Bilinska, Z.T.; et al. Evidence for troponin C (TNNC1) as a gene for autosomal recessive restrictive cardiomyopathy with fatal outcome in infancy. *Am. J. Med. Genet. Part A* **2016**, *170*, 3241–3248. [CrossRef] [PubMed]
37. Brodehl, A.; Ferrier, R.A.; Hamilton, S.J.; Greenway, S.C.; Brundler, M.A.; Yu, W.; Gibson, W.T.; McKinnon, M.L.; McGillivray, B.; Alvarez, N.; et al. Mutations in *FLNC* are associated with familial restrictive cardiomyopathy. *Hum. Mutat.* **2016**, *37*, 269–279. [CrossRef]
38. Yu, H.C.; Coughlin, C.R.; Geiger, E.A.; Salvador, B.J.; Elias, E.R.; Cavanaugh, J.L.; Chatfield, K.C.; Miyamoto, S.D.; Shaikh, T.H. Discovery of a potentially deleterious variant in TMEM87B in a patient with a hemizygous 2q13 microdeletion suggests a recessive condition characterized by congenital heart disease and restrictive cardiomyopathy. *Mol. Case Stud.* **2016**, *2*, a000844. [CrossRef]

39. Kostareva, A.; Kiselev, A.; Gudkova, A.; Frishman, G.; Ruepp, A.; Frishman, D.; Smolina, N.; Tarnovskaya, S.; Nilsson, D.; Zlotina, A.; et al. Genetic spectrum of idiopathic restrictive cardiomyopathy uncovered by next-generation sequencing. *PLoS ONE* **2016**, *11*, e0163362. [CrossRef]
40. Brodehl, A.; Gaertner-Rommel, A.; Klauke, B.; Grewe, S.A.; Schirmer, I.; Peterschroder, A.; Faber, L.; Vorgerd, M.; Gummert, J.; Anselmetti, D.; et al. The novel αB-crystallin (CRYAB) mutation p.D109G causes restrictive cardiomyopathy. *Hum. Mutat.* **2017**, *38*, 947–952. [CrossRef]
41. Paller, M.S.; Martin, C.M.; Pierpont, M.E. Restrictive cardiomyopathy: An unusual phenotype of a lamin A variant. *ESC Heart Fail.* **2018**, *5*, 724–726. [CrossRef]
42. Schanzer, A.; Rupp, S.; Graf, S.; Zengeler, D.; Jux, C.; Akinturk, H.; Gulatz, L.; Mazhari, N.; Acker, T.; Van Coster, R.; et al. Dysregulated autophagy in restrictive cardiomyopathy due to Pro209Leu mutation in BAG3. *Mol. Genet. Metab.* **2018**, *123*, 388–399. [CrossRef]
43. Alhamoudi, K.M.; Barhoumi, T.; Al-Eidi, H.; Asiri, A.; Nashabat, M.; Alaamery, M.; Alharbi, M.; Alhaidan, Y.; Tabarki, B.; Umair, M.; et al. A homozygous nonsense mutation in DCBLD2 is a candidate cause of developmental delay, dysmorphic features and restrictive cardiomyopathy. *Sci. Rep.* **2021**, *11*, 12861. [CrossRef]
44. Gordon, A.M.; Homsher, E.; Regnier, M. Regulation of contraction in striated muscle. *Physiol. Rev.* **2000**, *80*, 853–924. [CrossRef] [PubMed]
45. Thierfelder, L.; Watkins, H.; MacRae, C.; Lamas, R.; McKenna, W.; Vosberg, H.P.; Seidman, J.G.; Seidman, C.E. α-tropomyosin and cardiac troponin T mutations cause familial hypertrophic cardiomyopathy: A disease of the sarcomere. *Cell* **1994**, *77*, 701–712. [CrossRef]
46. Gomes, A.V.; Liang, J.; Potter, J.D. Mutations in human cardiac troponin I that are associated with restrictive cardiomyopathy affect basal ATPase activity and the calcium sensitivity of force development. *J. Biol. Chem.* **2005**, *280*, 30909–30915. [CrossRef] [PubMed]
47. Cimiotti, D.; Fujita-Becker, S.; Mohner, D.; Smolina, N.; Budde, H.; Wies, A.; Morgenstern, L.; Gudkova, A.; Sejersen, T.; Sjoberg, G.; et al. Infantile restrictive cardiomyopathy: cTnI-R170G/W impair the interplay of sarcomeric proteins and the integrity of thin filaments. *PLoS ONE* **2020**, *15*, e0229227. [CrossRef] [PubMed]
48. Davis, J.; Wen, H.; Edwards, T.; Metzger, J.M. Allele and species dependent contractile defects by restrictive and hypertrophic cardiomyopathy-linked troponin I mutants. *J. Mol. Cell. Cardiol.* **2008**, *44*, 891–904. [CrossRef]
49. Li, Y.; Charles, P.Y.; Nan, C.; Pinto, J.R.; Wang, Y.; Liang, J.; Wu, G.; Tian, J.; Feng, H.Z.; Potter, J.D.; et al. Correcting diastolic dysfunction by Ca^{2+} desensitizing troponin in a transgenic mouse model of restrictive cardiomyopathy. *J. Mol. Cell. Cardiol.* **2010**, *49*, 402–411. [CrossRef] [PubMed]
50. Li, Y.; Zhang, L.; Jean-Charles, P.Y.; Nan, C.; Chen, G.; Tian, J.; Jin, J.P.; Gelb, I.J.; Huang, X. Dose-dependent diastolic dysfunction and early death in a mouse model with cardiac troponin mutations. *J. Mol. Cell. Cardiol.* **2013**, *62*, 227–236. [CrossRef]
51. Kawai, M.; Johnston, J.R.; Karam, T.; Wang, L.; Singh, R.K.; Pinto, J.R. Myosin rod hypophosphorylation and CB kinetics in papillary muscles from a TnC-A8V KI mouse model. *Biophys. J.* **2017**, *112*, 1726–1736. [CrossRef]
52. Redwood, C.; Robinson, P. Alpha-tropomyosin mutations in inherited cardiomyopathies. *J. Muscle Res. Cell Motil.* **2013**, *34*, 285–294. [CrossRef]
53. Hassoun, R.; Budde, H.; Mannherz, H.G.; Lódi, M.; Fujita-Becker, S.; Laser, K.T.; Gärtner, A.; Klingel, K.; Möhner, D.; Stehle, R.; et al. De novo missense mutations in TNNC1 and TNNI3 causing severe infantile cardiomyopathy affect myofilament structure and function and are modulated by troponin targeting agents. *Int. J. Mol. Sci.* **2021**, *22*, 9625. [CrossRef]
54. Mouton, J.M.; Pellizzon, A.S.; Goosen, A.; Kinnear, C.J.; Herbst, P.G.; Brink, P.A.; Moolman-Smook, J.C. Diagnostic disparity and identification of two TNNI3 gene mutations, one novel and one arising de novo, in South African patients with restrictive cardiomyopathy and focal ventricular hypertrophy. *Cardiovasc. J. Afr.* **2015**, *26*, 63–69. [CrossRef] [PubMed]
55. Van den Wijngaard, A.; Volders, P.; Van Tintelen, J.P.; Jongbloed, J.D.; van den Berg, M.P.; Lekanne Deprez, R.H.; Mannens, M.M.; Hofmann, N.; Slegtenhorst, M.; Dooijes, D.; et al. Recurrent and founder mutations in the Netherlands: Cardiac Troponin I (TNNI3) gene mutations as a cause of severe forms of hypertrophic and restrictive cardiomyopathy. *Neth. Heart J.* **2011**, *19*, 344–351. [CrossRef] [PubMed]
56. Ruan, Y.P.; Lu, C.X.; Zhao, X.Y.; Liang, R.J.; Lian, H.; Routledge, M.; Wu, W.; Zhang, X.; Fan, Z.J. Restrictive cardiomyopathy resulting from a troponin I type 3 mutation in a Chinese family. *Chin. Med. Sci. J.* **2016**, *31*, 1–7. [CrossRef]
57. Kostareva, A.; Gudkova, A.; Sjöberg, G.; Mörner, S.; Semernin, E.; Krutikov, A.; Shlyakhto, E.; Sejersen, T. Deletion in TNNI3 gene is associated with restrictive cardiomyopathy. *Int. J. Cardiol.* **2009**, *131*, 410–412. [CrossRef]
58. Mogensen, J.; Hey, T.; Lambrecht, S. A Systematic Review of Phenotypic Features Associated With Cardiac Troponin I Mutations in Hereditary Cardiomyopathies. *Can. J. Cardiol.* **2015**, *31*, 1377–1385. [CrossRef]
59. Ding, W.H.; Han, L.; Xiao, Y.Y.; Mo, Y.; Yang, J.; Wang, X.F.; Jin, M. Role of Whole-exome sequencing in phenotype classification and clinical treatment of pediatric restrictive cardiomyopathy. *Chin. Med. J.* **2017**, *130*, 2823–2828. [CrossRef]
60. Rai, T.S.; Ahmad, S.; Ahluwalia, T.S.; Ahuja, M.; Bahl, A.; Saikia, U.N.; Singh, B.; Talwar, K.K.; Khullar, M. Genetic and clinical profile of Indian patients of idiopathic restrictive cardiomyopathy with and without hypertrophy. *Mol. Cell. Biochem.* **2009**, *331*, 187–192. [CrossRef]
61. Gerhardt, T.; Monserrat, L.; Landmesser, U.; Poller, W. A novel Troponin I mutation associated with severe restrictive cardiomyopathy-a case report of a 27-year-old woman with fatigue. *Eur. Heart J. Case Rep.* **2022**, *6*, ytac053. [CrossRef]

62. Shah, S.; Yogasundaram, H.; Basu, R.; Wang, F.; Paterson, D.I.; Alastalo, T.P.; Oudit, G.Y. Novel dominant-negative mutation in cardiac troponin I causes severe restrictive cardiomyopathy. *Circ. Heart Fail.* **2017**, *10*, e003820. [CrossRef]
63. Pantou, M.P.; Gourzi, P.; Gkouziouta, A.; Armenis, I.; Kaklamanis, L.; Zygouri, C.; Constantoulakis, P.; Adamopoulos, S.; Degiannis, D. A case report of recessive restrictive cardiomyopathy caused by a novel mutation in cardiac troponin I (TNNI3). *BMC Med. Genet.* **2019**, *20*, 61. [CrossRef]
64. Yang, S.W.; Hitz, M.P.; Andelfinger, G. Ventricular septal defect and restrictive cardiomyopathy in a paediatric TNNI3 mutation carrier. *Cardiol. Young* **2010**, *20*, 574–576. [CrossRef] [PubMed]
65. Gambarin, F.I.; Tagliani, M.; Arbustini, E. Pure restrictive cardiomyopathy associated with cardiac troponin I gene mutation: Mismatch between the lack of hypertrophy and the presence of disarray. *Heart* **2008**, *94*, 1257. [CrossRef] [PubMed]
66. Menon, S.C.; Michels, V.V.; Pellikka, P.A.; Ballew, J.D.; Karst, M.L.; Herron, K.J.; Nelson, S.M.; Rodeheffer, R.J.; Olson, T.M. Cardiac troponin T mutation in familial cardiomyopathy with variable remodeling and restrictive physiology. *Clin. Genet.* **2008**, *74*, 445–454. [CrossRef] [PubMed]
67. Ezekian, J.E.; Clippinger, S.R.; Garcia, J.M.; Yang, Q.; Denfield, S.; Jeewa, A.; Dreyer, W.J.; Zou, W.; Fan, Y.; Allen, H.D.; et al. Variant R94C in TNNT2-encoded troponin t predisposes to pediatric restrictive cardiomyopathy and sudden death through impaired thin filament relaxation resulting in myocardial diastolic dysfunction. *J. Am. Heart Assoc.* **2020**, *9*, e015111. [CrossRef] [PubMed]
68. Yamada, Y.; Namba, K.; Fujii, T. Cardiac muscle thin filament structures reveal calcium regulatory mechanism. *Nat. Commun.* **2020**, *11*, 153. [CrossRef] [PubMed]
69. Ueyama, H.; Inazawa, J.; Ariyama, T.; Nishino, H.; Ochiai, Y.; Ohkubo, I.; Miwa, T. Reexamination of chromosomal loci of human muscle actin genes by fluorescence in situ hybridization. *Jpn. J. Hum. Genet.* **1995**, *40*, 145–148. [CrossRef]
70. Gunning, P.; Ponte, P.; Kedes, L.; Eddy, R.; Shows, T. Chromosomal location of the co-expressed human skeletal and cardiac actin genes. *Proc. Natl. Acad. Sci. USA* **1984**, *81*, 1813–1817. [CrossRef]
71. Squire, J. Special issue: The actin-myosin interaction in muscle: Background and overview. *Int. J. Mol. Sci.* **2019**, *20*, 5715. [CrossRef]
72. Olson, T.M.; Michels, V.V.; Thibodeau, S.N.; Tai, Y.S.; Keating, M.T. Actin mutations in dilated cardiomyopathy, a heritable form of heart failure. *Science* **1998**, *280*, 750–752. [CrossRef]
73. Olson, T.M.; Doan, T.P.; Kishimoto, N.Y.; Whitby, F.G.; Ackerman, M.J.; Fananapazir, L. Inherited and de novo mutations in the cardiac actin gene cause hypertrophic cardiomyopathy. *J. Mol. Cell. Cardiol.* **2000**, *32*, 1687–1694. [CrossRef]
74. Klaassen, S.; Probst, S.; Oechslin, E.; Gerull, B.; Krings, G.; Schuler, P.; Greutmann, M.; Hurlimann, D.; Yegitbasi, M.; Pons, L.; et al. Mutations in sarcomere protein genes in left ventricular noncompaction. *Circulation* **2008**, *117*, 2893–2901. [CrossRef] [PubMed]
75. Greenway, S.C.; McLeod, R.; Hume, S.; Roslin, N.M.; Alvarez, N.; Giuffre, M.; Zhan, S.H.; Shen, Y.; Preuss, C.; Andelfinger, G.; et al. Exome sequencing identifies a novel variant in ACTC1 associated with familial atrial septal defect. *Can. J. Cardiol.* **2014**, *30*, 181–187. [CrossRef] [PubMed]
76. Sheikh, F.; Lyon, R.C.; Chen, J. Getting the skinny on thick filament regulation in cardiac muscle biology and disease. *Trends Cardiovasc. Med.* **2014**, *24*, 133–141. [CrossRef] [PubMed]
77. Warrick, H.M.; Spudich, J.A. Myosin structure and function in cell motility. *Annu. Rev. Cell Biol.* **1987**, *3*, 379–421. [CrossRef]
78. Alamo, L.; Ware, J.S.; Pinto, A.; Gillilan, R.E.; Seidman, J.G.; Seidman, C.E.; Padron, R. Effects of myosin variants on interacting-heads motif explain distinct hypertrophic and dilated cardiomyopathy phenotypes. *eLife* **2017**, *6*, e24634. [CrossRef]
79. Colegrave, M.; Peckham, M. Structural implications of beta-cardiac myosin heavy chain mutations in human disease. *Anat. Rec.* **2014**, *297*, 1670–1680. [CrossRef]
80. Vale, R.D.; Milligan, R.A. The way things move: Looking under the hood of molecular motor proteins. *Science* **2000**, *288*, 88–95. [CrossRef]
81. Trybus, K.M. Role of myosin light chains. *J. Muscle Res. Cell. Motil.* **1994**, *15*, 587–594. [CrossRef]
82. Wolny, M.; Colegrave, M.; Colman, L.; White, E.; Knight, P.J.; Peckham, M. Cardiomyopathy mutations in the tail of beta-cardiac myosin modify the coiled-coil structure and affect integration into thick filaments in muscle sarcomeres in adult cardiomyocytes. *J. Biol. Chem.* **2013**, *288*, 31952–31962. [CrossRef]
83. Geisterfer-Lowrance, A.A.; Kass, S.; Tanigawa, G.; Vosberg, H.P.; McKenna, W.; Seidman, C.E.; Seidman, J.G. A molecular basis for familial hypertrophic cardiomyopathy: A beta cardiac myosin heavy chain gene missense mutation. *Cell* **1990**, *62*, 999–1006. [CrossRef]
84. Moller, D.V.; Andersen, P.S.; Hedley, P.; Ersboll, M.K.; Bundgaard, H.; Moolman-Smook, J.; Christiansen, M.; Kober, L. The role of sarcomere gene mutations in patients with idiopathic dilated cardiomyopathy. *Eur. J. Hum. Genet.* **2009**, *17*, 1241–1249. [CrossRef] [PubMed]
85. Ferradini, V.; Parca, L.; Martino, A.; Lanzillo, C.; Silvetti, E.; Calo, L.; Caselli, S.; Novelli, G.; Helmer-Citterich, M.; Sangiuolo, F.C.; et al. Variants in MHY7 gene cause arrhythmogenic cardiomyopathy. *Genes* **2021**, *12*, 793. [CrossRef] [PubMed]
86. Olson, T.M.; Karst, M.L.; Whitby, F.G.; Driscoll, D.J. Myosin light chain mutation causes autosomal recessive cardiomyopathy with mid-cavitary hypertrophy and restrictive physiology. *Circulation* **2002**, *105*, 2337–2340. [CrossRef] [PubMed]
87. Yuan, C.C.; Kazmierczak, K.; Liang, J.; Kanashiro-Takeuchi, R.; Irving, T.C.; Gomes, A.V.; Wang, Y.; Burghardt, T.P.; Szczesna-Cordary, D. Hypercontractile mutant of ventricular myosin essential light chain leads to disruption of sarcomeric structure and function and results in restrictive cardiomyopathy in mice. *Cardiovasc. Res.* **2017**, *113*, 1124–1136. [CrossRef]

88. Poetter, K.; Jiang, H.; Hassanzadeh, S.; Master, S.R.; Chang, A.; Dalakas, M.C.; Rayment, I.; Sellers, J.R.; Fananapazir, L.; Epstein, N.D. Mutations in either the essential or regulatory light chains of myosin are associated with a rare myopathy in human heart and skeletal muscle. *Nat. Genet.* **1996**, *13*, 63–69. [CrossRef]
89. Flavigny, J.; Richard, P.; Isnard, R.; Carrier, L.; Charron, P.; Bonne, G.; Forissier, J.F.; Desnos, M.; Dubourg, O.; Komajda, M.; et al. Identification of two novel mutations in the ventricular regulatory myosin light chain gene (MYL2) associated with familial and classical forms of hypertrophic cardiomyopathy. *J. Mol. Med.* **1998**, *76*, 208–214. [CrossRef]
90. Osborn, D.P.S.; Emrahi, L.; Clayton, J.; Tabrizi, M.T.; Wan, A.Y.B.; Maroofian, R.; Yazdchi, M.; Garcia, M.L.E.; Galehdari, H.; Hesse, C.; et al. Autosomal recessive cardiomyopathy and sudden cardiac death associated with variants in MYL3. *Genet. Med.* **2021**, *23*, 787–792. [CrossRef]
91. Greenway, S.C.; Wilson, G.J.; Wilson, J.; George, K.; Kantor, P.F. Sudden death in an infant with angina, restrictive cardiomyopathy, and coronary artery bridging: An unusual phenotype for a beta-myosin heavy chain (MYH7) sarcomeric protein mutation. *Circ. Heart Fail.* **2012**, *5*, e92–e93. [CrossRef]
92. Neagoe, O.; Ciobanu, A.; Diaconu, R.; Mirea, O.; Donoiu, I.; Militaru, C. A rare case of familial restrictive cardiomyopathy, with mutations in MYH7 and ABCC9 genes. *Discoveries* **2019**, *7*, e99. [CrossRef]
93. Ware, S.M.; Quinn, M.E.; Ballard, E.T.; Miller, E.; Uzark, K.; Spicer, R.L. Pediatric restrictive cardiomyopathy associated with a mutation in beta-myosin heavy chain. *Clin. Genet.* **2008**, *73*, 165–170. [CrossRef]
94. Kawano, H.; Kawamura, K.; Kanda, M.; Ishijima, M.; Abe, K.; Hayashi, T.; Matsumoto, Y.; Kimura, A.; Maemura, K. Histopathological changes of myocytes in restrictive cardiomyopathy. *Med. Mol. Morphol.* **2021**, *54*, 289–295. [CrossRef] [PubMed]
95. Fan, L.L.; Guo, S.; Jin, J.Y.; He, Z.J.; Zhao, S.P.; Xiang, R.; Zhao, W. Whole exome sequencing identified a 13 base pair MYH7 deletion-mutation in a patient with restrictive cardiomyopathy and left ventricle hypertrophy. *Ann. Clin. Lab. Sci.* **2019**, *49*, 838–840. [PubMed]
96. Gerull, B. The rapidly evolving role of titin in cardiac physiology and cardiomyopathy. *Can. J. Cardiol.* **2015**, *31*, 1351–1359. [CrossRef] [PubMed]
97. Gerull, B.; Gramlich, M.; Atherton, J.; McNabb, M.; Trombitas, K.; Sasse-Klaassen, S.; Seidman, J.G.; Seidman, C.; Granzier, H.; Labeit, S.; et al. Mutations of TTN, encoding the giant muscle filament titin, cause familial dilated cardiomyopathy. *Nat. Genet.* **2002**, *30*, 201–204. [CrossRef]
98. Herman, D.S.; Lam, L.; Taylor, M.R.; Wang, L.; Teekakirikul, P.; Christodoulou, D.; Conner, L.; DePalma, S.R.; McDonough, B.; Sparks, E.; et al. Truncations of titin causing dilated cardiomyopathy. *N. Engl. J. Med.* **2012**, *366*, 619–628. [CrossRef]
99. Ware, J.S.; Cook, S.A. Role of titin in cardiomyopathy: From DNA variants to patient stratification. *Nat. Rev. Cardiol.* **2018**, *15*, 241–252. [CrossRef]
100. McAfee, Q.; Chen, C.Y.; Yang, Y.; Caporizzo, M.A.; Morley, M.; Babu, A.; Jeong, S.; Brandimarto, J.; Bedi, K.C., Jr.; Flam, E.; et al. Truncated titin proteins in dilated cardiomyopathy. *Sci. Transl. Med.* **2021**, *13*, eabd7287. [CrossRef]
101. Akinrinade, O.; Helio, T.; Lekanne Deprez, R.H.; Jongbloed, J.D.H.; Boven, L.G.; van den Berg, M.P.; Pinto, Y.M.; Alastalo, T.P.; Myllykangas, S.; Spaendonck-Zwarts, K.V.; et al. Relevance of titin missense and non-frameshifting insertions/deletions variants in dilated cardiomyopathy. *Sci. Rep.* **2019**, *9*, 4093. [CrossRef]
102. Brodehl, A.; Gaertner-Rommel, A.; Milting, H. Molecular insights into cardiomyopathies associated with desmin (DES) mutations. *Biophys. Rev.* **2018**, *10*, 983–1006. [CrossRef]
103. Dayal, A.A.; Medvedeva, N.V.; Nekrasova, T.M.; Duhalin, S.D.; Surin, A.K.; Minin, A.A. Desmin interacts directly with mitochondria. *Int. J. Mol. Sci.* **2020**, *21*, 8122. [CrossRef]
104. Patel, D.M.; Green, K.J. Desmosomes in the heart: A review of clinical and mechanistic analyses. *Cell Commun. Adhes.* **2014**, *21*, 109–128. [CrossRef] [PubMed]
105. Hatsell, S.; Cowin, P. Deconstructing desmoplakin. *Nat. Cell Biol.* **2001**, *3*, E270–E272. [CrossRef] [PubMed]
106. Gorza, L.; Sorge, M.; Secli, L.; Brancaccio, M. Master Regulators of muscle atrophy: Role of costamere components. *Cells* **2021**, *10*, 61. [CrossRef] [PubMed]
107. Wiche, G. Plectin-mediated intermediate filament functions: Why isoforms matter. *Cells* **2021**, *10*, 2154. [CrossRef] [PubMed]
108. Li, Z.; Colucci-Guyon, E.; Pincon-Raymond, M.; Mericskay, M.; Pournin, S.; Paulin, D.; Babinet, C. Cardiovascular lesions and skeletal myopathy in mice lacking desmin. *Dev. Biol.* **1996**, *175*, 362–366. [CrossRef]
109. Capetanaki, Y.; Milner, D.J.; Weitzer, G. Desmin in muscle formation and maintenance: Knockouts and consequences. *Cell Struct. Funct.* **1997**, *22*, 103–116. [CrossRef]
110. Schirmer, I.; Dieding, M.; Klauke, B.; Brodehl, A.; Gaertner-Rommel, A.; Walhorn, V.; Gummert, J.; Schulz, U.; Paluszkiewicz, L.; Anselmetti, D.; et al. A novel desmin (DES) indel mutation causes severe atypical cardiomyopathy in combination with atrioventricular block and skeletal myopathy. *Mol. Genet. Genom. Med.* **2018**, *6*, 288–293. [CrossRef]
111. Marakhonov, A.V.; Brodehl, A.; Myasnikov, R.P.; Sparber, P.A.; Kiseleva, A.V.; Kulikova, O.V.; Meshkov, A.N.; Zharikova, A.A.; Koretsky, S.N.; Kharlap, M.S.; et al. Noncompaction cardiomyopathy is caused by a novel in-frame desmin (DES) deletion mutation within the 1A coiled-coil rod segment leading to a severe filament assembly defect. *Hum. Mutat.* **2019**, *40*, 734–741. [CrossRef]
112. Kubanek, M.; Schimerova, T.; Piherova, L.; Brodehl, A.; Krebsova, A.; Ratnavadivel, S.; Stanasiuk, C.; Hansikova, H.; Zeman, J.; Palecek, T.; et al. Desminopathy: Novel desmin variants, a new cardiac phenotype, and further evidence for secondary mitochondrial dysfunction. *J. Clin. Med.* **2020**, *9*, 937. [CrossRef]

113. Protonotarios, A.; Brodehl, A.; Asimaki, A.; Jager, J.; Quinn, E.; Stanasiuk, C.; Ratnavadivel, S.; Futema, M.; Akhtar, M.M.; Gossios, T.D.; et al. The novel desmin variant p.Leu115Ile is associated with a unique form of biventricular arrhythmogenic cardiomyopathy. *Can. J. Cardiol.* **2021**, *37*, 857–866. [CrossRef]
114. Fischer, B.; Dittmann, S.; Brodehl, A.; Unger, A.; Stallmeyer, B.; Paul, M.; Seebohm, G.; Kayser, A.; Peischard, S.; Linke, W.A.; et al. Functional characterization of novel alpha-helical rod domain desmin (DES) pathogenic variants associated with dilated cardiomyopathy, atrioventricular block and a risk for sudden cardiac death. *Int. J. Cardiol.* **2021**, *329*, 167–174. [CrossRef] [PubMed]
115. Clemen, C.S.; Fischer, D.; Reimann, J.; Eichinger, L.; Muller, C.R.; Muller, H.D.; Goebel, H.H.; Schroder, R. How much mutant protein is needed to cause a protein aggregate myopathy in vivo? Lessons from an exceptional desminopathy. *Hum. Mutat.* **2009**, *30*, E490–E499. [CrossRef] [PubMed]
116. Brodehl, A.; Hain, C.; Flottmann, F.; Ratnavadivel, S.; Gaertner, A.; Klauke, B.; Kalinowski, J.; Körperich, H.; Gummert, J.; Paluszkiewicz, L.; et al. The desmin mutation DES-c.735G>C causes severe restrictive cardiomyopathy by inducing in-frame skipping of exon-3. *Biomedicines* **2021**, *9*, 1400. [CrossRef] [PubMed]
117. Chen, Z.; Li, R.; Wang, Y.; Cao, L.; Lin, C.; Liu, F.; Hu, R.; Nan, J.; Zhuang, X.; Lu, X.; et al. Features of myocardial injury detected by cardiac magnetic resonance in a patient with desmin-related restrictive cardiomyopathy. *ESC Heart Fail.* **2021**, *8*, 5560–5564. [CrossRef]
118. Herrmann, H.; Cabet, E.; Chevalier, N.R.; Moosmann, J.; Schultheis, D.; Haas, J.; Schowalter, M.; Berwanger, C.; Weyerer, V.; Agaimy, A.; et al. Dual Functional states of R406W-desmin assembly complexes cause cardiomyopathy with severe intercalated disc derangement in humans and in knock-in mice. *Circulation* **2020**, *142*, 2155–2171. [CrossRef]
119. Ojrzynska, N.; Bilinska, Z.T.; Franaszczyk, M.; Ploski, R.; Grzybowski, J. Restrictive cardiomyopathy due to novel desmin gene mutation. *Kardiol. Pol.* **2017**, *75*, 723. [CrossRef]
120. Jurcu, T.R.; Bastian, A.E.; Militaru, S.; Popa, A.; Manole, E.; Popescu, B.A.; Tallila, J.; Popescu, B.O.; Ginghina, C.D. Discovery of a new mutation in the desmin gene in a young patient with cardiomyopathy and muscular weakness. *Rom. J. Morphol. Embryol.* **2017**, *58*, 225–230.
121. Sharma, S.; Juneja, R.; Sharma, G.; Arava, S.; Ray, R. Desmin-related restrictive cardiomyopathy in a pediatric patient: A case report. *Indian J. Pathol. Microbiol.* **2013**, *56*, 402–404.
122. Pinol-Ripoll, G.; Shatunov, A.; Cabello, A.; Larrode, P.; de la Puerta, I.; Pelegrin, J.; Ramos, F.J.; Olive, M.; Goldfarb, L.G. Severe infantile-onset cardiomyopathy associated with a homozygous deletion in desmin. *Neuromuscul. Disord.* **2009**, *19*, 418–422. [CrossRef]
123. Bar, H.; Mucke, N.; Kostareva, A.; Sjoberg, G.; Aebi, U.; Herrmann, H. Severe muscle disease-causing desmin mutations interfere with in vitro filament assembly at distinct stages. *Proc. Natl. Acad. Sci. USA* **2005**, *102*, 15099–15104. [CrossRef]
124. Brodehl, A.; Hedde, P.N.; Dieding, M.; Fatima, A.; Walhorn, V.; Gayda, S.; Saric, T.; Klauke, B.; Gummert, J.; Anselmetti, D.; et al. Dual color photoactivation localization microscopy of cardiomyopathy-associated desmin mutants. *J. Biol. Chem.* **2012**, *287*, 16047–16057. [CrossRef] [PubMed]
125. Herrmann, H.; Aebi, U. Intermediate filaments: Structure and assembly. *Cold Spring Harb. Perspect. Biol.* **2016**, *8*, a018242. [CrossRef] [PubMed]
126. Quinlan, R.A.; Hatzfeld, M.; Franke, W.W.; Lustig, A.; Schulthess, T.; Engel, J. Characterization of dimer subunits of intermediate filament proteins. *J. Mol. Biol.* **1986**, *192*, 337–349. [CrossRef]
127. Parry, D.A.; Strelkov, S.V.; Burkhard, P.; Aebi, U.; Herrmann, H. Towards a molecular description of intermediate filament structure and assembly. *Exp. Cell Res.* **2007**, *313*, 2204–2216. [CrossRef]
128. Herrmann, H.; Haner, M.; Brettel, M.; Ku, N.O.; Aebi, U. Characterization of distinct early assembly units of different intermediate filament proteins. *J. Mol. Biol.* **1999**, *286*, 1403–1420. [CrossRef]
129. Herrmann, H.; Aebi, U. Intermediate filaments: Molecular structure, assembly mechanism, and integration into functionally distinct intracellular Scaffolds. *Annu. Rev. Biochem.* **2004**, *73*, 749–789. [CrossRef]
130. Colakoglu, G.; Brown, A. Intermediate filaments exchange subunits along their length and elongate by end-to-end annealing. *J. Cell Biol.* **2009**, *185*, 769–777. [CrossRef]
131. Winheim, S.; Hieb, A.R.; Silbermann, M.; Surmann, E.M.; Wedig, T.; Herrmann, H.; Langowski, J.; Mucke, N. Deconstructing the late phase of vimentin assembly by total internal reflection fluorescence microscopy (TIRFM). *PLoS ONE* **2011**, *6*, e19202. [CrossRef]
132. Noding, B.; Herrmann, H.; Koster, S. Direct observation of subunit exchange along mature vimentin intermediate filaments. *Biophys. J.* **2014**, *107*, 2923–2931. [CrossRef]
133. Park, K.Y.; Dalakas, M.C.; Goebel, H.H.; Ferrans, V.J.; Semino-Mora, C.; Litvak, S.; Takeda, K.; Goldfarb, L.G. Desmin splice variants causing cardiac and skeletal myopathy. *J. Med. Genet.* **2000**, *37*, 851–857. [CrossRef]
134. Arbustini, E.; Pasotti, M.; Pilotto, A.; Pellegrini, C.; Grasso, M.; Previtali, S.; Repetto, A.; Bellini, O.; Azan, G.; Scaffino, M.; et al. Desmin accumulation restrictive cardiomyopathy and atrioventricular block associated with desmin gene defects. *Eur. J. Heart Fail.* **2006**, *8*, 477–483. [CrossRef] [PubMed]
135. Olive, M.; Armstrong, J.; Miralles, F.; Pou, A.; Fardeau, M.; Gonzalez, L.; Martinez, F.; Fischer, D.; Martinez Matos, J.A.; Shatunov, A.; et al. Phenotypic patterns of desminopathy associated with three novel mutations in the desmin gene. *Neuromuscul. Disord.* **2007**, *17*, 443–450. [CrossRef] [PubMed]

136. Pruszczyk, P.; Kostera-Pruszczyk, A.; Shatunov, A.; Goudeau, B.; Draminska, A.; Takeda, K.; Sambuughin, N.; Vicart, P.; Strelkov, S.V.; Goldfarb, L.G.; et al. Restrictive cardiomyopathy with atrioventricular conduction block resulting from a desmin mutation. *Int. J. Cardiol.* **2007**, *117*, 244–253. [CrossRef] [PubMed]
137. Bar, H.; Goudeau, B.; Walde, S.; Casteras-Simon, M.; Mucke, N.; Shatunov, A.; Goldberg, Y.P.; Clarke, C.; Holton, J.L.; Eymard, B.; et al. Conspicuous involvement of desmin tail mutations in diverse cardiac and skeletal myopathies. *Hum. Mutat.* **2007**, *28*, 374–386. [CrossRef] [PubMed]
138. Bang, M.L.; Mudry, R.E.; McElhinny, A.S.; Trombitas, K.; Geach, A.J.; Yamasaki, R.; Sorimachi, H.; Granzier, H.; Gregorio, C.C.; Labeit, S. Myopalladin, a novel 145-kilodalton sarcomeric protein with multiple roles in Z-disc and I-band protein assemblies. *J. Cell Biol.* **2001**, *153*, 413–427. [CrossRef]
139. Filomena, M.C.; Yamamoto, D.L.; Carullo, P.; Medvedev, R.; Ghisleni, A.; Piroddi, N.; Scellini, B.; Crispino, R.; D'Autilia, F.; Zhang, J.; et al. Myopalladin knockout mice develop cardiac dilation and show a maladaptive response to mechanical pressure overload. *eLife* **2021**, *10*, e58313. [CrossRef]
140. Duboscq-Bidot, L.; Xu, P.; Charron, P.; Neyroud, N.; Dilanian, G.; Millaire, A.; Bors, V.; Komajda, M.; Villard, E. Mutations in the Z-band protein myopalladin gene and idiopathic dilated cardiomyopathy. *Cardiovasc. Res.* **2008**, *77*, 118–125. [CrossRef]
141. Bagnall, R.D.; Yeates, L.; Semsarian, C. Analysis of the Z-disc genes PDLIM3 and MYPN in patients with hypertrophic cardiomyopathy. *Int. J. Cardiol.* **2010**, *145*, 601–602. [CrossRef]
142. Miyatake, S.; Mitsuhashi, S.; Hayashi, Y.K.; Purevjav, E.; Nishikawa, A.; Koshimizu, E.; Suzuki, M.; Yatabe, K.; Tanaka, Y.; Ogata, K.; et al. Biallelic mutations in MYPN, encoding myopalladin, are associated with childhood-onset, slowly progressive nemaline myopathy. *Am. J. Hum. Genet.* **2017**, *100*, 169–178. [CrossRef]
143. Beggs, A.H.; Byers, T.J.; Knoll, J.H.; Boyce, F.M.; Bruns, G.A.; Kunkel, L.M. Cloning and characterization of two human skeletal muscle alpha-actinin genes located on chromosomes 1 and 11. *J. Biol. Chem.* **1992**, *267*, 9281–9288. [CrossRef]
144. Tiso, N.; Majetti, M.; Stanchi, F.; Rampazzo, A.; Zimbello, R.; Nava, A.; Danieli, G.A. Fine mapping and genomic structure of ACTN2, the human gene coding for the sarcomeric isoform of α-actinin-2, expressed in skeletal and cardiac muscle. *Biochem. Biophys. Res. Commun.* **1999**, *265*, 256–259. [CrossRef] [PubMed]
145. Wadmore, K.; Azad, A.J.; Gehmlich, K. The role of Z-disc proteins in myopathy and cardiomyopathy. *Int. J. Mol. Sci.* **2021**, *22*, 3058. [CrossRef] [PubMed]
146. Nicolas, A.; Delalande, O.; Hubert, J.F.; Le Rumeur, E. The spectrin family of proteins: A unique coiled-coil fold for various molecular surface properties. *J. Struct. Biol.* **2014**, *186*, 392–401. [CrossRef] [PubMed]
147. Davison, M.D.; Critchley, D.R. alpha-Actinins and the DMD protein contain spectrin-like repeats. *Cell* **1988**, *52*, 159–160. [CrossRef]
148. Djinovic-Carugo, K.; Gautel, M.; Ylanne, J.; Young, P. The spectrin repeat: A structural platform for cytoskeletal protein assemblies. *FEBS Lett.* **2002**, *513*, 119–123. [CrossRef]
149. Ribeiro Ede, A., Jr.; Pinotsis, N.; Ghisleni, A.; Salmazo, A.; Konarev, P.V.; Kostan, J.; Sjoblom, B.; Schreiner, C.; Polyansky, A.A.; Gkougkoulia, E.A.; et al. The structure and regulation of human muscle α-actinin. *Cell* **2014**, *159*, 1447–1460. [CrossRef]
150. Mohapatra, B.; Jimenez, S.; Lin, J.H.; Bowles, K.R.; Coveler, K.J.; Marx, J.G.; Chrisco, M.A.; Murphy, R.T.; Lurie, P.R.; Schwartz, R.J.; et al. Mutations in the muscle LIM protein and α-actinin-2 genes in dilated cardiomyopathy and endocardial fibroelastosis. *Mol. Genet. Metab.* **2003**, *80*, 207–215. [CrossRef]
151. Prondzynski, M.; Lemoine, M.D.; Zech, A.T.; Horvath, A.; Di Mauro, V.; Koivumaki, J.T.; Kresin, N.; Busch, J.; Krause, T.; Kramer, E.; et al. Disease modeling of a mutation in α-actinin 2 guides clinical therapy in hypertrophic cardiomyopathy. *EMBO Mol. Med.* **2019**, *11*, e11115. [CrossRef]
152. Park, J.; Cho, Y.G.; Park, H.W.; Cho, J.S. Case report: Novel likely pathogenic ACTN2 variant causing heterogeneous phenotype in a korean family with left ventricular non-compaction. *Front. Pediatr.* **2021**, *9*, 609389. [CrossRef]
153. Good, J.M.; Fellmann, F.; Bhuiyan, Z.A.; Rotman, S.; Pruvot, E.; Schlapfer, J. ACTN2 variant associated with a cardiac phenotype suggestive of left-dominant arrhythmogenic cardiomyopathy. *HeartRhythm Case Rep.* **2020**, *6*, 15–19. [CrossRef]
154. Inoue, M.; Noguchi, S.; Sonehara, K.; Nakamura-Shindo, K.; Taniguchi, A.; Kajikawa, H.; Nakamura, H.; Ishikawa, K.; Ogawa, M.; Hayashi, S.; et al. A recurrent homozygous ACTN2 variant associated with core myopathy. *Acta Neuropathol.* **2021**, *142*, 785–788. [CrossRef] [PubMed]
155. Vorgerd, M.; van der Ven, P.F.; Bruchertseifer, V.; Lowe, T.; Kley, R.A.; Schroder, R.; Lochmuller, H.; Himmel, M.; Koehler, K.; Furst, D.O.; et al. A mutation in the dimerization domain of filamin c causes a novel type of autosomal dominant myofibrillar myopathy. *Am. J. Hum. Genet.* **2005**, *77*, 297–304. [CrossRef]
156. Duff, R.M.; Tay, V.; Hackman, P.; Ravenscroft, G.; McLean, C.; Kennedy, P.; Steinbach, A.; Schoffler, W.; van der Ven, P.F.M.; Furst, D.O.; et al. Mutations in the N-terminal actin-binding domain of filamin C cause a distal myopathy. *Am. J. Hum. Genet.* **2011**, *88*, 729–740. [CrossRef]
157. Chakarova, C.; Wehnert, M.S.; Uhl, K.; Sakthivel, S.; Vosberg, H.P.; van der Ven, P.F.; Furst, D.O. Genomic structure and fine mapping of the two human filamin gene paralogues *FLNB* and *FLNC* and comparative analysis of the filamin gene family. *Hum. Genet.* **2000**, *107*, 597–611. [CrossRef] [PubMed]
158. Mao, Z.; Nakamura, F. Structure and function of filamin c in the muscle Z-disc. *Int. J. Mol. Sci.* **2020**, *21*, 2696. [CrossRef]
159. Pudas, R.; Kiema, T.R.; Butler, P.J.; Stewart, M.; Ylanne, J. Structural basis for vertebrate filamin dimerization. *Structure* **2005**, *13*, 111–119. [CrossRef] [PubMed]

160. van der Ven, P.F.; Obermann, W.M.; Lemke, B.; Gautel, M.; Weber, K.; Furst, D.O. Characterization of muscle filamin isoforms suggests a possible role of gamma-filamin/ABP-L in sarcomeric Z-disc formation. *Cell Motil. Cytoskelet.* **2000**, *45*, 149–162. [CrossRef]
161. Labeit, S.; Lahmers, S.; Burkart, C.; Fong, C.; McNabb, M.; Witt, S.; Witt, C.; Labeit, D.; Granzier, H. Expression of distinct classes of titin isoforms in striated and smooth muscles by alternative splicing, and their conserved interaction with filamins. *J. Mol. Biol.* **2006**, *362*, 664–681. [CrossRef]
162. Gonzalez-Morales, N.; Holenka, T.K.; Schock, F. Filamin actin-binding and titin-binding fulfill distinct functions in Z-disc cohesion. *PLoS Genet.* **2017**, *13*, e1006880. [CrossRef]
163. Gontier, Y.; Taivainen, A.; Fontao, L.; Sonnenberg, A.; van der Flier, A.; Carpen, O.; Faulkner, G.; Borradori, L. The Z-disc proteins myotilin and FATZ-1 interact with each other and are connected to the sarcolemma via muscle-specific filamins. *J. Cell Sci.* **2005**, *118 Pt 16*, 3739–3749. [CrossRef]
164. Thompson, T.G.; Chan, Y.M.; Hack, A.A.; Brosius, M.; Rajala, M.; Lidov, H.G.; McNally, E.M.; Watkins, S.; Kunkel, L.M. Filamin 2 (FLN2): A muscle-specific sarcoglycan interacting protein. *J. Cell Biol.* **2000**, *148*, 115–126. [CrossRef] [PubMed]
165. Valdes-Mas, R.; Gutierrez-Fernandez, A.; Gomez, J.; Coto, E.; Astudillo, A.; Puente, D.A.; Reguero, J.R.; Alvarez, V.; Moris, C.; Leon, D.; et al. Mutations in filamin C cause a new form of familial hypertrophic cardiomyopathy. *Nat. Commun.* **2014**, *5*, 5326. [CrossRef] [PubMed]
166. Begay, R.L.; Tharp, C.A.; Martin, A.; Graw, S.L.; Sinagra, G.; Miani, D.; Sweet, M.E.; Slavov, D.B.; Stafford, N.; Zeller, M.J.; et al. *FLNC* gene splice mutations cause dilated cardiomyopathy. *JACC Basic Transl. Sci.* **2016**, *1*, 344–359. [CrossRef] [PubMed]
167. Augusto, J.B.; Eiros, R.; Nakou, E.; Moura-Ferreira, S.; Treibel, T.A.; Captur, G.; Akhtar, M.M.; Protonotarios, A.; Gossios, T.D.; Savvatis, K.; et al. Dilated cardiomyopathy and arrhythmogenic left ventricular cardiomyopathy: A comprehensive genotype-imaging phenotype study. *Eur. Heart J. Cardiovasc. Imaging* **2020**, *21*, 326–336. [CrossRef]
168. Van Waning, J.I.; Hoedemaekers, Y.M.; te Rijdt, W.P.; Jpma, A.I.; Heijsman, D.; Caliskan, K.; Hoendermis, E.S.; Willems, T.P.; van den Wijngaard, A.; Suurmeijer, A. *FLNC* missense variants in familial noncompaction cardiomyopathy. *Cardiogenetics* **2019**, *9*, 9–13. [CrossRef]
169. Reinstein, E.; Gutierrez-Fernandez, A.; Tzur, S.; Bormans, C.; Marcu, S.; Tayeb-Fligelman, E.; Vinkler, C.; Raas-Rothschild, A.; Irge, D.; Landau, M.; et al. Congenital dilated cardiomyopathy caused by biallelic mutations in Filamin C. *Eur. J. Hum. Genet.* **2016**, *24*, 1792–1796. [CrossRef]
170. Chen, J.; Wu, J.; Han, C.; Li, Y.; Guo, Y.; Tong, X. A mutation in the filamin c gene causes myofibrillar myopathy with lower motor neuron syndrome: A case report. *BMC Neurol.* **2019**, *19*, 198. [CrossRef]
171. Dalkilic, I.; Schienda, J.; Thompson, T.G.; Kunkel, L.M. Loss of FilaminC (FLNc) results in severe defects in myogenesis and myotube structure. *Mol. Cell. Biol.* **2006**, *26*, 6522–6534. [CrossRef]
172. Ruparelia, A.A.; Zhao, M.; Currie, P.D.; Bryson-Richardson, R.J. Characterization and investigation of zebrafish models of filamin-related myofibrillar myopathy. *Hum. Mol. Genet.* **2012**, *21*, 4073–4083. [CrossRef]
173. Fujita, M.; Mitsuhashi, H.; Isogai, S.; Nakata, T.; Kawakami, A.; Nonaka, I.; Noguchi, S.; Hayashi, Y.K.; Nishino, I.; Kudo, A. *Filamin C* plays an essential role in the maintenance of the structural integrity of cardiac and skeletal muscles, revealed by the medaka mutant zacro. *Dev. Biol.* **2012**, *361*, 79–89. [CrossRef]
174. Deo, R.C.; Musso, G.; Tasan, M.; Tang, P.; Poon, A.; Yuan, C.; Felix, J.F.; Vasan, R.S.; Beroukhim, R.; De Marco, T.; et al. Prioritizing causal disease genes using unbiased genomic features. *Genome Biol.* **2014**, *15*, 534. [CrossRef] [PubMed]
175. Chevessier, F.; Schuld, J.; Orfanos, Z.; Plank, A.C.; Wolf, L.; Maerkens, A.; Unger, A.; Schlotzer-Schrehardt, U.; Kley, R.A.; Von Horsten, S.; et al. Myofibrillar instability exacerbated by acute exercise in filaminopathy. *Hum. Mol. Genet.* **2015**, *24*, 7207–7220. [CrossRef] [PubMed]
176. Kiselev, A.; Vaz, R.; Knyazeva, A.; Khudiakov, A.; Tarnovskaya, S.; Liu, J.; Sergushichev, A.; Kazakov, S.; Frishman, D.; Smolina, N.; et al. De novo mutations in *FLNC* leading to early-onset restrictive cardiomyopathy and congenital myopathy. *Hum. Mutat.* **2018**, *39*, 1161–1172. [CrossRef] [PubMed]
177. Ruparelia, A.A.; Oorschot, V.; Ramm, G.; Bryson-Richardson, R.J. *FLNC* myofibrillar myopathy results from impaired autophagy and protein insufficiency. *Hum. Mol. Genet.* **2016**, *25*, 2131–2142. [CrossRef]
178. Zhou, Y.; Chen, Z.; Zhang, L.; Zhu, M.; Tan, C.; Zhou, X.; Evans, S.M.; Fang, X.; Feng, W.; Chen, J. Loss of *Filamin C* is catastrophic for heart function. *Circulation* **2020**, *141*, 869–871. [CrossRef]
179. Rodina, N.; Khudiakov, A.; Perepelina, K.; Muravyev, A.; Boytsov, A.; Zlotina, A.; Sokolnikova, P.; Kostareva, A. Generation of iPSC line (FAMRCi009-A) from patient with familial progressive cardiac conduction disorder carrying genetic variant *FLNC* p.Val2264Met. *Stem Cell Res.* **2021**, *59*, 102640. [CrossRef]
180. Perepelina, K.; Khudiakov, A.; Rodina, N.; Boytsov, A.; Vavilova, T.; Zlotina, A.; Sokolnikova, P.; Kostareva, A. Generation of iPSC line FAMRCi010-A from patient with restrictive cardiomyopathy carrying genetic variant *FLNC* p.Gly2011Arg. *Stem Cell Res.* **2021**, *59*, 102639. [CrossRef]
181. Tucker, N.R.; McLellan, M.A.; Hu, D.; Ye, J.; Parsons, V.A.; Mills, R.W.; Clauss, S.; Dolmatova, E.; Shea, M.A.; Milan, D.J.; et al. Novel mutation in *FLNC* (*Filamin C*) causes familial restrictive cardiomyopathy. *Circ. Cardiovasc. Genet.* **2017**, *10*, e001780. [CrossRef]
182. Xiao, F.; Wei, Q.; Wu, B.; Liu, X.; Mading, A.; Yang, L.; Li, Y.; Liu, F.; Pan, X.; Wang, H. Clinical exome sequencing revealed that *FLNC* variants contribute to the early diagnosis of cardiomyopathies in infant patients. *Transl. Pediatr.* **2020**, *9*, 21–33. [CrossRef]

183. Roldan-Sevilla, A.; Palomino-Doza, J.; de Juan, J.; Sanchez, V.; Dominguez-Gonzalez, C.; Salguero-Bodes, R.; Arribas-Ynsaurriaga, F. Missense mutations in the *FLNC* gene causing familial restrictive cardiomyopathy. *Circ. Genom. Precis. Med.* **2019**, *12*, e002388. [CrossRef]
184. Schubert, J.; Tariq, M.; Geddes, G.; Kindel, S.; Miller, E.M.; Ware, S.M. Novel pathogenic variants in *Filamin C* identified in pediatric restrictive cardiomyopathy. *Hum. Mutat.* **2018**, *39*, 2083–2096. [CrossRef] [PubMed]
185. Aebi, U.; Cohn, J.; Buhle, L.; Gerace, L. The nuclear lamina is a meshwork of intermediate-type filaments. *Nature* **1986**, *323*, 560–564. [CrossRef] [PubMed]
186. Dobrzynska, A.; Gonzalo, S.; Shanahan, C.; Askjaer, P. The nuclear lamina in health and disease. *Nucleus* **2016**, *7*, 233–248. [CrossRef] [PubMed]
187. Fatkin, D.; MacRae, C.; Sasaki, T.; Wolff, M.R.; Porcu, M.; Frenneaux, M.; Atherton, J.; Vidaillet, H.J., Jr.; Spudich, S.; De Girolami, U.; et al. Missense mutations in the rod domain of the lamin A/C gene as causes of dilated cardiomyopathy and conduction-system disease. *N. Engl. J. Med.* **1999**, *341*, 1715–1724. [CrossRef]
188. Quarta, G.; Syrris, P.; Ashworth, M.; Jenkins, S.; Zuborne Alapi, K.; Morgan, J.; Muir, A.; Pantazis, A.; McKenna, W.J.; Elliott, P.M. Mutations in the Lamin A/C gene mimic arrhythmogenic right ventricular cardiomyopathy. *Eur. Heart J.* **2012**, *33*, 1128–1136. [CrossRef]
189. Liu, Z.; Shan, H.; Huang, J.; Li, N.; Hou, C.; Pu, J. A novel lamin A/C gene missense mutation (445 V > E) in immunoglobulin-like fold associated with left ventricular non-compaction. *Europace* **2016**, *18*, 617–622. [CrossRef]
190. Raffaele Di Barletta, M.; Ricci, E.; Galluzzi, G.; Tonali, P.; Mora, M.; Morandi, L.; Romorini, A.; Voit, T.; Orstavik, K.H.; Merlini, L.; et al. Different mutations in the LMNA gene cause autosomal dominant and autosomal recessive Emery-Dreifuss muscular dystrophy. *Am. J. Hum. Genet.* **2000**, *66*, 1407–1412. [CrossRef]
191. Shackleton, S.; Lloyd, D.J.; Jackson, S.N.; Evans, R.; Niermeijer, M.F.; Singh, B.M.; Schmidt, H.; Brabant, G.; Kumar, S.; Durrington, P.N.; et al. LMNA, encoding lamin A/C, is mutated in partial lipodystrophy. *Nat. Genet.* **2000**, *24*, 153–156. [CrossRef]
192. Eriksson, M.; Brown, W.T.; Gordon, L.B.; Glynn, M.W.; Singer, J.; Scott, L.; Erdos, M.R.; Robbins, C.M.; Moses, T.Y.; Berglund, P.; et al. Recurrent de novo point mutations in lamin A cause Hutchinson-Gilford progeria syndrome. *Nature* **2003**, *423*, 293–298. [CrossRef]
193. Merner, N.D.; Hodgkinson, K.A.; Haywood, A.F.; Connors, S.; French, V.M.; Drenckhahn, J.D.; Kupprion, C.; Ramadanova, K.; Thierfelder, L.; McKenna, W.; et al. Arrhythmogenic right ventricular cardiomyopathy type 5 is a fully penetrant, lethal arrhythmic disorder caused by a missense mutation in the TMEM43 gene. *Am. J. Hum. Genet.* **2008**, *82*, 809–821. [CrossRef]
194. Hirata, T.; Fujita, M.; Nakamura, S.; Gotoh, K.; Motooka, D.; Murakami, Y.; Maeda, Y.; Kinoshita, T. Post-Golgi anterograde transport requires GARP-dependent endosome-to-TGN retrograde transport. *Mol. Biol. Cell* **2015**, *26*, 3071–3084. [CrossRef] [PubMed]
195. Russell, M.W.; Raeker, M.O.; Geisler, S.B.; Thomas, P.E.; Simmons, T.A.; Bernat, J.A.; Thorsson, T.; Innis, J.W. Functional analysis of candidate genes in 2q13 deletion syndrome implicates FBLN7 and TMEM87B deficiency in congenital heart defects and FBLN7 in craniofacial malformations. *Hum. Mol. Genet.* **2014**, *23*, 4272–4284. [CrossRef] [PubMed]
196. Garrido, C.; Paul, C.; Seigneuric, R.; Kampinga, H.H. The small heat shock proteins family: The long forgotten chaperones. *Int. J. Biochem. Cell Biol.* **2012**, *44*, 1588–1592. [CrossRef] [PubMed]
197. Dubin, R.A.; Ally, A.H.; Chung, S.; Piatigorsky, J. Human αB-crystallin gene and preferential promoter function in lens. *Genomics* **1990**, *7*, 594–601. [CrossRef]
198. Dimauro, I.; Antonioni, A.; Mercatelli, N.; Caporossi, D. The role of αB-crystallin in skeletal and cardiac muscle tissues. *Cell Stress Chaperones* **2018**, *23*, 491–505. [CrossRef]
199. Chepelinsky, A.B.; Piatigorsky, J.; Pisano, M.M.; Dubin, R.A.; Wistow, G.; Limjoco, T.I.; Klement, J.F.; Jaworski, C.J. Lens protein gene expression: Alpha-crystallins and MIP. *Lens Eye Toxic Res.* **1991**, *8*, 319–344.
200. Sacconi, S.; Feasson, L.; Antoine, J.C.; Pecheux, C.; Bernard, R.; Cobo, A.M.; Casarin, A.; Salviati, L.; Desnuelle, C.; Urtizberea, A. A novel CRYAB mutation resulting in multisystemic disease. *Neuromuscul. Disord.* **2012**, *22*, 66–72. [CrossRef]
201. Safieh, L.A.; Khan, A.O.; Alkuraya, F.S. Identification of a novel CRYAB mutation associated with autosomal recessive juvenile cataract in a Saudi family. *Mol. Vis.* **2009**, *15*, 980–984.
202. Inagaki, N.; Hayashi, T.; Arimura, T.; Koga, Y.; Takahashi, M.; Shibata, H.; Teraoka, K.; Chikamori, T.; Yamashina, A.; Kimura, A. αB-crystallin mutation in dilated cardiomyopathy. *Biochem. Biophys. Res. Commun.* **2006**, *342*, 379–386. [CrossRef]
203. Peschek, J.; Braun, N.; Franzmann, T.M.; Georgalis, Y.; Haslbeck, M.; Weinkauf, S.; Buchner, J. The eye lens chaperone α-crystallin forms defined globular assemblies. *Proc. Natl. Acad. Sci. USA* **2009**, *106*, 13272–13277. [CrossRef]
204. Ganea, E. Chaperone-like activity of alpha-crystallin and other small heat shock proteins. *Curr. Protein Pept. Sci.* **2001**, *2*, 205–225. [CrossRef] [PubMed]
205. Bullard, B.; Ferguson, C.; Minajeva, A.; Leake, M.C.; Gautel, M.; Labeit, D.; Ding, L.; Labeit, S.; Horwitz, J.; Leonard, K.R.; et al. Association of the chaperone αB-crystallin with titin in heart muscle. *J. Biol. Chem.* **2004**, *279*, 7917–7924. [CrossRef] [PubMed]
206. Jehle, S.; Rajagopal, P.; Bardiaux, B.; Markovic, S.; Kuhne, R.; Stout, J.R.; Higman, V.A.; Klevit, R.E.; van Rossum, B.J.; Oschkinat, H. Solid-state NMR and SAXS studies provide a structural basis for the activation of αB-crystallin oligomers. *Nat. Struct. Mol. Biol.* **2010**, *17*, 1037–1042. [CrossRef] [PubMed]

207. Rajasekaran, N.S.; Connell, P.; Christians, E.S.; Yan, L.J.; Taylor, R.P.; Orosz, A.; Zhang, X.Q.; Stevenson, T.J.; Peshock, R.M.; Leopold, J.A.; et al. Human αB-crystallin mutation causes oxido-reductive stress and protein aggregation cardiomyopathy in mice. *Cell* **2007**, *130*, 427–439. [CrossRef] [PubMed]
208. Sturner, E.; Behl, C. The role of the multifunctional BAG3 protein in cellular protein quality control and in disease. *Front. Mol. Neurosci.* **2017**, *10*, 177. [CrossRef] [PubMed]
209. Takayama, S.; Xie, Z.; Reed, J.C. An evolutionarily conserved family of Hsp70/Hsc70 molecular chaperone regulators. *J. Biol. Chem.* **1999**, *274*, 781–786. [CrossRef] [PubMed]
210. Lin, H.; Koren, S.A.; Cvetojevic, G.; Girardi, P.; Johnson, G.V.W. The role of BAG3 in health and disease: A "Magic BAG of Tricks". *J. Cell. Biochem.* **2022**, *123*, 4–21. [CrossRef]
211. Kogel, D.; Linder, B.; Brunschweiger, A.; Chines, S.; Behl, C. At the crossroads of apoptosis and autophagy: Multiple roles of the Co-chaperone bag3 in stress and therapy resistance of cancer. *Cells* **2020**, *9*, 574. [CrossRef]
212. Takayama, S.; Reed, J.C. Molecular chaperone targeting and regulation by BAG family proteins. *Nat. Cell Biol.* **2001**, *3*, E237–E241. [CrossRef]
213. Sondermann, H.; Scheufler, C.; Schneider, C.; Hohfeld, J.; Hartl, F.U.; Moarefi, I. Structure of a Bag/Hsc70 complex: Convergent functional evolution of Hsp70 nucleotide exchange factors. *Science* **2001**, *291*, 1553–1557. [CrossRef]
214. Shemetov, A.A.; Gusev, N.B. Biochemical characterization of small heat shock protein HspB8 (Hsp22)-Bag3 interaction. *Arch. Biochem. Biophys.* **2011**, *513*, 1–9. [CrossRef] [PubMed]
215. Morelli, F.F.; Mediani, L.; Heldens, L.; Bertacchini, J.; Bigi, I.; Carra, A.D.; Vinet, J.; Carra, S. An interaction study in mammalian cells demonstrates weak binding of HSPB2 to BAG3, which is regulated by HSPB3 and abrogated by HSPB8. *Cell Stress Chaperones* **2017**, *22*, 531–540. [CrossRef] [PubMed]
216. Hishiya, A.; Salman, M.N.; Carra, S.; Kampinga, H.H.; Takayama, S. BAG3 directly interacts with mutated αB-crystallin to suppress its aggregation and toxicity. *PLoS ONE* **2011**, *6*, e16828. [CrossRef] [PubMed]
217. Rauch, J.N.; Tse, E.; Freilich, R.; Mok, S.A.; Makley, L.N.; Southworth, D.R.; Gestwicki, J.E. BAG3 is a modular, scaffolding protein that physically links heat shock protein 70 (Hsp70) to the small heat shock proteins. *J. Mol. Biol.* **2017**, *429*, 128–141. [CrossRef] [PubMed]
218. Fuchs, M.; Poirier, D.J.; Seguin, S.J.; Lambert, H.; Carra, S.; Charette, S.J.; Landry, J. Identification of the key structural motifs involved in HspB8/HspB6-Bag3 interaction. *Biochem. J.* **2009**, *425*, 245–255. [CrossRef] [PubMed]
219. Mizushima, W.; Sadoshima, J. BAG3 plays a central role in proteostasis in the heart. *J. Clin. Investig.* **2017**, *127*, 2900–2903. [CrossRef] [PubMed]
220. Norton, N.; Li, D.; Rieder, M.J.; Siegfried, J.D.; Rampersaud, E.; Zuchner, S.; Mangos, S.; Gonzalez-Quintana, J.; Wang, L.; McGee, S.; et al. Genome-wide studies of copy number variation and exome sequencing identify rare variants in BAG3 as a cause of dilated cardiomyopathy. *Am. J. Hum. Genet.* **2011**, *88*, 273–282. [CrossRef]
221. Semmler, A.L.; Sacconi, S.; Bach, J.E.; Liebe, C.; Burmann, J.; Kley, R.A.; Ferbert, A.; Anderheiden, R.; Van den Bergh, P.; Martin, J.J.; et al. Unusual multisystemic involvement and a novel BAG3 mutation revealed by NGS screening in a large cohort of myofibrillar myopathies. *Orphanet J. Rare Dis.* **2014**, *9*, 121. [CrossRef]
222. Kimura, K.; Ooms, A.; Graf-Riesen, K.; Kuppusamy, M.; Unger, A.; Schuld, J.; Daerr, J.; Lother, A.; Geisen, C.; Hein, L.; et al. Overexpression of human BAG3(P209L) in mice causes restrictive cardiomyopathy. *Nat. Commun.* **2021**, *12*, 3575. [CrossRef]
223. Fang, X.; Bogomolovas, J.; Zhou, P.S.; Mu, Y.; Ma, X.; Chen, Z.; Zhang, L.; Zhu, M.; Veevers, J.; Ouyang, K.; et al. P209L mutation in Bag3 does not cause cardiomyopathy in mice. *Am. J. Physiol. Heart Circ. Physiol.* **2019**, *316*, H392–H399. [CrossRef]
224. Kobuke, K.; Furukawa, Y.; Sugai, M.; Tanigaki, K.; Ohashi, N.; Matsumori, A.; Sasayama, S.; Honjo, T.; Tashiro, K. ESDN, a novel neuropilin-like membrane protein cloned from vascular cells with the longest secretory signal sequence among eukaryotes, is up-regulated after vascular injury. *J. Biol. Chem.* **2001**, *276*, 34105–34114. [CrossRef] [PubMed]
225. Schmoker, A.M.; Ebert, A.M.; Ballif, B.A. The DCBLD receptor family: Emerging signaling roles in development, homeostasis and disease. *Biochem. J.* **2019**, *476*, 931–950. [CrossRef] [PubMed]
226. Sadeghi, M.M.; Esmailzadeh, L.; Zhang, J.; Guo, X.; Asadi, A.; Krassilnikova, S.; Fassaei, H.R.; Luo, G.; Al-Lamki, R.S.; Takahashi, T.; et al. ESDN is a marker of vascular remodeling and regulator of cell proliferation in graft arteriosclerosis. *Am. J. Transplant.* **2007**, *7*, 2098–2105. [CrossRef]
227. Nie, L.; Guo, X.; Esmailzadeh, L.; Zhang, J.; Asadi, A.; Collinge, M.; Li, X.; Kim, J.D.; Woolls, M.; Jin, S.W.; et al. Transmembrane protein ESDN promotes endothelial VEGF signaling and regulates angiogenesis. *J. Clin. Investig.* **2013**, *123*, 5082–5097. [CrossRef]
228. Xie, P.; Yuan, F.Q.; Huang, M.S.; Zhang, W.; Zhou, H.H.; Li, X.; Liu, Z.Q. DCBLD2 affects the development of colorectal cancer via emt and angiogenesis and modulates 5-FU drug resistance. *Front. Cell Dev. Biol.* **2021**, *9*, 669285. [CrossRef] [PubMed]
229. Olivotto, I.; Oreziak, A.; Barriales-Villa, R.; Abraham, T.P.; Masri, A.; Garcia-Pavia, P.; Saberi, S.; Lakdawala, N.K.; Wheeler, M.T.; Owens, A.; et al. Mavacamten for treatment of symptomatic obstructive hypertrophic cardiomyopathy (EXPLORER-HCM): A randomised, double-blind, placebo-controlled, phase 3 trial. *Lancet* **2020**, *396*, 759–769. [CrossRef]
230. Teerlink, J.R.; Diaz, R.; Felker, G.M.; McMurray, J.J.V.; Metra, M.; Solomon, S.D.; Adams, K.F.; Anand, I.; Arias-Mendoza, A.; Biering-Sorensen, T.; et al. Cardiac myosin activation with omecamtiv mecarbil in systolic heart failure. *N. Engl. J. Med.* **2021**, *384*, 105–116. [CrossRef]
231. Jinek, M.; Chylinski, K.; Fonfara, I.; Hauer, M.; Doudna, J.A.; Charpentier, E. A programmable dual-RNA-guided DNA endonuclease in adaptive bacterial immunity. *Science* **2012**, *337*, 816–821. [CrossRef]

232. Ozcan, A.; Krajeski, R.; Ioannidi, E.; Lee, B.; Gardner, A.; Makarova, K.S.; Koonin, E.V.; Abudayyeh, O.O.; Gootenberg, J.S. Programmable RNA targeting with the single-protein CRISPR effector Cas7-11. *Nature* **2021**, *597*, 720–725. [CrossRef]
233. Jungmann, A.; Leuchs, B.; Rommelaere, J.; Katus, H.A.; Muller, O.J. Protocol for efficient generation and characterization of adeno-associated viral vectors. *Hum. Gene Ther. Methods* **2017**, *28*, 235–246. [CrossRef]
234. Weinmann, J.; Weis, S.; Sippel, J.; Tulalamba, W.; Remes, A.; El Andari, J.; Herrmann, A.K.; Pham, Q.H.; Borowski, C.; Hille, S.; et al. Identification of a myotropic AAV by massively parallel in vivo evaluation of barcoded capsid variants. *Nat. Commun.* **2020**, *11*, 5432. [CrossRef] [PubMed]
235. Fomin, A.; Gartner, A.; Cyganek, L.; Tiburcy, M.; Tuleta, I.; Wellers, L.; Folsche, L.; Hobbach, A.J.; von Frieling-Salewsky, M.; Unger, A.; et al. Truncated titin proteins and titin haploinsufficiency are targets for functional recovery in human cardiomyopathy due to TTN mutations. *Sci. Transl. Med.* **2021**, *13*, eabd3079. [CrossRef] [PubMed]

Journal of
Clinical Medicine

MDPI

Review

Treatment of Transthyretin Amyloid Cardiomyopathy: The Current Options, the Future, and the Challenges

Carsten Tschöpe [1,2,3,*] and Ahmed Elsanhoury [1,2]

1 Berlin Institute of Health (BIH) Center for Regenerative Therapies (BCRT), Campus Virchow Clinic, Charité–University Medicine Berlin, D-13353 Berlin, Germany; ahmed.elsanhoury@charite.de
2 German Centre for Cardiovascular Research (DZHK), Partner Site Berlin, D-13353 Berlin, Germany
3 Department of Cardiology, Campus Virchow Klinikum, Charité–University Medicine Berlin, D-13353 Berlin, Germany
* Correspondence: carsten.tschoepe@charite.de; Tel.: +49-(30)-450-553711

Abstract: Transthyretin amyloid cardiomyopathy (ATTR-CM) is a progressively debilitating, rare disease associated with high mortality. ATTR-CM occurs when TTR amyloid protein builds up in the myocardium along with different organs, most commonly the peripheral and the autonomic nervous systems. Managing the cardiac complications with standard heart failure medications is difficult due to the challenge to maintain a balance between the high filling pressure associated with restricted ventricular volume and the low cardiac output. To date, tafamidis is the only agent approved for ATTR-CM treatment. Besides, several agents, including green tea, tolcapone, and diflunisal, are used off-label in ATTR-CM patients. Novel therapies using RNA interference also offer clinical promise. Patisiran and inotersen are currently approved for ATTR-polyneuropathy of hereditary origin and are under investigation for ATTR-CM. Monoclonal antibodies in the early development phases carry hope for amyloid deposit clearance. Despite several drug candidates in the clinical development pipeline, the small ATTR-CM patient population raises several challenges. This review describes current and future therapies for ATTR-CM and sheds light on the clinical development hurdles facing them.

Keywords: transthyretin amyloid cardiomyopathy; TTR amyloid; cardiac amyloidosis; tafamidis; clinical development

Citation: Tschöpe, C.; Elsanhoury, A. Treatment of Transthyretin Amyloid Cardiomyopathy: The Current Options, the Future, and the Challenges. *J. Clin. Med.* **2022**, *11*, 2148. https://doi.org/10.3390/jcm11082148

Academic Editor: Stefan Peters

Received: 21 March 2022
Accepted: 8 April 2022
Published: 12 April 2022

1. Introduction

Amyloidosis is a rare disease in which amyloid fibrils misfold and aggregate into toxic oligomers that build up extracellularly in the tissue [1]. It can affect different organs, most commonly the heart, kidneys, liver, spleen, peripheral nerves, and gastrointestinal tract [1,2]. There are different types of amyloidosis according to the nature of the misfolded protein. Immunoglobulin light chain amyloidosis (AL) and transthyretin amyloidosis (ATTR) are the main two types of amyloidosis that affect the heart [2,3]. The first results from abnormal plasma cell production of monoclonal light chain fragments that misfold, causing myocardial toxicity [2,4]. The latter results from the dissociation and misfolding of the transthyretin (TTR), the protein that transports thyroxine (T4) and retinol-binding protein (RBP) in the serum and cerebrospinal fluid [2,5]. Both forms together account for nearly 95% of all cardiac amyloidosis cases [2,3,6]. TTR is mainly produced by the liver (90%) and circulates as a homotetramer. The choroid plexus and retinal epithelium produce the remaining 10% [7,8]. Destabilization of the tetramer results in the dissociation and aggregation of amyloid fibrils, which then accumulate in the interstitial space of various organs, causing progressive loss of function [9,10]. Transthyretin amyloid cardiomyopathy (ATTR-CM) is a rare, progressively debilitating disease that occurs when TTR builds up in the myocardium along with the peripheral and autonomic nervous systems [10].

ATTR-CM often presents with progressive heart failure with right- and left-sided symptoms, complicated by arrhythmias, most commonly atrial fibrillation, owing to conduction abnormalities [10,11]. However, cardiac symptoms are often proceeded by musculoskeletal manifestation (e.g., carpal tunnel syndrome) [12]. There are two forms of ATTR-CM, hereditary and wild type. Hereditary ATTR-CM (ATTRv) is characterized by a single amino acid substitution caused by a point mutation in the *TTR* gene, located on the long arm of chromosome 18 [13,14]. The most common mutation in ATTRv-CM is V122I, present in African Americans at a prevalence of 3.4% [15]. The prevalence of the V122I mutation in non-African American descents is low or possibly under-estimated. Wild-type ATTR-CM (ATTRwt), previously termed senile cardiac amyloidosis (SSA), is a non-familial form of the disease that predominantly presents in elderly male patients [16,17]. Both ATTR-CM forms are associated with impaired survival rates. The median survival of untreated ATTR-CM is 2.5 years for ATTRv V122I and 3.6 years for ATTRwt [18]. ATTR-CM is usually misdiagnosed, particularly early in its course owing to non-specific symptoms and multi-system involvement [19,20]. Lately, ATTR-CM is increasingly being recognized in clinical practice as a result of increased disease awareness and enhanced diagnostic techniques. Echocardiography-measured strain indices, advanced magnetic resonance imaging modalities, including T1 mapping and extracellular volume evaluation, as well as bone scintigraphy provide the necessary tools for the non-invasive diagnosis of ATTR-CM [20]. Moreover, genetic testing is instrumental to confirm the diagnosis of ATTRv. A definitive diagnosis could be reached with the aforementioned non-invasive tools, yet endomyocardial biopsy (EMB) evaluation is recommended in cases where AL amyloidosis cannot be ruled out via serum analysis [21]. However, histologic differentiation between ATTR and AL amyloidosis cannot be based solely on the Congo red staining. There is a compelling medical need to develop therapies for ATTR-CM, being an incapacitative illness that is eventually fatal if left untreated [22]. For many decades, the treatment of ATTRv-CM consisted of liver transplantation to remove the source of misfolded TTR or combined liver/heart transplantation, besides symptomatic treatments or solely heart transplantation in advanced ATTRwt-CM [23]. After the positive results of the ATTR-ACT study [24], the United States Food and Drug Administration (FDA) and the European Medicines Agency (EMA) have granted tafamidis 61 mg capsules marketing authorization for ATTRv and ATTRwt-CM. However, so far, no treatment can reverse the disease. This review discusses the current and future therapies for ATTR-CM and the hurdles facing their clinical development.

2. Symptomatic Treatments

The distinctive pathophysiology of ATTR-CM, characterized by both restrictive ventricular filling and reduced stroke volume, renders the use of standard heart failure medications difficult [18], summarized in Table 1. Loop diuretics are vital to reduce cardiac and peripheral congestion, especially in patients with right ventricular (RV) congestion and pulmonary edema, which subsequently relieves dyspnea [18,25,26], preferably taken in combination with aldosterone antagonists to prevent hypokalemia. However, blood pressure must be monitored adequately, since reducing preload may adversely affect renal perfusion and cardiac output [18]. Drugs acting on the renin-angiotensin system are poorly tolerated since they exacerbate hypotension, especially in patients with amyloid-associated autonomic dysfunction [18,26]. Beta-blockers are also poorly tolerated due to their negative chronotropic effect, given the restricted ventricular volume and the reliance of the cardiac output on the heart rate [18,26]. Calcium channel blockers and digoxin are generally contraindicated due to their profound binding to amyloid, which intensifies their pharmacologic effects and can result in cardiac rhythm disturbances or sudden death [18,26,27]. However, digoxin can be an option for pulse control in uncontrollable tachyarrhythmia absoluta. Alpha-1-adrenoreceptor agonists such as midodrine can treat orthostatic hypotension allowing higher doses of diuretics [28]. Amiodarone is the anti-arrhythmic agent of choice for patients with atrial fibrillation/flutter [28]. Oral anticoagulants are particularly required for patients with atrial fibrillation since blood stasis is a major source of thromboembolic events [18,29,30]. Pacemaker implantation is necessary for up to 25–36% of ATTRv patients and as many as 43% of ATTRwt patients [26,31]. However, in ATTR-CM patients pacemaker implantation is associated with high risk and worse survival [32]. There is no clear indication for prophylactic implantable cardioverter-defibrillator (ICD) therapy in ATTR-CM, since arrhythmias are not the primary cause of cardiac death in this population, except for patients with a high burden of ventricular tachycardias [33]. In general, the symptomatic management of ATTR-CM follows the CHAD-STOP concept: conduction and rhythm disorders prevention, high heart rate maintenance, anticoagulation, diuretics, and STOP ß-receptor and calcium-channel blockers, digoxin, and renin-angiotensin-aldosterone inhibitors [34].

Table 1. The use of standard heart failure therapies in transthyretin amyloid cardiomyopathy. * *except for* pulse control in uncontrollable tachyarrhythmia absoluta.

	Yes	*Sometimes*	*No*
Diuretics ± aldosterone antagonists	✓		
Renin-angiotensin system inhibitors		–	
Beta-adrenoreceptor blockers		–	
Alpha-1-adrenoreceptor agonists		–	
Calcium channel blockers			✗
Digoxin *			✗

3. Supportive Therapy with Epigallocatechin-3-Gallate (Green Tea)

Epigallocatechin-3-gallate (EGCG) is a polyphenolic natural compound most abundant in green tea [35]. EGCG is well tolerated, without major safety concerns. It has been shown to disaggregate amyloid fibrils and prevent TTR formation [36]. An observational study reported that the treatment of ATTR-CM patients with green tea extract for nine months was able to reduce left ventricular (LV) wall mass and thickness [36]. However, in a single-center retrospective study, patients who received a 675 mg daily dose of EGCG for a minimum of nine months did not gain any survival benefit compared to patients on solely symptomatic treatment [37].

4. Specific Treatments

For many decades, liver transplantation has been considered the only approach to halt the progression of ATTRv-CM. Although liver transplantation removes the main source of aberrant amyloid protein, it does not provide a complete cure for the disease. In a large collective of 2127 liver transplant patients who were included in Familial Amyloidotic Polyneuropathy World Transplant Registry (FAPWTR), the overall 20-year survival rate was 55.3%. The largest benefit was observed in ATTRv patients carrying the most common pVal50Met variant [38]. The reason behind the incomplete cure is the aggregation of newly formed amyloid around the preexisting amyloid seeds [39]. Combining liver and heart transplantation can overcome this setback [40]. Moreover, this treatment approach is restricted by the availability of transplant organs as well as the advanced age and comorbidities of most ATTR-CM patients, which limits the feasibility of undergoing surgery and the need for life-long immunosuppression therapy [41]. Accordingly, there is a great need for ATTR-CM-specific pharmacological treatments. In 2019, the U.S. Food and Drug

Administration (FDA) approved tafamidis at a dose-strength of 61 mg capsule as the first pharmacologic treatment for ATTR-CM of any kind. Different pharmacological treatments are used off-label or in the development pipeline. However, none of them is yet approved for ATTR-CM, as illustrated in Figure 1.

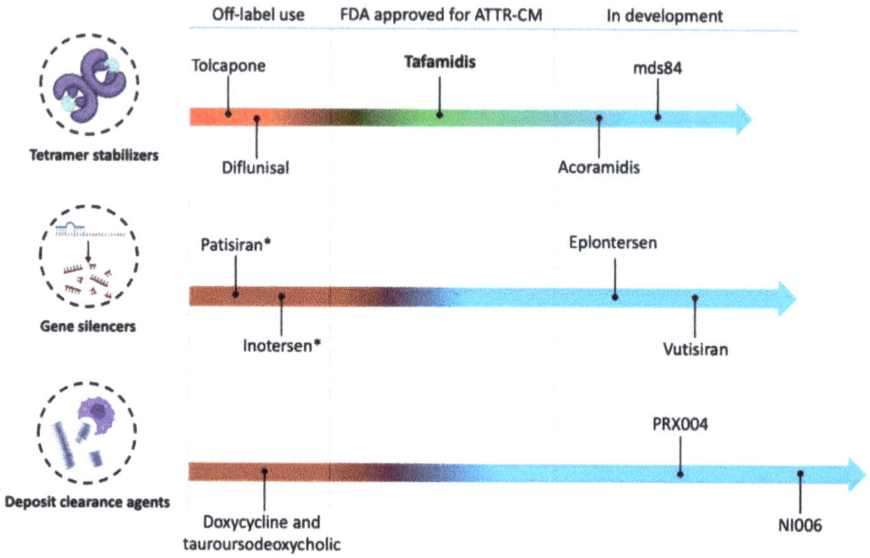

Figure 1. The clinical development pipeline of therapies for transthyretin amyloid cardiomyopathy (ATTR-CM). * Approved by the American food and drug administration and the European medicine agency for the treatment of ATTR-polyneuropathy. Figure cartoons were created with Biorender.com (accessed on 11 March 2022).

4.1. Transthyretin Tetramer Stabilization

Dissociation of the TTR tetramer is considered the rate-limiting step in the amyloidogenesis [42]. The binding of T4 into one of the two interdimeric binding pockets of TTE increases the stability of the tetramer. When both binding pockets are occupied, the tetramer becomes more stable. However, the binding of T4 to one of the pockets exerts a negative cooperativity effect that reduces the accessibility to the second binding pocket by undergoing a conformational change [43].

4.1.1. Tolcapone

Tolcapone is an orally available catechol-O-methyltransferase inhibitor used for the treatment of Parkinson's disease, usually in combination with levodopa and carbidopa. It has a high binding affinity to the TTR binding pockets, stabilizing the tetramer [44]. Tolcapone is used as an off-label medication for ATTR-CM. The results of a phase IIa study (NCT02191826) support the repurposing of tolcapone for both ATTRwt and ATTRv. The study showed that tolcapone increases TTR stability by 52% 2 h following a single 200 mg dose. Patients who received 100 mg of tolcapone every 4 h showed a 38.8% increase in TTR stability 2 h following the first dose, and this effect was maintained for 24 h [45]. Owing to its high central nervous system (CNS) penetrance, tolcapone was evaluated in a proof-of-concept study as a possible treatment for leptomeningeal ATTR, a rare CNS form of ATTR. The study was completed in April 2019, but the results are not yet published (NCT03591757). Despite these promising results, the clinical application of tolcapone in ATTR-CM is rather difficult. The drug has a short half-life, which mandates short dosing intervals. The side effects of tolcapone are severe, including hepatotoxicity, sleep disturbances, dyskinesia, and gastrointestinal disturbances. In addition, the drug is metabolized through the CYP2C9 enzyme which causes interactions with a wide range of medications, e.g., warfarin and sulfonylurea [46–48].

4.1.2. Diflunisal

Diflunisal is an FDA-approved non-steroidal anti-inflammatory agent (NSAID). Due to its structural match to T4, diflunisal can bind and stabilize the TTR tetramer [42]. A randomized placebo-controlled clinical trial showed that diflunisal significantly reduces the neurological impairment and preserved quality of life of familial amyloid polyneuropathy, a neurological phenotype of ATTR [49]. The results of an open-label observational study that monitored the effect of diflunisal 500 mg daily support its efficacy in ATTRv patients. However, around 19% of the patients dropped out due to typical NSAID side-effects of diflunisal, most prominently gastrolesivity, cardiotoxicity, and nephrotoxicity [50]. A retrospective cohort study of 35 patients with ATTRwt-CM showed that diflunisal administration improved survival and overall stability in clinical echocardiographic disease markers [51]. Another retrospective study on 81 ATTR-CM patients (54 with ATTRwt) showed that diflunisal treatment for a median of one year is associated with reductions in cardiac troponin, brain natriuretic peptide (BNP), and favourable differences in echocardiographic parameters [52]. Chemical-structure modification deprived diflunisal of its cyclooxygenase inhibitory action while maintaining its TTR stabilizing effect. The new similarly structured compound was later called tafamidis [53,54].

4.1.3. Tafamidis

Tafamidis meglumine (20 mg) was approved in 2011 by the EMA for stage I ATTRv polyneuropathy following the results of an 18-month phase III clinical trial (NCT00409175) where it was able to stop the disease progression in 60% of the treated compared to 38% of the placebo group [55,56]. The results of several open-label studies on patients with cardiac and neurological ATTR phenotypes warranted the investigation of tafamidis meglumine in ATTR-CM patients [57–59]. In 2018, the ATTR-ACT (NCT01994889) multicenter, international, double-blind, placebo-controlled, phase 3 trial, randomly assigned 441 patients with transthyretin amyloid cardiomyopathy (76% ATTRwt) in a 2:1:2 ratio to receive a daily dose of 80 mg of tafamidis meglumine, 20 mg of tafamidis meglumine, or placebo for 30 months [24]. In the composite endpoint based on a hierarchical analysis of all-cause mortality and the frequency of cardiovascular (CV) hospitalization, Tafamidis meglumine showed superiority versus placebo with a win ratio of 1.7 in a pooled approach of both doses at 18 months. Tafamidis meglumine was associated with 30% lower all-cause mortality than placebo (29.5% vs. 42.9%) and a lower rate of cardiovascular-related hospitalizations with a risk reduction of 32%. As secondary outcome parameters, tafamidis was associated with a lower rate of decline in the 6 min walk test distance and a lower rate of decline in the quality of life assessed by the score on the Kansas City Cardiomyopathy Questionnaire. Subgroup analysis showed the significant superiority of tafamidis meglumine over placebo except in patients with New York Heart Association (NYHA) class III at baseline, with an even more pronounced CV-hospitalization rate. Tafamidis meglumine was well tolerated with minor side effects, principally urinary tract infection. There was no meaningful difference in the safety of the two doses of tafamidis meglumine [24]. Higher tafamidis plasma concentrations, with doses > 60 mg tafamidis meglumine are required to achieve maximum TTR kinetic stability [60]. The results of the clinical trial supported the FDA and EMA ATTR-CM following bioequivalence studies, to grant marketing authorization of a once-daily dose of tafamidis 61 mg free acid single capsule [61]. More recently, an open-label long-term extension of the ATTR-ACT trial showed a significantly greater survival benefit with tafamidis meglumine 80 mg (4 × 20 mg) over 20 mg [62]. Further analyses from the ATTR-ACT trial showed that severely limited 6 min walk test distance (<269 m) at baseline is associated with lower mortality, but higher hospitalization compared to placebo, which can be designated clinically as the point of therapy reconciliation in NYHA

III [63]. A statistical post-hoc analysis taking deaths in NYHA III patients into account could also show a benefit in CV-hospitalization rates in the survivors [64]. Based on the primary analysis with reflections to significance, the ESC granted a 1B recommendation for tafamidis in patients with hereditary ATTRv-CM or ATTRwt-CM and NYHA class I or II symptoms to reduce symptoms, CV hospitalization, and mortality [65].

4.1.4. Acoramidis

Acoramidis (AG10) is an orally active TTR stabilizer under investigation. The small molecule mimics the protective TTR mutation Thr119Met by forming hydrogen bonds with the serine residues at position 117 [66]. In human plasma samples of ATTRwt, AG10 is slightly more potent as a TTR kinetic stabilizer compared to tafamidis and tolcapone. However, a dose of 1600 mg AG10 per day is required to reach the same effect of 80 mg tafamidis meglumine [67]. In a randomized, double-blind, placebo-controlled study, 49 patients with ATTRwt or ATTRm were treated with AG10 800 mg or 400 mg or placebo for 28 days. The mean changes in the serum concentration of TTR were 50%, 36%, and −7% compared to baseline, respectively. This result indicates TTR stabilization at high AG10 doses [66]. The currently ongoing ATTRibute-CM study (NCT03860935) evaluates the efficacy of AG10 800 mg b.i.d. against placebo. The study is designed to enroll 510 patients with symptomatic ATTR-CM, with an estimated completion date of May 2023. Recently, BridgeBio Pharma announced that the 12-month topline results of the ATTRibute-CM trial did not meet its primary endpoint [68].

4.1.5. Bivalent TTR Stabilizers

Mds84 is a bivalent TTR ligand that simultaneously binds both binding pockets. This property overcomes the monovalent agent's negative cooperativity binding effect [69]. In vitro, it exhibited more potent TTR stabilization compared to monovalent agents, including tolcapone and tafamidis [69,70]. However, mds84 has not been evaluated in clinical trials.

4.2. *Transthyretin Gene Silencers*

Replacing the source of aberrant TTR protein via liver transplantation has been the only effective treatment strategy for decades. ATTRv patients could only benefit from liver transplantation reaching a one-year survival rate of 74.3% and three- and five-year survival rates of 60.0% and 52.5%, respectively [71]. A paradigm-changing strategy is knocking down the gene responsible for TTR production in the liver. This is possible via small interfering RNA (siRNA) and antisense oligonucleotides (ASOs) targeting the TTR messenger RNA (mRNA) leading to its degradation before translation [72]. Knocking down the TTR gene suppresses the circulating TTR protein and disables retinol (vitamin A) transport around the body, mandating oral substitution [73]. In addition, siRNA and ASO therapies are associated with infusion-related reactions, requiring premedications or thrombopenia [71,73].

4.2.1. Patisiran

Patisiran is a siRNA encapsulated in lipid-based nanoparticles enabling hepatic uptake via micropinocytosis [74]. It is the first-ever FDA-approved RNA-interfering therapy and it is indicated for Coutinho stages I and II of hereditary ATTR-polyneuropathy. Following the results of the APOLLO study, the EMA approved patisiran for mild and moderate stages of the disease. The study enrolled 225 patients with ATTRv-polyneuropathy in a placebo-controlled design. Patients who received patisiran (0.3 mg/kg every two weeks for 18 months) showed improved neurological manifestation compared to those who received placebo [75]. Typical side effects included peripheral edema and infusion reactions, mandating pre-medication with dexamethasone and histamine receptor blocker. In a subpopulation of the APOLLO study comprised of 126 patients with cardiac involvement (56% of the total population, but defined only with LV-wall thickness >13 mm in the absence of hypertension or aortic valve disease), patisiran reduced the LV wall thickness by 0.9 ± 0.4 mm, decreased global longitudinal strain by −1.4 ± 0.6%, and increased cardiac output by 0.38 ± 0.19 L/min. However, in the main cohort, there were seven deaths, all cardiovascular related, five of which were due to sudden cardiac death. In contrast, there were six deaths in the placebo group, of which only three were cardiovascular-related. It has not been elucidated whether patisiran has a causal relationship with cardiac death [76]. Recently, a small cohort of 16 hereditary ATTR-CM patients on patisiran underwent serial monitoring using cardiac magnetic resonance, echocardiography, cardiac biomarkers, bone scintigraphy, and 6-min walk tests over 12 months. Twelve patients were on concomitant diflunisal 250 mg twice daily. The results were compared to 16 retrospectively matched ATTR-CM patients who did not receive patisiran. The median serum TTR gene knockdown among treated patients was 86%. Interestingly, 82% of patients demonstrated >80% gene knockdown. Moreover, the treatment was associated with a −6.2% reduction in cardiac extracellular volume (ECV), a fall in N-terminal pro-BNP (NT-proBNP) concentrations by 1342 ng/L, an increase in 6-min walk distances by 169 m, and a median reduction in cardiac uptake by bone scintigraphy of 19.6% [77]. The APOLLO-B study (NCT03997383) is a phase III, multicenter, randomized, placebo-controlled study that investigates patisiran in ATTR-CM patients. The primary outcome measure is only the change from baseline at month 12 in the 6-min walk distance. The estimated study completion date is June 2025.

4.2.2. Inotersen

Inotersen is a subcutaneously administered ASO, approved by the FDA and EMA for hereditary ATTR-polyneuropathy following the results of the NEURO-ATTR study. The approval of inotersen came two months after that of patisiran. The NEURO-ATTR study enrolled 172 patients who were randomized in a 2:1 ratio to inotrasine (300 mg every week) or placebo. Compared to placebo, the treatment group showed improved neurological manifestation, improved quality of life, and reduced mean serum TTR level by 75% from baseline [78]. Recently, Dasgupta et al. showed that long-term treatment with inotersen is safe and effective in inhibiting progression and potentially reversing the cardiac amyloid burden. Sixteen patients who completed two years of inotersen treatment showed a mean LV mass reduction of 8.4% as measured by magnetic resonance imaging, and a mean 6-min walk distance improvement by 20.2 m [79]. Today, inotersen is indicated for patients with primary hereditary ATTR-polyneuropathy stage (I–II), after the exclusion of significant ATTR-CM.

4.2.3. Revusiran

Revusiran is the first N-acetylgalactosamine (GalNAc) conjugated siRNA to enter clinical trials. GalNAc is a galactose derivative that binds to the asialoglycoprotein receptor (ASGPR) on hepatocytes leading to clathrin-mediated uptake. This advancement allows dose-reduction and enables subcutaneous administration [80]. The Phase 3 ENDEAVOUR study evaluated revusiran in patients with ATTR-CM [81]. The patients were randomized 2:1 to receive subcutaneous daily revusiran 500 mg (n = 140) or placebo (n = 66) for five days over a week followed by weekly doses. The study was prematurely terminated after 6.71 months due to high mortality in the revusiran-treated arm (18 deaths) compared to the placebo-treated arm (two deaths). The subsequent analysis did not reveal any causality [81].

4.2.4. Second Generation TTR Gene Silencers

Molecular modifications known as enhanced stabilization chemistry (ESC) patterns characterize second-generation RNA interference agents. ESC remarkably enhances the pharmacodynamic and pharmacokinetic properties of the RNA interference agents, allowing a significantly lower dose, with a markedly reduced dosing frequency compared to the first-generation agents [82].

Vutrisiran, formerly known as ALN-TTRsc02, is a long-acting, subcutaneously administered successor of patisiran. In a phase I, randomized, single-blind, placebo-controlled trial on 80 healthy subjects, vutrisiran demonstrated a favourable safety profile and sustained TTR plasma level reduction in a dose-dependent manner [83]. The drug is currently in a patisiran-controlled phase III trial for patients with hereditary ATTR- polyneuropathy (HELIOS-A, NCT03759379), and in a placebo-controlled phase III trial for patients with hereditary and wild-type ATTR-CM (HELIOS-B, NCT04153149). The phase III trials are estimated to be completed by May 2024 and June 2025, respectively. HELIOS-B is designed to evaluate the efficacy of vutisiran in the composite endpoint of all-cause Mortality and recurrent cardiovascular events at month 30. The study patients are 1:1 randomized to receive either vutrisiran 25 mg or placebo, subcutaneously once every three months. Recently, the drug developer announced that HELIOS-A has met all secondary endpoints measured at 18 months. In addition to improvements in exploratory cardiac endpoints including NT-proBNP, echocardiographic and scintigraphy parameters relative to placebo [84]. The FDA is currently evaluating the new drug application of vutisiran and has set an action date of April 2022.

Eplontersen, formerly known as AKCEA-TTR-LRx or IONIS-TTR-LRx, is the GalNAc-conjugated successor of inotersen. The global phase III NEURO-TTRansform study (NCT04136184) is currently evaluating eplontersen subcutaneous injections 45 mg every four weeks against inotersen 284 mg weekly in patients with hereditary ATTR-polyneuropathy [85]. In parallel, the CARDIO-TTRransform phase III study (NCT04136171) is evaluating eplontersen in ATTR-CM patients in a double-blind, randomized, placebo-controlled design. The primary endpoint is the composite cardiovascular mortality and cardiovascular event rate at week 120. The study completion date is estimated to be around June 2024.

4.3. Gene Editing

The recently introduced clustered regularly interspaced short palindromic repeats and associated Cas9 endonuclease (CRISPR-Cas9) gene-editing system has revolutionized biomedical research via allowing one-time treatment for deadly diseases including ATTR-CM [86]. NTLA-2001 is the first CRISPR-Cas9 therapy investigated in humans. Preclinical studies showed durable knockout of TTR after a single dose of NTLA-2001. Preliminary results from six hereditary ATTR-polyneuropathy patients enrolled in phase 1, open-label, multicenter study warrant further evaluation (NCT04601051) [87]. Three patients received a dose of 0.1 mg per kg and another three received 0.3 mg per kg. On day 28, NTLA-2001 was associated with mean TTR reductions of 52% in the first group and 87% in the second group, respectively. Mild adverse events were observed in three of the six patients [87]. The phase I study estimated completion date is August 2024.

4.4. Enhancing Amyloid Clearance

4.4.1. Doxycycline and Tauroursodeoxycholic Acid

Doxycycline is an FDA-approved broad-spectrum antibiotic that belongs to the tetracyclines family. Tetracyclines can bind to the ribosomal subunits disrupting the synthesis of aggregation-prone proteins [88,89]. Preclinical studies on familial amyloidotic polyneuropathy mice showed that a combination of doxycycline and tauroursodeoxycholic acid (TUDCA) could remove TTR amyloid deposits and lower associated tissue markers [90]. Clinical studies have conflicting results considering the tolerability of the combination therapy. A phase II study concluded that the doxycycline/TUDCA combination is effective to halt the progression of ATTR neuropathy and cardiomyopathy with an acceptable toxicity profile [91]. In contrast, another phase II study with 28 ATTR-CM patients could only retain 36% of the enrolled patients due to adverse events including sun hypersensitivity and gastrointestinal side effects, in addition to heart function deterioration indicated by NT-proBNP elevation in the evaluated patients [92].

4.4.2. Human Monoclonal Antibodies

Targeting pathological TTR amyloid deposits while sparing physiological TTR tetramers is conceivable via antibodies designed to recognize prefibrillar and fibrillar TTR-specific epitopes [93]. Antibody binding mediates the elimination of ATTR aggregates via phagocytes, which potentially leads to amyloid clearance [94]. Two drugs in this category have reached the clinical development pipeline, both designed to inhibit fibril formation via specifically targeting misfolded TTR, namely PRX004 and NI006. A phase I trial evaluating PRX004 in ATTRm patients has been recently terminated because of the COVID pandemic (NCT03336580). NI006 is currently under evaluation in a phase I, randomized, placebo-controlled, double-blind, dose-escalation trial, followed by an open-label extension phase in subjects with ATTR-CM (NCT04360434). The study completion date is estimated to be June 2022.

5. Discussion

ATTR-CM is an orphan disease characterized by a small patient population. The clinical development of therapies for ATTR-CM faces several challenges, as shown in Figure 2. Tafamidis (20 mg), patisiran, and inotersen are approved by the EMA (Patisiran and Inotersen by FDA also) for ATTR-polyneuropathy. Currently, only tafamidis (61 mg) is approved for ATTRv/wt-CM worldwide and recommended by the European society of cardiology guidelines as a class 1b indication in ATTR-CM patients with NYHA functional class I-II [65]. Up to now, no head-to-head comparison has been made between any of them. The three agents come at very high price tags exceeding €10,000 per month [95]. This can be attributed to the high research and development cost, the advanced technology involved in manufacturing, and most decisively the small market size. To generate sufficient revenue, orphan-designated therapeutics are high-priced [96]. The EMA offers 10 years of market exclusivity as an incentive to develop orphan-designated products. Tafamidis was granted orphan market exclusivity by the EMA based on designation EU/3/06/401. The initial price of tafamidis greatly exceeded the conventional cost-effectiveness thresholds in the US [97]. However, some price reductions are expected after the orphan market exclusivity and introduction of other stabilizers. The second wave of price reduction with generic drugs is not expected before 2026. Clinical trials in orphan diseases like ATTR-CM are challenging, the small target population results in limited power to detect the difference and greater outcome variability [98]. In part, developed treatments target the liver, being the main source of TTR. However, around 5–10% of TTR is produced in the choroid plexus and retina. A drug needs to be able to cross the blood–brain barrier (BBB) to target more neurological forms like leptomeningeal ATTR. Of the three approved medications, only tafamidis can cross the BBB. However, no more than 1.5% of the plasma-circulating drug reach the cerebrospinal fluid [99,100], which is a target of further research. Such patients may benefit from the off-label use of tolcapone. However, the use of tolcapone is limited by its hepatotoxicity and short half-life. Improving the kinetic properties of drug molecules to reduce the dose and/or the frequency of dosing has been achievable in some cases. The free acid tafamidis formulation of 61 mg allows a lower tablet consumption compared to the conventional tafamidis meglumine (4 × 20 mg). Efforts to increase the stability of the currently approved siRNA and ASOs would allow long-term TTR knock-down and less frequent dosing. Conformation-specific monoclonal antibodies are very promising and would allow clearance of the amyloid deposits without affecting the physiological TTR. Ongoing studies will determine whether ATTR-CM patients can benefit from hereditary ATTR-polyneuropathy targeting treatments. We suggest that future ATTR-polyneuropathy studies would need to include more cardiovascular-related inclusion criteria and endpoints. Direct comparative studies between different TTR-targeting treatments have been hampered by the sample size, different clinical endpoints, costs, and other reasons [101]. Post-marketing studies would be beneficial to compare the effectiveness of the different agents in the real world and to determine their superiority over each other's taking the cost into account. In conclusion, tafamidis is the current standard of care for ATTR-CM with

NYHA I-II. Patisiran and inotersen are currently used for hereditary ATTR-polyneuropathy on the way to being approved for ATTR-CM. Patients with contraindications to tafamidis or who have no insurance coverage may benefit from green tea or from the off-label use of diflunisal or tolcapone.

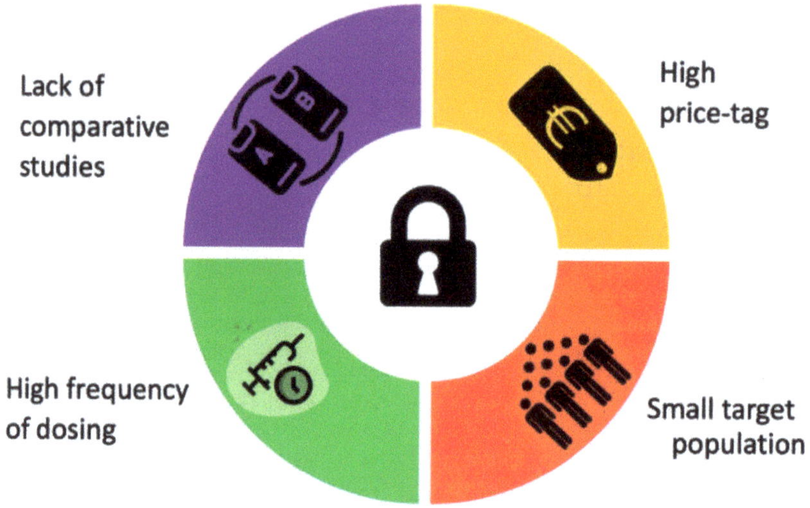

Figure 2. Challenges facing the clinical development of therapies for transthyretin amyloid cardiomyopathy.

Author Contributions: C.T. and A.E. have contributed equally to this manuscript. All authors have read and agreed to the published version of the manuscript.

Funding: This research received no external funding.

Data Availability Statement: Not applicable.

Conflicts of Interest: C.T. has received speaker fees and/or contributions to congresses from Abbott, Abiomed, Astra Zeneca, Bayer, Böhringer-Ingelheim, Novartis, and Pfizer.

References

1. Gillmore, J.D.; Hawkins, P.N. Pathophysiology and treatment of systemic amyloidosis. *Nat. Rev. Nephrol.* **2013**, *9*, 574–586. [CrossRef] [PubMed]
2. Donnelly, J.; Hanna, M. Cardiac amyloidosis: An update on diagnosis and treatment. *Cleve Clin. J. Med.* **2017**, *84* (Suppl. S3), 12–26. [CrossRef] [PubMed]
3. Kholova, I.; Niessen, H.W. Amyloid in the cardiovascular system: A review. *J. Clin. Pathol.* **2005**, *58*, 125–133. [CrossRef] [PubMed]
4. Muchtar, E.; Buadi, F.K.; Dispenzieri, A.; Gertz, M.A. Immunoglobulin Light-Chain Amyloidosis: From Basics to New Developments in Diagnosis, Prognosis and Therapy. *Acta Haematol.* **2016**, *135*, 172–190. [CrossRef] [PubMed]
5. Liz, M.A.; Mar, F.M.; Franquinho, F.; Sousa, M.M. Aboard transthyretin: From transport to cleavage. *IUBMB Life* **2010**, *62*, 429–435. [CrossRef]
6. Maleszewski, J.J. Cardiac amyloidosis: Pathology, nomenclature, and typing. *Cardiovasc. Pathol.* **2015**, *24*, 343–350. [CrossRef]
7. Kelly, J.W.; Colon, W.; Lai, Z.; Lashuel, H.A.; Mcculloch, J.; Mccutchen, S.L.; Miroy, G.J.; Peterson, S.A. Transthyretin quaternary and tertiary structural changes facilitate misassembly into amyloid. *Adv. Protein Chem.* **1997**, *50*, 161–181.
8. Herbert, J.; Wilcox, J.N.; Pham, K.-T.C.; Fremeau, R.T.; Zeviani, M.; Dwork, A.; Soprano, D.R.; Makover, A.; Goodman, D.S.; Zimmerman, E.A.; et al. Transthyretin: A choroid plexus-specific transport protein in human brain. The 1986 S. Weir Mitchell award. *Neurology* **1986**, *36*, 900–911. [CrossRef]
9. Merlini, G.; Bellotti, V. Molecular mechanisms of amyloidosis. *N. Engl. J. Med.* **2003**, *349*, 583–596. [CrossRef]
10. Nativi-Nicolau, J.N.; Karam, C.; Khella, S.; Maurer, M.S. Screening for ATTR amyloidosis in the clinic: Overlapping disorders, misdiagnosis, and multiorgan awareness. *Heart Fail. Rev.* **2021**, 1–9. [CrossRef]

11. Rapezzi, C.; Merlini, G.; Quarta, C.C.; Riva, L.; Longhi, S.; Leone, O.; Salvi, F.; Ciliberti, P.; Pastorelli, F.; Biagini, E.; et al. Systemic cardiac amyloidoses: Disease profiles and clinical courses of the 3 main types. *Circulation* **2009**, *120*, 1203–1212. [CrossRef] [PubMed]
12. Sperry, B.W.; Reyes, B.A.; Ikram, A.; Donnelly, J.; Phelan, D.; Jaber, W.A.; Shapiro, D.; Evans, P.J.; Maschke, S.; Kilpatrick, S.E.; et al. Tenosynovial and Cardiac Amyloidosis in Patients Undergoing Carpal Tunnel Release. *J. Am. Coll. Cardiol.* **2018**, *72*, 2040–2050. [CrossRef] [PubMed]
13. Ando, Y.; Coelho, T.; Berk, J.L.; Cruz, M.W.; Ericzon, B.-G.; Ikeda, S.-i.; Lewis, W.D.; Obici, L.; Planté-Bordeneuve, V.; Rapezzi, C.; et al. Guideline of transthyretin-related hereditary amyloidosis for clinicians. *Orphanet J. Rare Dis.* **2013**, *8*, 31. [CrossRef] [PubMed]
14. Maurer, M.S.; Hanna, M.; Grogan, M.; Dispenzieri, A.; Witteles, R.; Drachman, B.; Judge, D.P.; Lenihan, D.J.; Gottlieb, S.S.; Shah, S.J.; et al. Genotype and Phenotype of Transthyretin Cardiac Amyloidosis: THAOS (Transthyretin Amyloid Outcome Survey). *J. Am. Coll. Cardiol.* **2016**, *68*, 161–172. [CrossRef] [PubMed]
15. Buxbaum, J.N.; Ruberg, F.L. Transthyretin V122I (pV142I)* cardiac amyloidosis: An age-dependent autosomal dominant cardiomyopathy too common to be overlooked as a cause of significant heart disease in elderly African Americans. *Genet. Med.* **2017**, *19*, 733–742. [CrossRef] [PubMed]
16. Ruberg, F.L.; Berk, J.L. Transthyretin (TTR) cardiac amyloidosis. *Circulation* **2012**, *126*, 1286–1300. [CrossRef]
17. Westermark, P.; Sletten, K.; Johansson, B.; Cornwell, G.G., 3rd. Fibril in senile systemic amyloidosis is derived from normal transthyretin. *Proc. Natl. Acad. Sci. USA* **1990**, *87*, 2843–2845. [CrossRef]
18. Kittleson, M.M.; Maurer, M.S.; Ambardekar, A.V.; Bullock-Palmer, R.P.; Chang, P.P.; Eisen, H.J.; Nair, A.P.; Nativi-Nicolau, J.; Ruberg, F.L.; American Heart Association Heart Failure and Transplantation Committee of the Council on Clinical Cardiology. Cardiac. Amyloidosis: Evolving Diagnosis and Management: A Scientific Statement From the American Heart Association. *Circulation* **2020**, *142*, e7–e22. [CrossRef]
19. Conceição, I.; González-Duarte, A.; Obici, L.; Schmidt, H.H.J.; Simoneau, D.; Ong, M.L.; Amass, L. "Red-flag" symptom clusters in transthyretin familial amyloid polyneuropathy. *J. Peripher. Nerv. Syst.* **2016**, *21*, 5–9. [CrossRef]
20. Nativi-Nicolau, J.; Maurer, M.S. Amyloidosis cardiomyopathy: Update in the diagnosis and treatment of the most common types. *Curr. Opin. Cardiol.* **2018**, *33*, 571–579. [CrossRef]
21. Witteles, R.M.; Bokhari, S.; Damy, T.; Elliott, P.; Falk, R.H.; Fine, N.M.; Gospodinova, M.; Obici, L.; Rapezzi, C.; Garcia-Pavia, P. Screening for Transthyretin Amyloid Cardiomyopathy in Everyday Practice. *JACC Heart Fail.* **2019**, *7*, 709–716. [CrossRef] [PubMed]
22. Rintell, D.; Heath, D.; Braga Mendendez, F.; Cross, E.; Cross, T.; Knobel, V.; Gagnon, B.; Turtle, C.; Cohen, A.; Kalmykov, E.; et al. Patient and family experience with transthyretin amyloid cardiomyopathy (ATTR-CM) and polyneuropathy (ATTR-PN) amyloidosis: Results of two focus groups. *Orphanet J. Rare Dis.* **2021**, *16*, 70. [CrossRef] [PubMed]
23. Grande-Trillo, A.; Baliellas, C.; Lladó, L.; Casasnovas, C.; Franco-Baux, J.V.; Gracia-Sánchez, L.; Bravo, M.G.; González-Vilatarsana, E.; Caballero-Gullón, L.; Echeverri, E.; et al. Transthyretin amyloidosis with cardiomyopathy after domino liver transplantation: Results of a cross-sectional study. *Am. J. Transplant.* **2021**, *21*, 372–381. [CrossRef] [PubMed]
24. Maurer, M.S.; Schwartz, J.H.; Gundapaneni, B.; Elliott, P.M.; Merlini, G.; Waddington-Cruz, M.; Kristen, A.V.; Grogan, M.; Witteles, R.; Damy, T.; et al. Tafamidis Treatment for Patients with Transthyretin Amyloid Cardiomyopathy. *N. Engl. J. Med.* **2018**, *379*, 1007–1016. [CrossRef]
25. Falk, R.H.; Alexander, K.M.; Liao, R.; Dorbala, S. AL (Light-Chain) Cardiac Amyloidosis: A Review of Diagnosis and Therapy. *J. Am. Coll. Cardiol.* **2016**, *68*, 1323–1341. [CrossRef]
26. Castaño, A.; Drachman, B.M.; Judge, D.; Maurer, M.S. Natural history and therapy of TTR-cardiac amyloidosis: Emerging disease-modifying therapies from organ transplantation to stabilizer and silencer drugs. *Heart Fail. Rev.* **2015**, *20*, 163–178. [CrossRef]
27. Cassidy, J.T. Cardiac amyloidosis. Two cases with digitalis sensitivity. *Ann. Intern. Med.* **1961**, *55*, 989–994. [CrossRef]
28. Palma, J.A.; Gonzalez-Duarte, A.; Kaufmann, H. Orthostatic hypotension in hereditary transthyretin amyloidosis: Epidemiology, diagnosis and management. *Clin. Auton. Res.* **2019**, *29* (Suppl. S1), 33–44. [CrossRef]
29. Aimo, A.; Rapezzi, C.; Vergaro, G.; Giannoni, A.; Spini, V.; Passino, C.; Emdin, M. Management of complications of cardiac amyloidosis: 10 questions and answers. *Eur. J. Prev. Cardiol.* **2021**, *28*, 1000–1005. [CrossRef]
30. Mitrani, L.R.; Santos, J.D.L.; Driggin, E.; Kogan, R.; Helmke, S.; Goldsmith, J.; Biviano, A.B.; Maurer, M.S. Anticoagulation with warfarin compared to novel oral anticoagulants for atrial fibrillation in adults with transthyretin cardiac amyloidosis: Comparison of thromboembolic events and major bleeding. *Amyloid* **2021**, *28*, 30–34. [CrossRef]
31. Givens, R.C.; Russo, C.; Green, P.; Maurer, M.S. Comparison of cardiac amyloidosis due to wild-type and V122I transthyretin in older adults referred to an academic medical center. *Aging Health* **2013**, *9*, 229–235. [CrossRef] [PubMed]
32. Pinney, J.H.; Whelan, C.J.; Petrie, A.; Dungu, J.; Banypersad, S.M.; Sattianayagam, P.; Wechalekar, A.; Gibbs, S.D.J.; Venner, C.P.; Wassef, N.; et al. Senile systemic amyloidosis: Clinical features at presentation and outcome. *J. Am. Heart Assoc.* **2013**, *2*, e000098. [CrossRef] [PubMed]
33. Varr, B.C.; Zarafshar, S.; Coakley, T.; Liedtke, M.; Lafayette, R.A.; Arai, S.; Schrier, S.L.; Witteles, R.M. Implantable cardioverter-defibrillator placement in patients with cardiac amyloidosis. *Heart Rhythm.* **2014**, *11*, 158–162. [CrossRef] [PubMed]

34. Ternacle, J.; Krapf, L.; Mohty, D.; Magne, J.; Nguyen, A.; Galat, A.; Gallet, R.; Teiger, E.; Côté, N.; Clavel, M.A.; et al. Aortic Stenosis and Cardiac Amyloidosis: JACC Review Topic of the Week. *J. Am. Coll. Cardiol.* **2019**, *74*, 2638–2651. [CrossRef]
35. Nagle, D.G.; Ferreira, D.; Zhou, Y.-D. Epigallocatechin-3-gallate (EGCG): Chemical and biomedical perspectives. *Phytochemistry* **2006**, *67*, 1849–1855. [CrossRef]
36. Kristen, A.V.; Lehrke, S.; Buss, S.; Mereles, D.; Steen, H.; Ehlermann, P.; Hardt, S.; Giannitsis, E.; Schreiner, R.; Haberkorn, U.; et al. Green tea halts progression of cardiac transthyretin amyloidosis: An observational report. *Clin. Res. Cardiol.* **2012**, *101*, 805–813. [CrossRef] [PubMed]
37. Cappelli, F.; Martone, R.; Taborchi, G.; Morini, S.; Bartolini, S.; Angelotti, P.; Farsetti, S.; Di Mario, C.; Perfetto, F. Epigallocatechin-3-gallate tolerability and impact on survival in a cohort of patients with transthyretin-related cardiac amyloidosis. A single-center retrospective study. *Intern. Emerg. Med.* **2018**, *13*, 873–880. [CrossRef]
38. Ericzon, B.G.; Wilczek, H.E.; Larsson, M.; Wijayatunga, P.; Stangou, A.; Pena, J.R.; Furtado, E.; Barroso, E.; Daniel, J.; Samuel, D.; et al. Liver Transplantation for Hereditary Transthyretin Amyloidosis: After 20 Years Still the Best Therapeutic Alternative? *Transplantation* **2015**, *99*, 1847–1854. [CrossRef]
39. Liepnieks, J.J.; Zhang, L.Q.; Benson, M.D. Progression of transthyretin amyloid neuropathy after liver transplantation. *Neurology* **2010**, *75*, 324–327. [CrossRef]
40. Barreiros, A.-P.; Post, F.; Hoppe-Lotichius, M.; Linke, R.P.; Vahl, C.F.; Schäfers, H.-J.; Galle, P.R.; Otto, G. Liver transplantation and combined liver-heart transplantation in patients with familial amyloid polyneuropathy: A single-center experience. *Liver Transpl.* **2010**, *16*, 314–323. [CrossRef]
41. González-López, E.; Sainz, A.L.; Garcia-Pavia, P. Diagnosis and Treatment of Transthyretin Cardiac Amyloidosis. *Prog. Hope Rev. Esp. Cardiol. Engl. Ed.* **2017**, *70*, 991–1004. [CrossRef]
42. Almeida, M.; Gales, L.; Damas, A.M.; Cardoso, I.; Saraiva, M.J. Small transthyretin (TTR) ligands as possible therapeutic agents in TTR amyloidoses. *Curr. Drug Targets CNS Neurol. Disord.* **2005**, *4*, 587–596. [CrossRef] [PubMed]
43. Mangione, P.P.; Verona, G.; Corazza, A.; Marcoux, J.; Canetti, D.; Giorgetti, S.; Raimondi, S.; Stoppini, M.; Esposito, M.; Relini, A.; et al. Plasminogen activation triggers transthyretin amyloidogenesis in vitro. *J. Biol. Chem.* **2018**, *293*, 14192–14199. [CrossRef] [PubMed]
44. Almeida, M.; Macedo, B.; Cardoso, I.; Alves, I.; Valencia, G.; Arsequell, G.; Planas, A.; Saraiva, M.J. Selective binding to transthyretin and tetramer stabilization in serum from patients with familial amyloidotic polyneuropathy by an iodinated diflunisal derivative. *Biochem. J.* **2004**, *381 Pt 2*, 351–356. [CrossRef]
45. Gamez, J.; Salvadó, M.; Reig, N.; Suñé, P.; Casasnovas, C.; Rojas-Garcia, R.; Insa, R. Transthyretin stabilization activity of the catechol-O-methyltransferase inhibitor tolcapone (SOM0226) in hereditary ATTR amyloidosis patients and asymptomatic carriers: Proof-of-concept study. *Amyloid* **2019**, *26*, 74–84. [CrossRef]
46. Larsen, K.R.; Dajani, E.Z.; Dajani, N.E.; Dayton, M.T.; Moore, J.G. Effects of tolcapone, a catechol-O-methyltransferase inhibitor, and Sinemet on intestinal electrolyte and fluid transport in conscious dogs. *Dig. Dis. Sci.* **1998**, *43*, 1806–1813. [CrossRef]
47. Kaakkola, S. Clinical pharmacology, therapeutic use and potential of COMT inhibitors in Parkinson's disease. *Drugs* **2000**, *59*, 1233–1250. [CrossRef]
48. Van Booven, D.; Marsh, S.; McLeod, H.; Whirl-Carrillo, M.; Sangkuhl, K.; Klein, T.E.; Altman, R.B. Cytochrome P450 2C9-CYP2C9. *Pharm. Genom.* **2010**, *20*, 277–281. [CrossRef]
49. Berk, J.L.; Suhr, O.B.; Obici, L.; Sekijima, Y.; Zeldenrust, S.R.; Yamashita, T.; Heneghan, M.A.; Gorevic, P.D.; Litchy, W.J.; Wiesman, J.F.; et al. Repurposing diflunisal for familial amyloid polyneuropathy: A randomized clinical trial. *JAMA* **2013**, *310*, 2658–2667. [CrossRef]
50. Wixner, J.; Westermark, P.; Ihse, E.; Pilebro, B.; Lundgren, H.-E.; Anan, I. The Swedish open-label diflunisal trial (DFNS01) on hereditary transthyretin amyloidosis and the impact of amyloid fibril composition. *Amyloid* **2019**, *26* (Suppl. S1), 39–40. [CrossRef]
51. Siddiqi, O.K.; Mints, Y.Y.; Berk, J.L.; Connors, L.; Doros, G.; Gopal, D.M.; Kataria, S.; Lohrmann, G.; Pipilas, A.R.; Ruberg, F.L. Diflunisal treatment is associated with improved survival for patients with early stage wild-type transthyretin (ATTR) amyloid cardiomyopathy: The Boston University Amyloidosis Center experience. *Amyloid* **2022**, 1–8. [CrossRef] [PubMed]
52. Lohrmann, G.; Pipilas, A.; Mussinelli, R.; Gopal, D.M.; Berk, J.L.; Connors, L.H.; Vellanki, N.; Hellawell, J.; Siddiqi, O.K.; Fox, J.; et al. Stabilization of Cardiac Function With Diflunisal in Transthyretin (ATTR) Cardiac Amyloidosis. *J. Card. Fail.* **2020**, *26*, 753–759. [CrossRef] [PubMed]
53. Razavi, H.; Palaninathan, S.K.; Powers, E.T.; Wiseman, R.L.; Purkey, H.E.; Mohamedmohaideen, N.N.; Deechongkit, S.; Chiang, K.P.; Dendle, M.T.A.; Sacchettini, J.C.; et al. Benzoxazoles as transthyretin amyloid fibril inhibitors: Synthesis, evaluation, and mechanism of action. *Angew. Chem. Int. Ed. Engl.* **2003**, *42*, 2758–2761. [CrossRef] [PubMed]
54. Park, J.; Egolum, U.; Parker, S.; Andrews, E.; Ombengi, D.; Ling, H. Tafamidis: A First-in-Class Transthyretin Stabilizer for Transthyretin Amyloid Cardiomyopathy. *Ann. Pharmacother.* **2020**, *54*, 470–477. [CrossRef]
55. Coelho, T.; Maia, L.; Da Silva, A.M.; Cruz, M.W.; Planté-Bordeneuve, V.; Lozeron, P.; Suhr, O.; Campistol, J.M.; Conceicao, I.; Schmidt, H.H.-J.; et al. Tafamidis for transthyretin familial amyloid polyneuropathy: A randomized, controlled trial. *Neurology* **2012**, *79*, 785–792. [CrossRef]
56. Lozeron, P.; Theaudin, M.; Mincheva, Z.; Ducot, B.; Lacroix, C.; Adams, D.; French Network for FAP (CORNAMYL). Effect on disability and safety of Tafamidis in late onset of Met30 transthyretin familial amyloid polyneuropathy. *Eur. J. Neurol.* **2013**, *20*, 1539–1545. [CrossRef]

57. Merlini, G.; Planté-Bordeneuve, V.; Judge, D.; Schmidt, H.; Obici, L.; Perlini, S.; Packman, J.; Tripp, T.; Grogan, D.R. Effects of tafamidis on transthyretin stabilization and clinical outcomes in patients with non-Val30Met transthyretin amyloidosis. *J. Cardiovasc. Transl. Res.* **2013**, *6*, 1011–1020. [CrossRef]
58. Maurer, M.S.; Grogan, D.R.; Judge, D.P.; Mundayat, R.; Packman, J.; Lombardo, I.; Quyyumi, A.A.; Aarts, J.; Falk, R.H. Tafamidis in transthyretin amyloid cardiomyopathy: Effects on transthyretin stabilization and clinical outcomes. *Circ. Heart Fail.* **2015**, *8*, 519–526. [CrossRef]
59. Bézard, M.; Kharoubi, M.; Galat, A.; Poullot, E.; Guendouz, S.; Fanen, P.; Funalot, B.; Moktefi, A.; Lefaucheur, J.; Abulizi, M.; et al. Natural history and impact of treatment with tafamidis on major cardiovascular outcome-free survival time in a cohort of patients with transthyretin amyloidosis. *Eur. J. Heart Fail.* **2021**, *23*, 264–274. [CrossRef]
60. Cho, Y.; Baranczak, A.; Helmke, S.; Teruya, S.; Horn, E.M.; Maurer, M.S.; Kelly, J.W. Personalized medicine approach for optimizing the dose of tafamidis to potentially ameliorate wild-type transthyretin amyloidosis (cardiomyopathy). *Amyloid* **2015**, *22*, 175–180. [CrossRef]
61. Lockwood, P.A.; Le, V.H.; O'Gorman, M.T.; Patterson, T.A.; Sultan, M.B.; Tankisheva, E.; Wang, Q.; Riley, S. The Bioequivalence of Tafamidis 61-mg Free Acid Capsules and Tafamidis Meglumine 4 x 20-mg Capsules in Healthy Volunteers. *Clin. Pharmacol. Drug Dev.* **2020**, *9*, 849–854. [CrossRef] [PubMed]
62. Damy, T.; Garcia-Pavia, P.; Hanna, M.; Judge, D.P.; Merlini, G.; Gundapaneni, B.; Patterson, T.A.; Riley, S.; Schwartz, J.H.; Sultan, M.B.; et al. Efficacy and safety of tafamidis doses in the Tafamidis in Transthyretin Cardiomyopathy Clinical Trial (ATTR-ACT) and long-term extension study. *Eur. J. Heart Fail.* **2021**, *23*, 277–285. [CrossRef] [PubMed]
63. Rapezzi, C.; Kristen, A.; Gundapaneni, B.; Sultan, M.; Hanna, M. Benefits of tafamidis in patients with advanced transthyretin amyloid cardiomyopathy. *Eur. Heart J.* **2020**, *41* (Suppl. S2). [CrossRef]
64. Li, H.; Rozenbaum, M.; Casey, M.; Sultan, M. Estimating treatment effect of tafamidis on hospitalisation in NYHA class III ATTR-CM patients in the presence of death using principal stratification. *Eur. Heart J.* **2021**, *42* (Suppl. S1), ehab724.0829. [CrossRef]
65. McDonagh, T.A.; Metra, M.; Adamo, M.; Gardner, R.S.; Baumbach, A.; Böhm, M.; Burri, H.; Butler, J.; Čelutkienė, J.; Chioncel, O.; et al. 2021 ESC Guidelines for the diagnosis and treatment of acute and chronic heart failure. *Eur. Heart J.* **2021**, *42*, 3599–3726. [CrossRef]
66. Judge, D.; Heitner, S.B.; Falk, R.H.; Maurer, M.S.; Shah, S.; Witteles, R.M.; Grogan, M.; Selby, V.N.; Jacoby, D.; Hanna, M.; et al. Transthyretin Stabilization by AG10 in Symptomatic Transthyretin Amyloid Cardiomyopathy. *J. Am. Coll. Cardiol.* **2019**, *74*, 285–295. [CrossRef]
67. Nelson, L.T.; Paxman, R.J.; Xu, J.; Webb, B.; Powers, E.T.; Kelly, J.W. Blinded potency comparison of transthyretin kinetic stabilisers by subunit exchange in human plasma. *Amyloid* **2021**, *28*, 24–29. [CrossRef]
68. Trial of Acoramidis for Transthyretin Amyloid Cardiomyopathy Misses Primary Endpoint. 2021. Available online: https://www.healio.com/news/cardiology/20211228/trial-of-acoramidis-for-transthyretin-amyloid-cardiomyopathy-misses-primary-endpoint (accessed on 21 March 2022).
69. Corazza, A.; Verona, G.; Waudby, C.A.; Mangione, P.P.; Bingham, R.; Uings, I.; Canetti, D.; Nocerino, P.; Taylor, G.W.; Pepys, M.B.; et al. Binding of Monovalent and Bivalent Ligands by Transthyretin Causes Different Short- and Long-Distance Conformational Changes. *J. Med. Chem.* **2019**, *62*, 8274–8283. [CrossRef]
70. Verona, G.; Mangione, P.P.; Raimondi, S.; Giorgetti, S.; Faravelli, G.; Porcari, R.; Corazza, A.; Gillmore, J.D.; Hawkins, P.N.; Pepys, M.B.; et al. Inhibition of the mechano-enzymatic amyloidogenesis of transthyretin: Role of ligand affinity, binding cooperativity and occupancy of the inner channel. *Sci. Rep.* **2017**, *7*, 182. [CrossRef]
71. Franz, C.; Hoffmann, K.; Hinz, U.; Singer, R.; Hund, E.; Gotthardt, D.N.; Ganten, T.; Kristen, A.V.; Hegenbart, U.; Schönland, S.; et al. Modified body mass index and time interval between diagnosis and operation affect survival after liver transplantation for hereditary amyloidosis: A single-center analysis. *Clin. Transplant.* **2013**, *27* (Suppl. S25), 40–48. [CrossRef]
72. Crooke, S.T.; Witztum, J.L.; Bennett, C.F.; Baker, B.F. RNA-Targeted Therapeutics. *Cell Metab.* **2018**, *27*, 714–739. [CrossRef] [PubMed]
73. Rizk, M.; Tuzmen, S. Update on the clinical utility of an RNA interference-based treatment: Focus on Patisiran. *Pharmgenom. Pers. Med.* **2017**, *10*, 267–278. [CrossRef] [PubMed]
74. Yonezawa, S.; Koide, H.; Asai, T. Recent advances in siRNA delivery mediated by lipid-based nanoparticles. *Adv. Drug Deliv. Rev.* **2020**, *154–155*, 64–78. [CrossRef] [PubMed]
75. Adams, D.; Gonzalez-Duarte, A.; O'Riordan, W.D.; Yang, C.C.; Ueda, M.; Kristen, A.V.; Tournev, I.; Schmidt, H.H.; Coelho, T.; Berk, J.L.; et al. Patisiran, an RNAi Therapeutic, for Hereditary Transthyretin Amyloidosis. *N. Engl. J. Med.* **2018**, *379*, 11–21. [CrossRef] [PubMed]
76. Solomon, S.D.; Adams, D.; Kristen, A.; Grogan, M.; González-Duarte, A.; Maurer, M.S.; Merlini, G.; Damy, T.; Slama, M.S.; Brannagan, I.I.I.; et al. Effects of Patisiran, an RNA Interference Therapeutic, on Cardiac Parameters in Patients With Hereditary Transthyretin-Mediated Amyloidosis. *Circulation* **2019**, *139*, 431–443. [CrossRef]
77. Fontana, M.; Martinez Naharro, A.; Chacko, L.; Rowczenio, D.; Gilbertson, J.A.; Whelan, C.J.; Strehina, S.; Lane, T., Moon, J., Hutt, D.F.; et al. Reduction in CMR Derived Extracellular Volume With Patisiran Indicates Cardiac Amyloid Regression. *JACC Cardiovasc. Imaging* **2021**, *14*, 189–199. [CrossRef]

78. Benson, M.D.; Waddington-Cruz, M.; Berk, J.L.; Polydefkis, M.; Dyck, P.J.; Wang, A.K.; Planté-Bordeneuve, V.; Barroso, F.A.; Merlini, G.; Obici, L.; et al. Inotersen Treatment for Patients with Hereditary Transthyretin Amyloidosis. *N. Engl. J. Med.* **2018**, *379*, 22–31. [CrossRef]
79. Dasgupta, N.R.; Rissing, S.M.; Smith, J.; Jung, J.; Benson, M.D. Inotersen therapy of transthyretin amyloid cardiomyopathy. *Amyloid* **2020**, *27*, 52–58. [CrossRef]
80. Zimmermann, T.S.; Karsten, V.; Chan, A.; Chiesa, J.; Boyce, M.; Bettencourt, B.R.; Hutabarat, R.; Nochur, S.; Vaishnaw, A.; Gollob, J. Clinical Proof of Concept for a Novel Hepatocyte-Targeting GalNAc-siRNA Conjugate. *Mol. Ther.* **2017**, *25*, 71–78. [CrossRef]
81. Judge, D.P.; Kristen, A.V.; Grogan, M.; Maurer, M.S.; Falk, R.H.; Hanna, M.; Gillmore, J.; Garg, P.; Vaishnaw, A.K.; Harrop, J.; et al. Phase 3 Multicenter Study of Revusiran in Patients with Hereditary Transthyretin-Mediated (hATTR) Amyloidosis with Cardiomyopathy (ENDEAVOUR). *Cardiovasc. Drugs Ther.* **2020**, *34*, 357–370. [CrossRef]
82. Hu, B.; Zhong, L.; Weng, Y.; Peng, L.; Huang, Y.; Zhao, Y.; Liang, X.-J. Therapeutic siRNA: State of the art. *Signal. Transduct. Target. Ther.* **2020**, *5*, 101. [CrossRef] [PubMed]
83. Habtemariam, B.A.; Karsten, V.; Attarwala, H.; Goel, V.; Melch, M.; Clausen, V.A.; Garg, P.; Vaishnaw, A.K.; Sweetser, M.T.; Robbie, G.J.; et al. Single-Dose Pharmacokinetics and Pharmacodynamics of Transthyretin Targeting N-acetylgalactosamine-Small Interfering Ribonucleic Acid Conjugate, Vutrisiran, in Healthy Subjects. *Clin. Pharmacol. Ther.* **2021**, *109*, 372–382. [CrossRef] [PubMed]
84. Alnylam Pharmaceuticals. Alnylam Presents Positive 18-Month Results from HELIOS-A Phase 3 Study of Investigational Vutrisiran in Patients with hATTR Amyloidosis with Polyneuropathy. Available online: https://investors.alnylam.com/press-release?id=26396 (accessed on 21 January 2022).
85. Coelho, T.; Ando, Y.; Benson, M.D.; Berk, J.L.; Waddington-Cruz, M.; Dyck, P.J.; Gillmore, J.D.; Khella, S.L.; Litchy, W.J.; Obici, L.; et al. Design and Rationale of the Global Phase 3 NEURO-TTRansform Study of Antisense Oligonucleotide AKCEA-TTR-LRx (ION-682884-CS3) in Hereditary Transthyretin-Mediated Amyloid Polyneuropathy. *Neurol. Ther.* **2021**, *10*, 375–389. [CrossRef] [PubMed]
86. Ledford, H. Landmark CRISPR trial shows promise against deadly disease. *Nature* **2021**. [CrossRef]
87. Gillmore, J.D.; Gane, E.; Taubel, J.; Kao, J.; Fontana, M.; Maitland, M.L.; Seitzer, J.; O'Connell, D.; Walsh, K.R.; Wood, K.; et al. CRISPR-Cas9 In Vivo Gene Editing for Transthyretin Amyloidosis. *N. Engl. J. Med.* **2021**, *385*, 493–502. [CrossRef]
88. Chukwudi, C.U. rRNA Binding Sites and the Molecular Mechanism of Action of the Tetracyclines. *Antimicrob. Agents Chemother* **2016**, *60*, 4433–4441. [CrossRef]
89. Medina, L.; González-Lizárraga, F.; Dominguez-Meijide, A.; Ploper, D.; Parrales, V.; Sequeira, S.; Cima-Omori, M.-S.; Zweckstetter, M.; Del Bel, E.; Michel, P.P.; et al. Doxycycline Interferes With Tau Aggregation and Reduces Its Neuronal Toxicity. *Front. Aging Neurosci.* **2021**, *13*, 635760. [CrossRef]
90. Cardoso, I.; Martins, D.; Ribeiro, T.; Merlini, G.; Saraiva, M.J. Synergy of combined doxycycline/TUDCA treatment in lowering Transthyretin deposition and associated biomarkers: Studies in FAP mouse models. *J. Transl. Med.* **2010**, *8*, 74. [CrossRef]
91. Obici, L.; Cortese, A.; Lozza, A.; Lucchetti, J.; Gobbi, M.; Palladini, G.; Perlini, S.; Saraiva, M.J.; Merlini, G. Doxycycline plus tauroursodeoxycholic acid for transthyretin amyloidosis: A phase II study. *Amyloid* **2012**, *19* (Suppl. S1), 34–36. [CrossRef]
92. Wixner, J.; Pilebro, B.; Lundgren, H.-E.; Olsson, M.; Anan, I. Effect of doxycycline and ursodeoxycholic acid on transthyretin amyloidosis. *Amyloid* **2017**, *24* (Suppl. S1), 78–79. [CrossRef]
93. Higaki, J.N.; Chakrabartty, A.; Galant, N.J.; Hadley, K.C.; Hammerson, B.; Nijjar, T.; Torres, R.; Tapia, J.R.; Salmans, J.; Barbour, R.; et al. Novel conformation-specific monoclonal antibodies against amyloidogenic forms of transthyretin. *Amyloid* **2016**, *23*, 86–97. [CrossRef] [PubMed]
94. Michalon, A.; Hagenbuch, A.; Huy, C.; Varela, E.; Combaluzier, B.; Damy, T.; Suhr, O.B.; Saraiva, M.J.; Hock, C.; Nitsch, R.M.; et al. A human antibody selective for transthyretin amyloid removes cardiac amyloid through phagocytic immune cells. *Nat. Commun.* **2021**, *12*, 3142. [CrossRef] [PubMed]
95. Yadav, J.D.; Othee, H.; Chan, K.A.; Man, D.C.; Belliveau, P.P.; Towle, J. Transthyretin Amyloid Cardiomyopathy-Current and Future Therapies. *Ann. Pharmacother.* **2021**, *55*, 1502–1514. [CrossRef] [PubMed]
96. Abou-El-Enein, M.; Elsanhoury, A.; Reinke, P. Overcoming Challenges Facing Advanced Therapies in the EU Market. *Cell Stem Cell* **2016**, *19*, 293–297. [CrossRef]
97. Kazi, D.S.; Bellows, B.K.; Baron, S.J.; Shen, C.; Cohen, D.J.; Spertus, J.A.; Yeh, R.W.; Arnold, S.V.; Sperry, B.W.; Maurer, M.S.; et al. Cost-Effectiveness of Tafamidis Therapy for Transthyretin Amyloid Cardiomyopathy. *Circulation* **2020**, *141*, 1214–1224. [CrossRef]
98. Rapezzi, C.; Elliott, P.; Damy, T.; Nativi-Nicolau, J.; Berk, J.L.; Velazquez, E.J.; Boman, K.; Gundapaneni, B.; Patterson, T.A.; Schwartz, J.H.; et al. Efficacy of Tafamidis in Patients With Hereditary and Wild-Type Transthyretin Amyloid Cardiomyopathy: Further Analyses From ATTR-ACT. *JACC Heart Fail.* **2021**, *9*, 115–123. [CrossRef]
99. Monteiro, C.; Martins da Silva, A.; Ferreira, N.; Mesgarzadeh, J.; Novais, M.; Coelho, T.; Kelly, J.W. Cerebrospinal fluid and vitreous body exposure to orally administered tafamidis in hereditary ATTRV30M (p.TTRV50M) amyloidosis patients. *Amyloid* **2018**, *25*, 120–128. [CrossRef]
100. Dohrn, M.F.; Medina, J.; Dague, K.R.O.; Hund, E. Are we creating a new phenotype? Physiological barriers and ethical considerations in the treatment of hereditary transthyretin-amyloidosis. *Neurol. Res. Pract.* **2021**, *3*, 57. [CrossRef]
101. Magrinelli, F.; Fabrizi, G.M.; Santoro, L.; Manganelli, F.; Zanette, G.; Cavallaro, T.; Tamburin, S. Pharmacological treatment for familial amyloid polyneuropathy. *Cochrane Database Syst. Rev.* **2020**, *4*, CD012395. [CrossRef]

Journal of
Clinical Medicine

MDPI

Article

Pregnancy in Women with Arrhythmogenic Left Ventricular Cardiomyopathy

Riccardo Bariani [1], Maria Bueno Marinas [1], Ilaria Rigato [2], Paola Veronese [2], Rudy Celeghin [1], Alberto Cipriani [1], Marco Cason [1], Valeria Pergola [2], Giulia Mattesi [2], Petra Deola [1], Alessandro Zorzi [1], Giuseppe Limongelli [3], Sabino Iliceto [1], Domenico Corrado [1], Cristina Basso [1], Kalliopi Pilichou [1,*] and Barbara Bauce [1,*]

1 Department of Cardiac, Thoracic, Vascular Sciences and Public Health, University of Padua, 35122 Padua, Italy
2 Azienda Ospedaliera di Padova, Via Giustiniani, 2, 35128 Padova, Italy
3 Department of Translational Sciences, University della Campania "Luigi Vanvitelli", 80138 Naples, Italy
* Correspondence: kalliopi.pilichou@unipd.it (K.P.); barbara.bauce@unipd.it (B.B.)

Abstract: Background: In the last few years, a phenotypic variant of arrhythmogenic cardiomyopathy (ACM) labeled arrhythmogenic left ventricular cardiomyopathy (ALVC) has been defined and researched. This type of cardiomyopathy is characterized by a predominant left ventricular (LV) involvement with no or minor right ventricular (RV) abnormalities. Data on the specific risk and management of pregnancy in women affected by ALVC are, thus far, not available. We have sought to characterize pregnancy course and outcomes in women affected by ALVC through the evaluation of a series of childbearing patients. Methods: A series of consecutive female ALVC patients were analyzed in a cross-sectional, retrospective study. Study protocol included 12-lead ECG assessments, 24-h Holter ECG evaluations, 2D-echocardiogram tests, cardiac magnetic resonance assessments, and genetic analysis. Furthermore, the long-term disease course of childbearing patients was compared with a group of nulliparous ALVC women. Results: A total of 35 patients (mean age 45 ± 9 years, 51% probands) were analyzed. Sixteen women (46%) reported a pregnancy, for a total of 27 singleton viable pregnancies (mean age at first childbirth 30 ± 9 years). Before pregnancy, all patients were in the NYHA class I and none of the patients reported a previous heart failure (HF) episode. No significant differences were found between childbearing and nulliparous women regarding ECG features, LV dimensions, function, and extent of late enhancement. Overall, 7 patients (20%, 4 belonging to the childbearing group) experienced a sustained ventricular tachycardia and 2 (6%)—one for each group—showed heart failure (HF) episodes. The analysis of arrhythmia-free survival patients did not show significant differences between childbearing and nulliparous women. Conclusions: In a cohort of ALVC patients without previous episodes of HF, pregnancy was well tolerated, with no significant influence on disease progression and degree of electrical instability. Further studies on a larger cohort of women with different degrees of disease extent and genetic background are needed in order to achieve a more comprehensive knowledge regarding the outcome of pregnancy in ALVC patients.

Keywords: arrhythmogenic left ventricular cardiomyopathy; pregnancy; desmoplakin; filamin C; plakofillin-2

Citation: Bariani, R.; Bueno Marinas, M.; Rigato, I.; Veronese, P.; Celeghin, R.; Cipriani, A.; Cason, M.; Pergola, V.; Mattesi, G.; Deola, P.; et al. Pregnancy in Women with Arrhythmogenic Left Ventricular Cardiomyopathy. *J. Clin. Med.* **2022**, *11*, 6735. https://doi.org/10.3390/jcm11226735

Academic Editor: Stefan Peters

Received: 9 October 2022
Accepted: 9 November 2022
Published: 14 November 2022

1. Introduction

Arrhythmogenic cardiomyopathy (ACM) is an inherited cardiac disease that is characterized by myocardial necrosis and fibro-fatty replacement that predisposes patients to ventricular arrhythmias (VAs), which can even lead to sudden cardiac death (SCD) [1].

Different from the original descriptions—which considered ACM a disease of the right ventricle (RV) with left ventricular (LV) involvement, usually mild when relevant mainly due to a disease progression in association with an advanced RV disease—in the last years it has become evident that LV involvement can be present in early stages of the disease, independently or concurrently with RV involvement [2,3].

Furthermore, recently a left dominant variant of the disease (arrhythmogenic left ventricular cardiomyopathy: ALVC) has been described [3,4]. In this form, the diagnosis can be challenging and it is usually made on the basis of ECG features (inferolateral T-wave inversion and low QRS voltages); VAs of LV origin; prominent LV dilatation/dysfunction in the setting of relatively mild or absent right-sided disease; and in the presence of subepicardial or ring-like late gadolinium enhancement (LGE) following a cardiac magnetic resonance (CMR) assessment [4–6]. Genotype–phenotype correlation studies demonstrated that desmoplakin (DSP) and filamin C (FLNC) are the most common disease genes in ALVC [7]. However, many cases are still gene elusive [5,8].

Recent studies on pregnancy in women affected by ACM demonstrated a low rate of major cardiac events during pregnancy [9]. Nonetheless, data on the specific risk and management of pregnancy in women affected by ALVC are not yet available.

In this study, we sought to characterize pregnancy course and outcome in women affected by ALVC through a retrospective evaluation of a series of childbearing patients. Moreover, in order to better characterize the effect of pregnancy in this population we compared the clinical and instrumental data of these patients to those of a group of nulliparous ALVC women.

2. Materials and Methods

2.1. Study Population

From the entire cohort of probands and family members followed at the Cardiomyopathy Unit of the University of Padua, from 1990 to 2020, we selected a consecutive cohort of 35 female patients diagnosed with ALVC. All patients provided written informed consent before inclusion in the study, in accordance with the protocol approved by the local ethics committee. All clinical investigations were conducted according to the principles expressed in the Declaration of Helsinki. Inclusion criteria for the diagnosis of ALVC were as follows: 1. The presence of a subepicardial LGE pattern with non-ischemic distribution and fatty infiltration at CMR assessment affecting exclusively or predominantly the LV, plus one of the following diagnostic features: A. positive genetic testing for likely pathogenic (LP, class IV)/pathogenic (P, class V) variants associated with ACM; B. presence of family history of ACM, ALVC, or dilated cardiomyopathy (DCM) and/or family history of SCD with autoptic findings in keeping with an ACM form. Moreover, three women belonging to two ALVC families showing LV dimensional, kinetic abnormalities, and carrying DSP P/LP variants who had already received an ICD without a previous CMR evaluation were enrolled.

The study protocol included familial and personal anamneses, 12-lead ECGs, two-dimensional Doppler echocardiograms, 24-h Holter ECGs, CMR assessments, and genetic tests. A comparison of the phenotypic expression and degree of electrical instability of childbearing and nulliparous patients was also performed.

2.2. Twelve-Lead Electrocardiograms

Twelve-lead ECGs were performed on a standard speed paper (25 mm/s, 10 mm/mV, and 0.05–150 Hz) and the following parameters were considered: duration of PQ interval, mean QRS duration, right bundle branch block (RBBB—incomplete or complete), left anterior fascicular block, complete left bundle branch block (LBBB), ST-segment alteration (ST elevation > 1.5–2 mm), pathological Q wave, T-wave inversion, and QRS voltages in both precordial and peripheral leads (low voltages were defined when QRS was <5 mm in peripheral leads or <10 mm in precordial leads).

2.3. Ventricular Arrhythmias and Heart Failure

Recorded VAs were classified in ventricular fibrillation (VF); sustained ventricular tachycardia (defined as a tachycardia that lasted >30 s) (sVT); (3) non-sustained ventricular tachycardia (defined as three or more consecutive ventricular beats, lasting <30 s, at a rate >120 beats/min) (NSVT); and (4) premature ventricular beats (PVBs). Heart failure (HF) was considered in the presence of the signs and symptoms requiring hospitalization or outpatient clinic evaluation.

2.4. Two-Dimensional and Doppler Echocardiography

Two-dimensional echocardiograms were performed with a commercially available Hewlett Packard model 5500 and GE S6 ultrasound machine equipped with a M5S probe. Parasternal, apical, and subcostal views were obtained. In addition, LV function, LV end diastolic volume, RV area, RV function were calculated on an apical four chambers view. Echocardiographic measurements were evaluated according to international recommendations [10].

2.5. Cardiac Magnetic Resonance

CMR assessment was performed via a 1.5-T scanner (Magnetom Avanto, Siemens Medical Solutions, Erlangen, Germany). All patients underwent a study protocol for myocarditis, including balanced steady-state free precession sequence cine images for morpho-functional evaluation, triple inversion recovery sequences for the detection of myocardial edema, and two-dimensional segmented breath-held fast low-angle shot inversion recovery sequences within 3 min after the administration of intravenous contrast agent (gadobenate dimeglumine; 0.2 mmol/kg of body weight) for the purposes of detecting early gadolinium enhancement (EGE) and 10–15 min for late gadolinium enhancement (LGE). Additionally, we used T1-weighted turbo spin-echo sequences for the purposes of detecting myocardial fat infiltration. The technical details of the CMR sequences and image post-processing analyses have been previously reported [11,12].

2.6. Genetic Analysis

Genetic testing was carried out as previously described [13,14].

2.7. Childbearing Group Evaluation

Among the 35 ALVC patients, 16 (45%) were childbearing and the obstetric courses were assessed through analyses of medical records. For each pregnancy's gestational duration, type of delivery, birth weight, obstetric complications, and perinatal health were evaluated.

2.8. Statistical Analysis

Data were presented as mean ± standard deviation, median with range, or frequencies with percentages, as appropriate. The normality of the quantitative variables was evaluated through the Shapiro–Wilk test, while their comparison was conducted through the application of the Student's *t*-test or the Mann–Whitney test, when appropriate. Categorical variables were compared by the chi-square test and Fisher's exact test, when appropriate. Kaplan–Meier curves were constructed, and a log-rank test was performed in order to assess cumulative lifetime sVT-free survival. The association between pregnancy and major VA (MVA) was tested using Cox regression analysis. The statistical significance for all tests was set for probability values $p < 0.05$. Statistical analyses were performed using SPSS version 27 software for MAC (SPSS, Inc., Chicago, IL, USA).

3. Results

A total of 35 women (age at evaluation 45 ± 9 years) were included in the study, of which 18 (51%) were probands. In 18 (51%) a family history of SCD was determined and in 11 (31%) instances of HF were present. The reasons for first evaluation were detection of VAs (n = 18, 51%), family history of cardiomyopathy or SCD (n = 13, 37%) and chest pain episodes with cardiac enzyme release (n = 4, 11%) (Table 1). Regarding medical therapy, 14 (88%) patients used beta-blockers (mainly metoprolol), 7 (50%) patients utilized ACE inhibitors, 1 patient used amiodarone (6%), and 1 patient utilized sotalol with ACE inhibitors (6%). Among the 16 childbearing women, 9 were diagnosed with ALVC after the last pregnancy. In the 7 patients diagnosed before pregnancy, therapy was modified by discontinuing the ACE inhibitor, while beta-blocker therapy was maintained.

Table 1. Clinical and ECG features of the 35 ALVC female patients.

	Overall $n = 35$	Childbearing Women $n = 16$	Nulliparous Women $n = 19$	p
Probands	18 (51%)	8 (50%)	10 (53%)	0.573
Age at evaluation	40 ± 11	45 ± 9	36 ± 11	0.050
Family history of SCD	18 (51%)	7 (44%)	11 (58%)	0.505
Family history of DCM	9 (26%)	5 (31%)	4 (21%)	0.700
Family history of ALVC	18 (51%)	8 (50%)	10 (52%)	1.000
Family history of ARVC	11 (31%)	5 (31%)	6 (32%)	1.000
Family history of HF	11 (31%)	8 (50%)	3 (16%)	0.065
Myocarditis-like episodes	4 (11%)	1 (6%)	3 (16%)	0.608
Ventricular arrhythmias	32 (91%)	15 (94%)	17 (89%)	1.000
Frequent PVBs	13 (37%)	4 (25%)	9 (42%)	0.311
NSVT	12(41%)	7 (50%)	5 (32%)	0.468
Sustained VT	7 (20%)	3 (19%)	4 (21%)	0.799
ICD	10 (29%)	5 (31%)	5 (32%)	0.747
Normal ECG	10 (28%)	4 (25%)	6 (31%)	0.099
Low QRS voltages (limb leads)	23 (65%)	13 (81%)	10 (53%)	0.152
Low QRS voltages (precordial leads)	11 (31%)	5 (31%)	6 (32%)	1.000
Negative T wave V1-V3	4 (11%)	1 (6%)	3 (16%)	0.608
Negative T wave V4-V6	7 (20%)	3 (19%)	4 (21%)	1.000
Negative T wave inferior leads	6 (17%)	2 (12%)	4 (21%)	0.666

SCD: sudden cardiac death; DCM: dilated cardiomyopathy; ALVC: arrhythmogenic left ventricular cardiomyopathy; ACM: arrhythmogenic right ventricular cardiomyopathy; HF: heart failure; PVBs: premature ventricular beats; VT: ventricular tachycardia; NSVT: non-sustained VT; and ICD: implantable cardioverter–defibrillator.

3.1. Genetic Data

Genetic screening was performed in 34 cases (97%) and genetic variants were identified in 29 (83%). In more detail, 21 (62%) patients carried a DSP, 5 (15%) a FLNC, 2 (6%) a PKP2, and one possessed a DSG2 (3%) genetic variant (Table 2). Moreover, in 5 cases (15%) the genetic test was negative.

Table 2. ACM genetic variants identified in 29 women affected with ALVC (see text).

Pt	Cohort	Gene	cDNA Change	Amino Acid Change	ACMG Classification	Reference
#1	*NW*	*DSP*	c.3465G > A	p.Trp1155*	P (PVS1, PM2, PP5)	
#2 and #3	*NW, CW*	*DSP*	c.939 + 1G > A	/	P (PVS1, PM2, PP5)	Whittock et al., 1999 [15]
#4	*NW*	*DSP*	c.3475G > T	p.Glu1159*	P (PVS1, PM2, PP5)	Bariani et al., 2021 [16]
#5	*NW*	*DSP*	c.132delG	p.Arg45Alafs*3	LP (PVS1, PM2)	
#6	*NW*	*DSP*	c.897C > G	p.Ser299Arg	LP (PM2, PP3, PP5, PS3)	Rampazzo et al., 2002 [17]
#7	*NW*	*DSP*	c.2821C > T	p.Arg941*	P (PVS1, PM2, PP5)	Quarta et al., 2011 [18]
#8	*CW*	*DSP*	c.939 + 1G > A	/	P (PVS1, PM2, PP5)	Whittock et al., 1999 [15]
#9 and #10	*NW, NW*	*DSP*	c.3891_3894dupGGTC	p.Met1299Glyfs*7	P (PVS1, PM2, PP5)	Bariani et al., 2022 [14]
#11	*NW*	*DSP*	c.337C > T	p.Gln113*	P (PVS1, PM2, PP5)	Bariani et al., 2022 [14]
#12	*NW*	*DSP*	c.2297 + 1G > T	/	P (PVS1, PM2, PP5)	Bariani et al., 2022 [14]
#13	*NW*	*DSP*	c.974_975delAG	p.Glu325Alafs*3	P (PVS1, PM2, PP5)	Bariani et al., 2022 [14]
#14 and #15	*CW, CW*	*DSP*	c.3889C > T	p.Gln1297*	P (PVS1, PM2, PP5)	Bariani et al., 2021 [14]
#16	*CW*	*DSP*	c.6850C > T	p.Arg2284*	P (PVS1, PM2, PP5)	Fressart V et al., 2010 [19]
#17 and #18	*CW, CW*	*DSP*	c.3416dupA	p.Tyr1139*	P (PVS1, PM2, PP5)	Bariani et al., 2022 [14]
#19	*CW*	*DSP*	c.423-1G > A	/	P (PVS1, PM2, PP5)	Bariani et al., 2022 [14]

Table 2. *Cont.*

Pt	Cohort	Gene	cDNA Change	Amino Acid Change	ACMG Classification	Reference
#20	*CW*	*DSP*	c.4207_4208delAG	p.Arg1403Glufs*4	LP (PVS1, PM2)	
#21	*NW*	*DSP*	c.1067C > T	p.Thr356Met	VUS (PM2, PP3)	
#22	*NW*	*DSG2*	c.3059_3062delAGAG	p.Glu1020Alafs*18	VUS (PVS1, BS2)	Christensen et al., 2010 [20]
#23	*NW*	*FLNC*	c.5926C > T	p.Gln1976*	P (PVS1, PM2, PP5)	Celeghin et al., 2021 [13]
#24 and #25	*NW, CW*	*FLNC*	c.5398 + 1G > T	/	P (PVS1, PM2)	Celeghin et al., 2021 [13]
#26	*NW*	*FLNC*	c.376_392delAACCTGAAGCTGATGCT	p.Asn126Glyfs*20	P (PVS1, PM2)	Celeghin et al., 2021 [13]
#27	*CW*	*FLNC*	c.7037dup	p.Leu2347Profs*9	P (PVS1, PM2, PP5)	Celeghin et al., 2021 [13]
#28	*NW*	*PKP2*	c.1521G > A	p.Trp507*	LP (PVS1, PM2)	
#29	*CW*	*PKP2*	c.2443_2448delAACACCinsGAAA	p.Asn815Glufs*11	P (PVS1, PM2, PP5)	

ACMG: American College of Medical Genetics and Genomics; P: pathogenic; LP; likely pathogenic; DSP: desmoplakin; PKP2: plakofillin-2; DSG2: desmoglein-2; FLNC: filamin-C; CW: childbearing woman; and NW: nulliparous woman.

3.2. Electrocardiographic Findings

ECG assessment showed abnormal features in 25 patients (71%). The most common findings were low QRS voltages in limb (n = 23, 65%) and precordial leads (n = 11, 31%), followed by negative T waves in left precordial leads (20%). All data on the ECG findings are reported in Table 1. In Figure 1, panel A, the ECG evaluation of a patient with ALVC is present, where low QRS voltages can be observed in the peripheral leads.

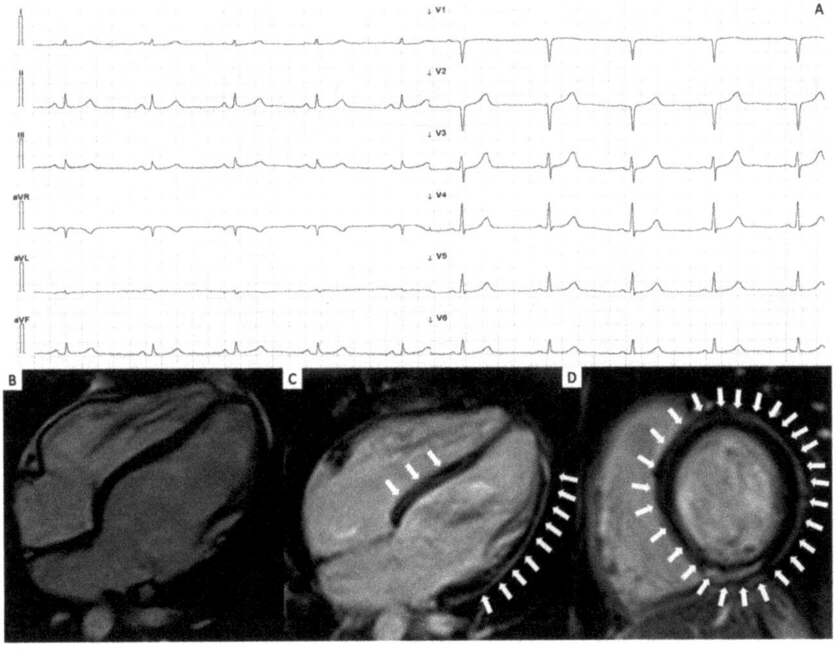

Figure 1. ECG and CMR assessments of a childbearing patient carrying a likely pathogenic variant of PKP2. The ECG assessment showed the presence of low QRS voltages (panel (**A**)). CMR evaluation demonstrated normal size and biventricular function (panel (**B**)), as well as extensive signs of fibrous infiltration with sub-epicardial "ring-like" distribution in LGE sequences (panels (**C**,**D**)). ECG: electrocardiogram; CMR: cardiac magnetic resonance; and LGE: late gadolinium enhancement.

3.3. Echocardiographic Features

2D-echocardiogram was performed on all subjects. Data on their ventricular functions and dimensions are available in Table 3. LV end diastolic volume (EDVi) was increased in 24 patients (89%) and LV ejection fraction (LV-EF) was reduced in 18 (51%), with the presence of regional kinetic abnormalities in 15 (43%). RV was dilated in 2 patients (6%) and RV systolic function was within limits in all cases.

Table 3. Imaging findings of the 35 ALVC female patients.

	Overall n = 35	Childbearing Women n = 16	Nulliparous Women n = 19	p
Echocardiographic findings				
LVEDVi (mL/m^2)	76 ± 15	80 ± 15	73 ± 15	0.104
LVESVi (mL/m^2)	39 ± 13	42 ± 12	36 ± 12	0.088
LVEF (%)	50 ± 7	48 ± 7	52 ± 7	0.230
LV kinetic abnormalities	17 (49%)	8 (50%)	9 (47%)	0.370
RVA (cm^2)	15,5 ± 3	16 ± 3	15 ± 3	0.092
RVAC (%)	40 ± 5	39 ± 6	41 ± 4	0.147
CMR findings	n = 32	n = 13	n = 19	
LVEDVi (mL/m^2)	89 ± 17	93 ± 19	88 ± 14	0.377
LVESVi (mL/m^2)	53 ± 8	45 ± 16	42 ± 6	0.734
LVEF (%)	52 ± 8	53 ± 9,8	53 ± 7	0.827
LV WMA	17 (49%)	10 (63%)	7 (37%)	0.181
CMR RVEDVi (mL/m^2)	77 ± 15	74 ± 14	79 ± 16	0.472
CMR RVEF (%)	60 ± 9	55 ± 6	58 ± 11	0.384
WMA RV	13 (37%)	6 (46%)	7 (37%)	0.720
FAT LV	12 (38%)	5 (39%)	7 (37%)	1.000
LGE LV	32 (100%)	13 (100%)	19 (100%)	1.000
LGE LV > 2 segments	25 (78%)	10 (77%)	15 (79%)	1.000
FAT RV	5 (16%)	4 (31%)	1 (5%)	0.132
LGE RV	2 (6%)	1 (8%)	1 (5%)	0.780
LGE RV > 2 segments	1 (3%)	1 (8%)	0 (0%)	0.406

CMR: cardiac magnetic resonance; LV: left ventricular; RV: right ventricular; LVEDVi: indexed LV end-diastolic volume; LVESVi: indexed LV end-systolic volume; LVEF: LV ejection fraction; RVA: RV area; RVAC: RV area change; WMA: wall motion abnormalities; and LGE: late enhancement.

3.4. CMR Findings

CMR assessment was performed on 32 patients (91%). The data on their biventricular dimensions, functions, wall motion alterations (WMAs), and tissue characterization are reported in Table 3.

In the overall population, EDVi was increased in 20 (63%) patients, while LV-EF was reduced in 24 (75%). In 17 cases (49%) LV-WMA was present, mainly involving the infero-posterior wall. RV dimensions and function were within limits in 28 patients (87%), while 4 (12%) showed a mildly increased RV-EDVi, whereas 1 (3%) possessed a mild systolic dysfunction. LV-EF was below 35% in 2 patients, 1 for each group. LV-LGE was detected in all patients with the most common pattern of distribution being the subepicardial stria, mostly located in the basal segments of the inferolateral wall (see Table 3). An example is shown in Figure 1, the description of which is in the caption.

3.5. Outcomes of ALVC Pregnancies

Overall, 16 patients experienced 27 singleton viable pregnancies (range 1–3 and mean age at first pregnancy 30 ± 3.9). All patients were on NYHA I functional class before pregnancy and none had a history of HF before pregnancy. During pregnancy, 3 patients (19%) complained of palpitations.

All viable pregnancies resulted in live-born children. Twenty-five (93%) were delivered full term, and two preterm at 37 and 38 weeks. A total of four cesarean sections (25%) were performed: two for ALVC-related reasons and two for primarily obstetric indications (i.e., fetal growth delay, who were both in therapy with beta-blockers). No major obstetric complications occurred during pregnancy. Patients diagnosed with ALVC before pregnancy underwent a close cardiac and obstetrical monitoring. From the cardiological point of view, each patient underwent a cardiological examination including an echocardiographic examination and a 24-h Holter ECG monitoring.

3.6. Comparison between Childbearing and Nulliparous Subjects

Genetic analysis identified a P/LP genetic variant in 11 (69%) childbearing women and in 15 (79%) nulliparous women (p = 0.490); however, this was without significant differences regarding the prevalence of specific disease genes in the two groups. The age of nulliparous women was significantly lower when compared to women with previous pregnancies (Table 1). There were no differences between the two groups regarding the ratio of probands, the family history of cardiomyopathies, HF, or ECG features. Regarding morphological abnormalities, a two-D echocardiogram comparison of RV dimensions was not significant (p = 0.060) (see Table 2). CMR assessment showed no differences between the two groups regarding LV and RV dimensions and function; however, WMA and the presence of LGE were reported. The 24-h ECG Holter evaluation of 32 patients (91%) showed VAs (isolated PVBs in 20 patients, 57%, and NSVT in 12 patients, 34%) without significant differences between the nulliparous and childbearing women.

3.7. Follow-Up Analysis

The follow-up period had a mean duration in the overall cohort of 7.80 ± 6.69 years (min 1–max 30 years). In detail, the mean duration for childbearing women was 8.31 ± 6.07 (min 2–max 20 years), while for nulliparous women it was 8.31 ± 7.37 (min 1–max 30 years), which demonstrated a p = 0.684. Considering overall events, seven patients (20%) experienced an sVT. Of these, four (57%) belonged to the childbearing group and all episodes occurred after the last pregnancy, with a median time interval of 11.5 years (min 2 months–max 27 years). Furthermore, the age at sVT onset did not differ significantly between the groups of nulliparous (median 33, min 29, max 36 years) and childbearing women (median 45, min 33, max 59 years), which demonstrated a p = 0.100. In a total of ten patients (29%) an ICD was implanted (age at implant 36 ± 7 years, min 25, max 45 years), whereas five (50%) patients possessed primary prevention (3 belonging to childbearing and 2 to nulliparous group). Two patients, one belonging to each group, had HF episodes at the age of 42 and 38 years, respectively. Kaplan–Meir analysis of the VT-free survival curves showed no significant difference between the groups of pregnant and nulliparous women (Log Rank p = 0.220). Furthermore, no association was found between pregnancy and MVA (HR 0.77, C.I. 95% 0.17–3.46, and p = 0.728).

4. Discussion

ALVC is a recently described clinical entity in which clinical manifestations, effective therapy, outcome, and risk stratification are not completely understood [5]. To the best of our knowledge, this is the first study that describes pregnancy course and outcome in a cohort of female patients that are diagnosed with this disease. Furthermore, our purpose was to characterize the effect of pregnancy on this type of cardiomyopathy through the comparison of a series of ALVC women who underwent a pregnancy with a group of affected nulliparous patients. We found that pregnancy is well tolerated in ALVC patients, and that history of pregnancy does not seem to modify the outcome in terms of either electrical instability or HF.

4.1. Physiological Cardiac Changes in Pregnancy

Different physiological changes in the cardiovascular system occur during pregnancy. The maternal blood volume increases significantly starting at around 6 weeks of gestation and reaches a maximal volume by the 32 weeks period with a comprehensive increase of 45% [21]. Furthermore, there is a comparable increase in cardiac output, which is achieved by a rise in stroke volume, and later in pregnancy with an increase in heart rate. The growth in plasma volume and cardiac output are triggered by vasodilation, which occurs early in pregnancy due to hormonal influences. The above circulatory changes are matched by an increase in the LV wall muscle and EDV, with end-systolic volume and end-diastolic pressure that remain unchanged [21]. Overall, LV systolic function improves early in pregnancy and progresses gradually until 20 weeks' gestation due to LV afterload reduction. Hemodynamic changes are fully reset after 6 months [22].

4.2. Pregnancy in Patients with ACM

Available data seem to indicate that in the majority of women with ACM the course of pregnancy and postpartum are uneventful with regard to pregnancy-related mortality and complications [23]. Depending on the number of patients enrolled in the study, individual risk profile, and duration of follow-up, the rates of maternal death from all causes varied from 0 to 4%. Moreover, the comparison of ACM patients who experienced a pregnancy with nulliparous affected patients demonstrated no difference in clinical event rates and acceleration of VA and HF, either during pregnancy or after childbirth, both early and long after [9,24,25]. Thus, published data appears to prove that pregnancy does not constitute a driving force for disease progression in ACM [23]. Furthermore, the number of pregnancies appear to have no impact on the outcome and incidence of maternal complications [9].

4.3. Pregnancy in Patients with DCM

DCM is characterized by dilation and impaired contraction, primarily of the left ventricle (LV). ALVC may overlap with DCM when LV dilation and systolic dysfunction are present in both conditions. Further, CMR assessment has an important role in providing a differential diagnosis of the extent of LV-LGE. Moreover, this predominantly affects the inferolateral segments and is, also, significantly greater in ALVC [3]. Only a few studies on the pregnancy outcomes of women with idiopathic DCM have been published so far [26–29]. Having said that, pregnancy in asymptomatic or mildly symptomatic DCM patients appears to be associated with a low risk of adverse maternal events. However, pregnancy is poorly tolerated in some women with pre-existing DCM, with the potential for significant deterioration in LV function. In addition, the predictors of maternal mortality are found in the NYHA class III/IV as well as at EF <40%. Highly adverse risk factors include EF <20%, the presence of mitral regurgitation, as well as RV failure and/or hypotension [30]. Furthermore, pregnant women with DCM experience more adverse events compared to non-pregnant women [28,31], and this could be partially explained by the increased hemodynamic challenge that occurs in pregnant patients and by the need to discontinue ACE-inhibitors during pregnancy due to their teratogenic effects.

4.4. Pregnancy Outcome in Patients with ALVC

In our patients, pregnancies were well tolerated, and none experienced adverse events. Nonetheless, it is important to underline that in our series LV systolic function was found to be severely reduced before pregnancy (EF < 35%) in only 1 of the 16 women belonging to the childbearing group, thus further data on a larger cohort are required for more comprehensive knowledge. One patient showed an sVT episode two months after the third pregnancy, however the same arrhythmic events also occurred two years later, thus a clear relationship between sVT and pregnancy cannot be proved. Furthermore, pregnancies do not seem to have a role on the degree of electrical instability, considering that the number of patients with sVT, as well as age of patients at the time of arrhythmic episodes, did not differ significantly in the two groups.

4.5. Pregnancy Management in ALVC Patients

As in other cardiomyopathies, women with ALVC who wish to have a baby require a pre-pregnancy risk assessment, counselling, and should be reviewed by a pregnancy heart team with a cardiologist and a gynecologist. Considering the lack of data on pregnancy tolerance in ALVC patients, we should also consider the existing data on DCM, which demonstrate that the NYHA class III/IV and EF <40% are predictors of maternal mortality, with highly adverse risk factors when EF <20%. Pre-pregnancy management should include modification of the existing medications in order to avoid teratogenicity and to minimize harm to the fetus. Even if the appropriate management strategy for ALVC is not completely established, in the presence of LV dilation/dysfunction ACE-inhibitors and angiotensin receptor blockers are frequently prescribed, as well as ARNI or mineralocorticoid receptor inhibitors; these are contraindicated during pregnancy and should be discontinued prior to conception, with close clinical and echocardiographic monitoring. Beta-adrenergic blocking agents are generally safe in pregnancy even if they are associated with increased rates of fetal growth restriction [30]. Flecainide has been safely used to treat maternal and fetal arrhythmias; however, although rare, neonatal toxicity can occur [31]. Patients should be monitored during pregnancy and postpartum with periodic cardiac evaluation with ECG assessments, 2-D-echocardiogram tests, and 24-h Holter ECG evaluations, and close cooperation with gynecologists. Additionally, if indicated, ICD implant is safe during pregnancy [32,33].

4.6. Possible Role of Pregnancy in Disease Progression in ALVC Patients

As expected, at the time of evaluation, patients with previous pregnancies were significantly older than nulliparous ones. Thus, considering that we are dealing with a progressive myocardial disease, the specific role of pregnancies in disease progression is difficult to estimate. Nonetheless, despite a significant age difference, the two groups of patients did not differ significantly regarding LV dimensions and function, as well as in the degree of electrical instability, thus suggesting the absence of a clear role of pregnancy in disease progression.

5. Conclusions

Pregnancy in ALVC patients with normal or mildly reduced systolic function, and without previous HF episodes, appear to be well tolerated and do not appear to have a role in disease progression, either in terms of ventricular dilatation/dysfunction or in the degree of electrical instability. Further studies on a larger cohort of patients with different degrees of disease extent and genetic background are needed in order to achieve a more comprehensive knowledge on the outcome of pregnancy in this disease.

Author Contributions: Conceptualization: B.B.; methodology: R.B., K.P., B.B. and D.C.; formal analysis: R.B., G.M. and B.B.; investigation: R.B., I.R., M.B.M., P.V., V.P., A.Z. and A.C.; resources: C.B. and S.I.; data curation: R.B. and P.D.; writing—original draft preparation: R.B., B.B., I.R., R.C. and M.C.; review and editing: R.B., B.B. and G.L.; supervision: K.P. and B.B.; and administration: B.B. All authors have read and agreed to the published version of the manuscript.

Funding: This research received no external funding.

Institutional Review Board Statement: The study was conducted in accordance with the guidelines in the Declaration of Helsinki and was approved by the local ethics committee (Ethics Committee of the University Hospital of Padua, ID:1967P, 1 October 2010).

Informed Consent Statement: Informed consent was obtained from all subjects involved in the study.

Data Availability Statement: The data presented in this study are available on request from the corresponding author.

Acknowledgments: The authors thank Alison Garside for assisting with the English version of this paper.

Conflicts of Interest: The authors declare no conflict of interest.

References

1. Thiene, G.; Nava, A.; Corrado, D.; Rossi, L.; Pennelli, N. Right Ventricular Cardiomyopathy and Sudden Death in Young People. *N. Engl. J. Med.* **1988**, *318*, 129–133. [CrossRef] [PubMed]
2. Sen-Chowdhry, S.; Syrris, P.; Ward, D.; Asimaki, A.; Sevdalis, E.; McKenna, W.J. Clinical and genetic characterization of families with arrhythmogenic right ventricular dysplasia/cardiomyopathy provides novel insights into patterns of disease expression. *Circulation* **2007**, *115*, 1710–1720. [CrossRef] [PubMed]
3. Cipriani, A.; Bauce, B.; De Lazzari, M.; Rigato, I.; Bariani, R.; Meneghin, S.; Pilichou, K.; Motta, R.; Aliberti, C.; Thiene, G.; et al. Arrhythmogenic Right Ventricular Cardiomyopathy: Characterization of Left Ventricular Phenotype and Differential Diagnosis With Dilated Cardiomyopathy. *J. Am. Heart Assoc.* **2020**, *9*, e014628. [CrossRef] [PubMed]
4. Sen-Chowdhry, S.; Syrris, P.; McKenna, W.J. Role of Genetic Analysis in the Management of Patients With Arrhythmogenic Right Ventricular Dysplasia/Cardiomyopathy. *J. Am. Coll. Cardiol.* **2007**, *50*, 1813–1821. [CrossRef] [PubMed]
5. Corrado, D.; Basso, C. Arrhythmogenic left ventricular cardiomyopathy. *Heart* **2022**, *108*, 733. [CrossRef] [PubMed]
6. Augusto, J.B.; Eiros, R.; Nakou, E.; Moura-Ferreira, S.; Treibel, T.A.; Captur, G.; Akhtar, M.M.; Protonotarios, A.; Gossios, T.D.; Savvatis, K.; et al. Dilated cardiomyopathy and arrhythmogenic left ventricular cardiomyopathy: A comprehensive genotype-imaging phenotype study. *Eur. Heart J. Cardiovasc. Imaging* **2020**, *21*, 326–336. [CrossRef] [PubMed]
7. Bariani, R.; Rigato, I.; Cason, M.; Bueno Marinas, M.; Celeghin, R.; Pilichou, K.; Bauce, B. Genetic Background and Clinical Features in Arrhythmogenic Left Ventricular Cardiomyopathy: A Systematic Review. *J. Clin. Med.* **2022**, *11*, 4313. [CrossRef]
8. Casella, M.; Gasperetti, A.; Sicuso, R.; Conte, E.; Catto, V.; Sommariva, E.; Bergonti, M.; Vettor, G.; Rizzo, S.; Pompilio, G.; et al. Characteristics of Patients With Arrhythmogenic Left Ventricular Cardiomyopathy. *Circ. Arrhythm. Electrophysiol.* **2020**, *13*, e009005. [CrossRef]
9. Hodes, A.R.; Tichnell, C.; te Riele, A.S.J.M.; Murray, B.; Groeneweg, J.A.; Sawant, A.C.; Russell, S.D.; van Spaendonck-Zwarts, K.Y.; van den Berg, M.P.; Wilde, A.A.; et al. Pregnancy course and outcomes in women with arrhythmogenic right ventricular cardiomyopathy. *Heart* **2016**, *102*, 303. [CrossRef]
10. Lang, R.M.; Badano, L.P.; Mor-Avi, V.; Afilalo, J.; Armstrong, A.; Ernande, L.; Flachskampf, F.A.; Foster, E.; Goldstein, S.A.; Kuznetsova, T.; et al. Recommendations for Cardiac Chamber Quantification by Echocardiography in Adults: An Update from the American Society of Echocardiography and the European Association of Cardiovascular Imaging. *Eur. Heart J. Cardiovasc. Imaging* **2015**, *16*, 233–271. [CrossRef]
11. Friedrich, M.G.; Sechtem, U.; Schulz-Menger, J.; Holmvang, G.; Alakija, P.; Cooper, L.T.; White, J.A.; Abdel-Aty, H.; Gutberlet, M.; Prasad, S.; et al. Cardiovascular Magnetic Resonance in Myocarditis: A JACC White Paper. *J. Am. Coll. Cardiol.* **2009**, *53*, 1475–1487. [CrossRef] [PubMed]
12. De Lazzari, M.; Zorzi, A.; Cipriani, A.; Susana, A.; Mastella, G.; Rizzo, A.; Rigato, I.; Bauce, B.; Giorgi, B.; Lacognata, C.; et al. Relationship Between Electrocardiographic Findings and Cardiac Magnetic Resonance Phenotypes in Arrhythmogenic Cardiomyopathy. *J. Am. Heart Assoc.* **2018**, *7*, e009855. [CrossRef] [PubMed]
13. Celeghin, R.; Cipriani, A.; Bariani, R.; Marinas, M.B.; Cason, M.; Bevilacqua, M.; Gaspari, M.D.; Rizzo, S.; Rigato, I.; Pozzo, S.D.; et al. Filamin-C variant-associated cardiomyopathy: A pooled analysis of individual patient data to evaluate the clinical profile and risk of sudden cardiac death. *Heart Rhythm* **2022**, *19*, 235–243. [CrossRef] [PubMed]
14. Bariani, R.; Cason, M.; Rigato, I.; Cipriani, A.; Celeghin, R.; De Gaspari, M.; Bueno Marinas, M.; Mattesi, G.; Pergola, V.; Rizzo, S.; et al. Clinical profile and long-term follow-up of a cohort of patients with desmoplakin cardiomyopathy. *Heart Rhythm* **2022**, *19*, 1315–1324. [CrossRef]
15. Whittock, N.V.; Ashton, G.H.; Dopping-Hepenstal, P.J.; Gratian, M.J.; Keane, F.M.; Eady, R.A.; McGrath, J.A. Striate Palmoplantar Keratoderma Resulting from Desmoplakin Haploinsufficiency. *J. Investig. Dermatol.* **1999**, *113*, 940–946. [CrossRef] [PubMed]
16. Bariani, R.; Cipriani, A.; Rizzo, S.; Celeghin, R.; Bueno Marinas, M.; Giorgi, B.; De Gaspari, M.; Rigato, I.; Leoni, L.; Zorzi, A.; et al. 'Hot Phase' Clinical Presentation in Arrhythmogenic Cardiomyopathy. *EP Eur.* **2021**, *23*, 907–917. [CrossRef] [PubMed]
17. Rampazzo, A.; Nava, A.; Malacrida, S.; Beffagna, G.; Bauce, B.; Rossi, V.; Zimbello, R.; Simionati, B.; Basso, C.; Thiene, G.; et al. Mutation in Human Desmoplakin Domain Binding to Plakoglobin Causes a Dominant Form of Arrhythmogenic Right Ventricular Cardiomyopathy. *Am. J. Hum. Genet.* **2002**, *71*, 1200–1206. [CrossRef]
18. Quarta, G.; Muir, A.; Pantazis, A.; Syrris, P.; Gehmlich, K.; Garcia-Pavia, P.; Ward, D.; Sen-Chowdhry, S.; Elliott, P.M.; McKenna, W.J. Familial Evaluation in Arrhythmogenic Right Ventricular Cardiomyopathy: Impact of Genetics and Revised Task Force Criteria. *Circulation* **2011**, *123*, 2701–2709. [CrossRef]
19. Fressart, V.; Duthoit, G.; Donal, E.; Probst, V.; Deharo, J.C.; Chevalier, P.; Klug, D.; Dubourg, O.; Delacretaz, E.; Cosnay, P.; et al. Desmosomal Gene Analysis in Arrhythmogenic Right Ventricular Dysplasia/Cardiomyopathy: Spectrum of Mutations and Clinical Impact in Practice. *Europace* **2010**, *12*, 861–868. [CrossRef]

20. Christensen, A.H.; Benn, M.; Bundgaard, H.; Tybjaerg-Hansen, A.; Haunso, S.; Svendsen, J.H. Wide Spectrum of Desmosomal Mutations in Danish Patients with Arrhythmogenic Right Ventricular Cardiomyopathy. *J. Med. Genet.* **2010**, *47*, 736–744. [CrossRef]
21. Ouzounian, J.G.; Elkayam, U. Physiologic Changes During Normal Pregnancy and Delivery. *Cardiol. Clin.* **2012**, *30*, 317–329. [CrossRef] [PubMed]
22. Schaufelberger, M. Cardiomyopathy and pregnancy. *Heart* **2019**, *105*, 1543–1551. [CrossRef] [PubMed]
23. Wichter, T.; Milberg, P.; Wichter, H.D.; Dechering, D.G. Pregnancy in arrhythmogenic cardiomyopathy. *Herzschrittmachertherapie Elektrophysiologie* **2021**, *32*, 186–198. [CrossRef] [PubMed]
24. Castrini, A.I.; Lie, Ø.H.; Leren, I.S.; Estensen, M.E.; Stokke, M.K.; Klæboe, L.G.; Edvardsen, T.; Haugaa, K.H. Number of pregnancies and subsequent phenotype in a cross-sectional cohort of women with arrhythmogenic cardiomyopathy. *Eur. Heart J. Cardiovasc. Imaging* **2019**, *20*, 192–198. [CrossRef] [PubMed]
25. Platonov, P.G.; Castrini, A.I.; Svensson, A.; Christiansen, M.K.; Gilljam, T.; Bundgaard, H.; Madsen, T.; Heliö, T.; Christensen, A.H.; Åström, M.A.; et al. Pregnancies, ventricular arrhythmias, and substrate progression in women with arrhythmogenic right ventricular cardiomyopathy in the Nordic ARVC Registry. *EP Eur.* **2020**, *22*, 1873–1879. [CrossRef] [PubMed]
26. Grewal, J.; Siu, S.C.; Ross, H.J.; Mason, J.; Balint, O.H.; Sermer, M.; Colman, J.M.; Silversides, C.K. Pregnancy Outcomes in Women With Dilated Cardiomyopathy. *J. Am. Coll. Cardiol.* **2009**, *55*, 45–52. [CrossRef] [PubMed]
27. Palojoki, E.; Kaartinen, M.; Kaaja, R.; Reissell, E.; Kärkkäinen, S.; Kuusisto, J.; Heliö, T. Pregnancy and childbirth in carriers of the lamin A/C-gene mutation. *Eur. J. Heart Fail.* **2010**, *12*, 630–633. [CrossRef]
28. Katsuragi, S.; Omoto, A.; Kamiya, C.; Ueda, K.; Sasaki, Y.; Yamanaka, K.; Neki, R.; Yoshimatsu, J.; Niwa, K.; Ikeda, T. Risk factors for maternal outcome in pregnancy complicated with dilated cardiomyopathy. *J. Perinatol.* **2012**, *32*, 170–175. [CrossRef]
29. Boyle, S.; Nicolae, M.; Kostner, K.; Davies, K.; Cukovski, I.; Cunliffe, A.; Morton, A. Dilated Cardiomyopathy in Pregnancy: Outcomes From an Australian Tertiary Centre for Maternal Medicine and Review of the Current Literature. *Heart Lung Circ.* **2019**, *28*, 591–597. [CrossRef]
30. Sliwa, K.; Meer, P.; Petrie, M.C.; Frogoudaki, A.; Johnson, M.R.; Hilfiker-Kleiner, D.; Hamdan, R.; Jackson, A.M.; Ibrahim, B.; Mbakwem, A.; et al. Risk stratification and management of women with cardiomyopathy/heart failure planning pregnancy or presenting during/after pregnancy: A position statement from the Heart Failure Association of the European Society of Cardiology Study Group on Peripartum Cardiomyopathy. *Eur. J. Heart Fail.* **2021**, *23*, 527–540. [CrossRef]
31. Tamirisa, K.P.; Elkayam, U.; Briller, J.E.; Mason, P.K.; Pillarisetti, J.; Merchant, F.M.; Patel, H.; Lakkireddy, D.R.; Russo, A.M.; Volgman, A.S.; et al. Arrhythmias in Pregnancy. *JACC Clin. Electrophysiol.* **2022**, *8*, 120–135. [CrossRef] [PubMed]
32. Regitz-Zagrosek, V.; Roos-Hesselink, J.W.; Bauersachs, J.; Blomström-Lundqvist, C.; Cífková, R.; De Bonis, M.; Iung, B.; Johnson, M.R.; Kintscher, U.; Kranke, P.; et al. 2018 ESC Guidelines for the management of cardiovascular diseases during pregnancy: The Task Force for the Management of Cardiovascular Diseases during Pregnancy of the European Society of Cardiology (ESC). *Eur. Heart J.* **2018**, *39*, 3165–3241. [CrossRef] [PubMed]
33. Seth, R.; Moss, A.J.; McNitt, S.; Zareba, W.; Andrews, M.L.; Qi, M.; Robinson, J.L.; Goldenberg, I.; Ackerman, M.J.; Benhorin, J.; et al. Long QT Syndrome and Pregnancy. *J. Am. Coll. Cardiol.* **2007**, *49*, 1092–1098. [CrossRef] [PubMed]

Journal of
Clinical Medicine

MDPI

Article

The Role of Stress in Stable Patients with Takotsubo Syndrome—Does the Trigger Matter?

Gassan Moady [1,2,*], Otman Ali [3], Rania Sweid [4] and Shaul Atar [1,2]

1 Department of Cardiology, Galilee Medical Center, Nahariya 2210001, Israel
2 Azrieli Faculty of Medicine, Bar Ilan University, Safed 5290002, Israel
3 Department of Internal Medicine, Galilee Medical Center, Nahariya 2210001, Israel
4 Biostatistics Unit, Galilee Medical Center, Nahariya 2210001, Israel
* Correspondence: gassanm@gmc.gov.il; Tel.: +972-4-9107273; Fax: +972-4-9107279

Abstract: Background: Takotsubo syndrome (TTS) is a unique type of reversible cardiomyopathy that predominantly affects elderly women. The role of physical and emotional stress in the pathophysiology of TTS is well established. However, the association between preceding emotional triggers and clinical outcomes in stable patients has not yet been fully investigated. We aimed to investigate the association between emotional triggers before symptom onset and clinical outcomes in stable patients with TTS. Methods: This is a retrospective cohort study based on the data of patients with ICD-9 discharge diagnosis of TTS between 2017 and 2022. Patients were divided into two groups: with and without obvious emotional trigger before symptom onset. Demographic, laboratory, echocardiographic, and clinical outcomes were obtained and compared between the two groups. Results: We included 86 patients (93% were women, mean age 68.8 $\pm$ 12.3 years). Of them, 64 (74.4%) reported an emotional trigger before symptom onset. Patients with a previous emotional trigger had a longer hospital stay (4.3 + 2.0 days vs. 3.0 + 1.4, $p = 0.002$) with no difference in in-hospital complications (32.8% vs. 13.6%, $p = 0.069$), with no difference in 30-day mortality, readmissions, or recurrence rate between the groups. Conclusions: Patients with TTS related to an emotional trigger may represent a different population from patients without a preceding trigger by having more symptomatic disease and longer hospital stay, yet with no difference in the 30-day outcomes.

Keywords: takotsubo; cardiomyopathy; trigger; stress; outcome

Citation: Moady, G.; Ali, O.; Sweid, R.; Atar, S. The Role of Stress in Stable Patients with Takotsubo Syndrome—Does the Trigger Matter? *J. Clin. Med.* **2022**, *11*, 7304. https://doi.org/10.3390/jcm11247304

Academic Editor: Stefan Peters

Received: 13 October 2022
Accepted: 7 December 2022
Published: 9 December 2022

1. Introduction

Takotsubo syndrome (TTS), also known as stress cardiomyopathy or apical ballooning syndrome, is a unique type of reversible cardiac dysfunction mediated by various neurohormonal processes, often preceded by a physical or emotional trigger [1–3]. According to previous studies, about two thirds of patients report a physical or mental trigger before symptom onset [1–3]. Several echocardiographic patterns have been reported, with apical ballooning being the most common variant [4]. The presentation of TTS often mimics acute coronary syndrome (ACS) by sharing similar clinical and laboratory characteristics, making the differentiation between the two conditions very challenging. In both conditions, the patient presents with chest pain, ECG changes, elevated troponin, and wall motion abnormality by echocardiography [5–7]. The underlying mechanism of TTS is not fully understood, but several pathways, including catecholamine surge, epicardial coronary spasm, microvascular dysfunction, and genetic predisposition are involved in the pathogenesis of the disease [8–11]. Most patients are hemodynamically stable and exhibit complete echocardiographic recovery of the cardiac function; however, fulminant course with cardiogenic shock or intractable pulmonary edema may occur in rare cases [1,12]. Major complications include QT segment prolongation and ventricular arrhythmia, cardiogenic shock, dynamic mitral regurgitation secondary to left ventricular (LV) outflow tract obstruction, and systemic embolism such as stroke or transient ischemic attack [1]. In one study, male sex, reduced LV function on admission, and acute neurologic events were associated with less LV function recovery and subsequently with less favorable 1-year outcomes [13]. It is now well established that long-term prognosis of TTS is comparable to that of ACS [1]. In the current study, we aimed to compare the baseline characteristics and the clinical outcomes of hemodynamically stable TTS, with and without an emotional trigger before symptom onset.

2. Methods

2.1. Study Design and Population

In this retrospective cohort study, we included patients with ICD-9 diagnosis of takotsubo syndrome on discharge between 2017 and 2022 in the cardiology department at Galilee Medical Center. We included only cases of confirmed diagnosis of TTS. The diagnosis was confirmed finally by a senior cardiologist according to the appropriate criteria based on the clinical presentation, electrocardiographic changes, biomarkers, echocardiography, and coronary angiography or CCT showing no obstructive coronary disease. Based on history taking, we divided the cohort into two groups, patients with an obvious emotional trigger before symptom onset (with trigger), and patients with confirmed TTS without any identified trigger before hospitalization (without trigger).

2.2. Definitions

The revised Mayo Clinic diagnostic criteria are used when the diagnosis of TTS is suspected, based on the following:

1. Transient dyskinesia of the left ventricular midsegment.
2. Regional wall motion abnormality, beyond single coronary artery.
3. Absence of obstructive coronary artery disease or acute plaque rupture.
4. New electrocardiographic abnormalities or modest troponin elevation.
5. Absence of pheochromocytoma and myocarditis.

In most cases, coronary angiography is performed to rule out obstructive coronary artery disease, and a ventriculogram is performed for further confirmation of the diagnosis; however, cardiac computed tomography (CCT) may also be used. CCT may be preferred when another non-coronary condition is suspected, such as aortic dissection, or when the patient is not interested in invasive angiography.

2.3. Data Collection

Baseline characteristics, laboratory, and echocardiographic data were obtained based on the computerized files of the hospitalized patients. The presence or absence of an emotional trigger was clearly identified in all patients based on history taking (repeat focused history taking is usually performed after confirming the diagnosis). Electrocardiographic changes were reported in the case of the following findings: ST-segment elevation or depression, T-wave inversion, and QT segment prolongation. Maximal troponin, C reactive protein (CRP), and white blood cells (WBC) are presented. High sensitivity troponin I (Hs-TnI) level was measured using ARCHITECT assay (Abbott). Cut-off values for abnormal hs-TnI levels were above 20 ng/L and 30 ng/L for men and women, respectively. The patients were divided into two groups: with and without trigger based on the reported history. Triggers were also classified by negative, positive, or other (related to surgery or infection). Cases of "without trigger" were defined by ruling out any obvious trigger after comprehensive investigation. In all cases of TTS, a physician reevaluated the patients with a focus on identifying potential triggers.

2.4. Clinical Outcomes

Retrospectively, we included the following outcomes: length of stay of the index hospitalization, TTS-related complications (including atrial fibrillation, pulmonary congestion, and non-sustained ventricular tachycardia), 30-day recurrence, and 30-day death. Clinical outcomes were retrieved retrospectively based on the computerized files of the patients.

2.5. Statistical Analysis

Categorical variables are presented as percentages, while continuous variables are presented as median with interquartile range (IQR) or mean with standard deviation (SD). We used Fisher's exact test and Chi square test to compare categorical variables between the two groups. Independent sample t-test or Mann–Whitney tests were used for continuous variables. The choice between those tests was made according to the distribution of the data; the Mann–Whitney test was used when a significant deviation from the normal distribution was found. To test the correlation between non-normal continuous variables we used Spearman's test. All tests were conducted at a two-sided overall 5% significance level ($\alpha = 0.05$). Multivariable logistic regression analysis and multivariable linear analysis were performed to examine the correlation between the trigger and complications and length of stay, respectively, adjusted to diabetes mellitus, neurological disease, and CRP. Odds ratio (OR) with 95% confidence interval (CI) were presented. To estimate time to recurrence, survival analysis was presented using the Kaplan–Meier method and Log-Rank test for the invariable analysis and Cox-regression with Hazard ratio (HR) and 95% CI for the multivariable analysis.

Statistical analysis was performed using R-IBM SPSS statistics (R-studio, V.4.0.3, Vienna, Austria). The study was approved by the local ethical committee of Galilee Medical Center.

3. Results

3.1. Baseline Characteristics

Among 86 patients with final diagnosis of TTS (93% female, mean age 68.8), 64 patients (74.4%) reported an emotional stress before admission. Table 1 summarizes the clinical characteristics and laboratory data of the study population.

Table 1. Baseline clinical characteristics and laboratory data of the study population.

n	86
Age (mean + SD)	68.8 + 12.3
Female (*n*, %)	80 (93)
Preceding trigger (*n*, %)	64 (74.4)
Tobacco use (*n*, %)	18 (20.9)
Diabetes Mellitus (*n*, %)	24 (27.9)
Hypertension (*n*, %)	55 (64)
Hyperlipidemia (*n*, %)	49 (57)
Psychological disease (*n*, %)	12 (14)
Neurological disease (*n*, %)	15 (17.4)
ECG changes (*n*, %)	51 (59.3)
SBP (mmHg, mean ± SD)	122.6 ± 25.7
DBP (mmHg, mean ± SD)	74.0 ± 15.5
Heart rate (bpm, mean ± SD)	80.2 ± 17.7
O_2 saturation (mean ± SD)	95.3 ± 5.3
WBC ($\times 10^9$/L, mean ± SD)	10.5 ± 4.8
CRP [(mg/L), median, IQR]	17.4 (6.1, 40.1)
Hemoglobin (gr/dL, mean ± SD)	12.2 ± 1.6
Hs-TnI [(ng/L), median, IQR]	1922.5 (852, 5382.5)
Creatinine (mg/dL, mean ± SD)	0.9 ± 0.4

IQR, interquartile range; CRP, C-reactive protein; DBP, diastolic blood pressure; ECG, electrocardiogram; Hs-TnI, high sensitivity troponin I; IQR, interquartile range; SBP, systolic blood pressure; SD, standard deviation; WBC, white blood cells.

Normal values: WBC (4.5–11.0); CRP (0.2–5.0); Hemoglobin (12.0–16.0); Hs-TnI (<20 for female, <30 for males); Creatinine (0.5–1.2).

The classification of the various triggers is provided in Table 2.

Table 2. Classification of the various triggers.

Negative Stress	**48 (75.0%)**
Positive stress	3 (4.7%)
Post-surgery	6 (9.4%)
Stress related to work	4 (6.3%)
COVID-19 related	3 (4.7%)

Examples of negative stress include grief or stressful arguments; stress related to work—the patient reported abrupt increase of required tasks; COVID-19, coronavirus disease-2019. Positive triggers may include a wedding, or a promotion at work

Overall, there was no statistical difference between groups, though some imbalance in proportions was present (e.g., for diabetes) (Table 3).

Table 3. Baseline characteristics in the two groups.

	with Trigger N = 64	**without Trigger N = 22**	***p* Value**
Age (years)	68.3 ± 11.9	70.1 ± 13.6	0.56
Female %	59 (92.2)	21 (95.5)	1
Tobacco use (*n*, %)	13 (20.3)	5 (22.7)	0.77
Diabetes Mellitus (*n*, %)	21 (32.8)	3 (13.6)	0.07
Hypertension (*n*, %)	43 (67.2)	12 (54.5)	0.31
Hyperlipidemia (*n*, %)	38 (59.4)	11 (50.0)	0.47
Psychological disease (*n*, %)	9 (14.1)	3 (13.6)	1
Neurological disease (*n*, %)	14 (21.9)	1 (4.5)	0.056

3.2. Clinical and Laboratory Parameters during the Index Hospitalization

During the index hospitalization, patients were monitored in the cardiology or cardiac care units. Hemodynamic and laboratory parameters are shown in Table 4. Of note, for patients in whom coronary angiography was not performed, coronary anatomy was demonstrated by cardiac computed tomography.

Table 4. Hemodynamic and laboratory parameters in the two groups.

	with Trigger N = 64	**without Trigger N = 22**	***p* Value**
ECG changes (%)	62.5	50	0.325
SBP (mmHg, mean ± SD)	122.3 ± 26.9	123.5 ± 22.2	0.881
DBP (mmHg, mean ± SD)	72.5 ± 16.1	78.5 ± 13.1	0.118
Heart rate (bpm, mean ± SD)	82.2 ± 18.3	74.6 ± 14.4	0.058
O_2 saturation (mean ± SD)	95.2 ± 5.8	95.5 ± 3.3	0.624
WBC ($\times 10^9$/L, mean ± SD)	10.7 ± 5.1	9.7 ± 3.7	0.793
CRP [(mg/L), median, IQR]	21.55 (7.93, 51.5)	9.55 (2.9, 25.25)	0.005
Hemoglobin (gr/dL, mean ± SD)	12.0 ± 1.6	12.9 ± 1.4	0.028
Hs-TnI [(ng/L), median, IQR]	2315 (889.75, 5790.5)	1232 (753.25, 4797.25)	0.252
Creatinine (mg/dL, mean ± SD)	0.92 ± 0.4	0.92 ± 0.4	0.939
LVEF (mean ± SD)	42 (38.5, 50.0)	40.5 (37.5, 51.25)	0.604

CRP, C-reactive protein; DBP, diastolic blood pressure; ECG, electrocardiogram; Hs-TnI, high sensitivity troponin I; IQR, interquartile range; LVEF, left ventricular ejection fraction; SBP, systolic blood pressure; SD, standard deviation; WBC, white blood cells. Normal values: WBC (4.5–11.0); CRP (0.2–5.0); Hemoglobin (12.0–16.0); Hs-TnI (<20 for female, <30 for males); Creatinine (0.5–1.2).

3.3. Outcomes

Overall, complications were reported in 27.9% of the study population (including atrial fibrillation, pulmonary congestion, and non-sustained ventricular tachycardia), with a trend for higher rates in the group with an emotional trigger, albeit it was not statistically significant (p = 0.069). Although QT-segment prolongation was documented in more than 50% of the patients, no events of Torsades de pointes were reported. The length of stay was significantly longer in the group with trigger before symptom onset. Beta-blockers and angiotensin converting enzyme inhibitors are often used when there is evidence of left ventricular dysfunction. Diuretic therapy was used in cases of volume overload. The outcomes during the index hospitalization and during 1 month after discharge are presented in Table 5.

Table 5. Outcomes during the index hospitalization and 30-day mortality.

	with Trigger N = 64	**without Trigger N = 22**	***p*-Value**
ICA (n, %)	51 (79.7)	21 (95.5)	0.074
Normal angiography (n, %)	40 (78.4)	18 (85.7)	0.47
Non-significant disease (n, %)	11 (21.6)	3 (14.3)	
Length of stay (days, mean ± SD)	4.28 + 1.98	3.0 + 1.38	0.002
Complications (n, %)	21 (32.8)	3 (13.6)	0.069
QT_C segment prolongation (n, %)	37 (57.8)	12 (54.5)	0.78
Use of medications			
Beta blockers (n, %)	19 (29.7)	7 (31.8)	0.85
ACE inhibitors (n, %)	10 (15.6)	3 (13.6)	0.82
Furosemide (n, %)	15 (23.4)	5 (22.7)	0.94
Inotropic support (n, %)	0	0	N/A
Mechanical ventilation	0	0	N/A
Recurrence within five years (n, %)	5 (7.8)	2 (9)	0.84
30-day mortality (%)	0	0	N/A
30-day readmission (%)	1	0	N/A

ACE, Angiotensin-converting enzyme; ICA, invasive coronary angiography; N/A not applicable; SD, standard deviation. Non-significant disease was defined as coronary artery stenosis ≤ 50%. Prolonged QTc was defined as >450 msec for men and >470 msec for women.

In a multivariable regression model for the presence of trigger, diabetes mellitus (OR 0.63, 95% CI 0.2–1.96), neurological disease (OR 1.07, 95% CI 0.31–3.66), and CRP level (OR 1.0, 95% CI 0.99–1.01) were not associated with increased in-hospital complications. In linear regression adjusted to diabetes mellitus, neurological disease, and CRP level with the length of stay, only CRP was associated with increased hospital stay (p = 0.42, p = 0.64, and p = 0.003 respectively).

In univariable survival analysis (Log-Rank, Mantel Cox), triggers were not associated with higher recurrence rate (p = 0.086), Similar results were obtained using the Cox regression model [HR 4.53, 95% CI 0.74–27.63, p = 0.101], also when the multivariable model was adjusted to diabetes, neurological disease, and CRP level. The Kaplan–Meier curve is presented in Figure 1.

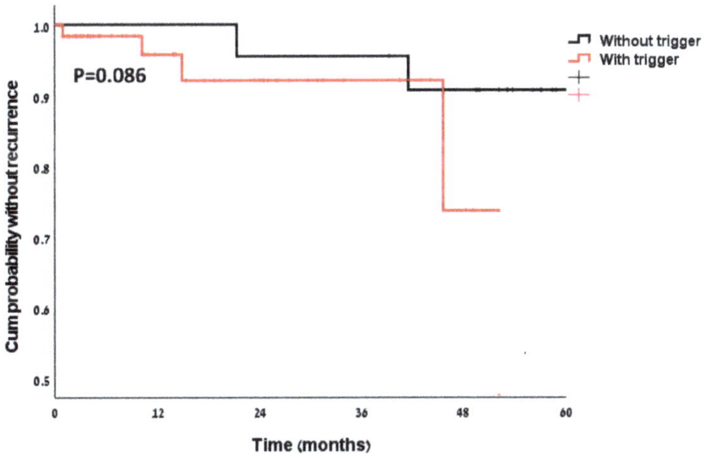

Figure 1. Kaplan–Meier curve for recurrence in the two groups.

3.4. Echocardiographic Follow Up

Forty-eight patients with reduced LV function (left ventricular ejection fraction (LVEF) < 50%) had repeated echocardiography after discharge. Of them, 41 (85.4%) experienced complete recovery of cardiac function (LVEF > 50%) within a range of 2–8 weeks, while a residual cardiac dysfunction was observed in 7 (14.6%) of them. Of note, all patients with residual cardiac dysfunction had an initial LVEF of 25% or less.

The flow diagram of the study is illustrated in Figure 2.

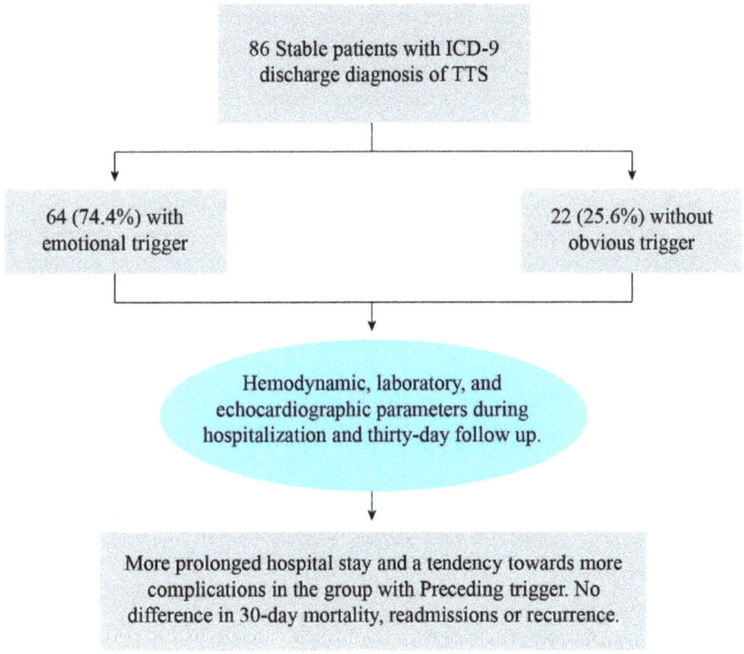

Figure 2. Flow diagram of the study.

4. Discussion

The role of stress in the pathogenesis of TTS is well established. In the current study, we aimed to compare the clinical outcomes of patients with TTS with and without a trigger before symptoms onset. The length of stay was longer in the group with a preceding trigger, probably driven by more prolonged symptoms. The impact of triggers on outcomes in TTS has been evaluated in previous studies, and a clear association was demonstrated between medical illness as the preceding trigger, and in-hospital mortality [2]. This association probably reflects the impact of the underlying disease on outcomes rather than the consequences of TTS. Some of the complications of TTS (such as arrhythmia and LVOT obstruction) may be explained by the abrupt surge of catecholamines during the acute phase of the disease [14–18]. Although there was no significant difference in the rate of complications between the two groups in the current study, this may be attributed to the small study population. We assume that all reported complications were related to TTS itself, because we included patients with stable hemodynamic and respiratory parameters without underlying severe illness during the index hospitalization, and without need for respiratory or circulatory mechanical support. TTS is mistakenly considered a benign condition, though the outcome is comparable to that of ACS. In the study by Templin et al., the mortality rate and major complications of patients with TTS were similar to those of patients with ACS [1]. Previous studies showed that TTS triggered by illness is associated with higher mortality rates in long-term follow up than acute coronary syndrome (ACS), while emotional stress-related TTS had better outcomes [2,19,20]. Thus, a new classification for prognostic purpose was proposed based on the preceding trigger [21]. It should be noted that, in all the patients in the study, the presence or absence of an emotional trigger was confirmed following a focused interview aimed at identifying possible triggers once the diagnosis of TTS had been suspected. We cannot claim that TTS with an emotional trigger represents a different disease with a different course and outcome because we could not eliminate all potential confounders. Therefore, we can rather conclude that TTS patients with a trigger may represent a different population from those presenting without a preceding trigger, and this may in part explain the difference in the clinical course. In our small study, the recurrence rate within five years was similar between the groups; however, large cohort studies are needed to address this issue. Overall, we found no correlation between the presence of an emotional trigger and short-term outcomes (30-day mortality or recurrence).

Despite the small sample size, we believe that our study provides some new insights.

First, we included only patients with emotional triggers before symptom onset and we excluded cases of TTS secondary to medical conditions that may mascaraed the course of TTS by dictating the outcome of the patient. Therefore, we tried to isolate the role of emotional stress in TTS and its implications on outcomes.

Second, we have provided 5-year outcomes. The relatively low recurrence rate that was observed (regardless of triggers) may strengthen other previous studies [22]. Further, studies including the measurement of catecholamines during the acute phase of different types of TTS (with and without trigger) are warranted.

5. Study Limitations

Our study has several limitations. First, the level of natriuretic peptide was not presented due to high missing values. Natriuretic peptide was shown in several studies as being a leading prognostic biomarker in TTS, in addition to its diagnostic role. Second, our small cohort exhibits a relatively stable course of the disease, with a relatively low rate of severe complications. Third, we do not have the long-term outcomes.

6. Conclusions

Patients with TTS presenting with an emotional trigger before symptoms onset may represent a different population from patients with TTS without a preceding trigger, characterized by a longer hospital stay without, however, a difference in 30-day mortality or recurrence rate.

Author Contributions: Conceptualization, G.M.; methodology, G.M., S.A. and O.A.; software, O.A. and G.M.; formal analysis, R.S.; writing, G.M., S.A. and O.A. All authors have read and agreed to the published version of the manuscript.

Funding: This research received no external funding.

Institutional Review Board Statement: The study was approved by the Institutional Review Board of Galilee Medical Center.

Informed Consent Statement: Patients were not involved in the design, conduct, reporting, or dissemination plans of this research.

Data Availability Statement: The data supporting this study's findings are available from the corresponding author upon reasonable request.

Conflicts of Interest: The authors declare no conflict of interest.

References

1. Templin, C.; Ghadri, J.R.; Diekmann, J.; Napp, L.C.; Bataiosu, D.R.; Jaguszewski, M.; Cammann, V.L.; Sarcon, A.; Geyer, V.; Neumann, C.A.; et al. Clinical Features and Outcomes of Takotsubo (Stress) Cardiomyopathy. *N. Engl. J. Med.* **2015**, *373*, 929–938. [CrossRef] [PubMed]
2. Uribarri, A.; Núñez-Gil, I.J.; Conty, D.A.; Vedia, O.; Almendro-Delia, M.; Duran Cambra, A.; Martin-Garcia, A.C.; Barrionuevo-Sánchez, M.; Martínez-Sellés, M.; Raposeiras-Roubín, S.; et al. Short- and Long-Term Prognosis of Patients With Takotsubo Syndrome Based on Different Triggers: Importance of the Physical Nature. *J. Am. Heart Assoc.* **2019**, *8*, e013701. [CrossRef] [PubMed]
3. Lyon, A.R.; Citro, R.; Schneider, B.; Morel, O.; Ghadri, J.R.; Templin, C.; Omerovic, E. Pathophysiology of Takotsubo Syndrome: JACC State-of-the-Art Review. *J. Am. Coll Cardiol.* **2021**, *77*, 902–921. [CrossRef]
4. Lyon, A.R.; Bossone, E.; Schneider, B.; Sechtem, U.; Citro, R.; Underwood, S.R.; Sheppard, M.N.; Figtree, G.A.; Parodi, G.; Akashi, Y.J.; et al. Current state of knowledge on Takotsubo syndrome: A Position Statement from the Taskforce on Takotsubo Syndrome of the Heart Failure Association of the European Society of Cardiology. *Eur. J. Heart Fail* **2016**, *18*, 8–27. [CrossRef] [PubMed]
5. Prasad, A.; Dangas, G.; Srinivasan, M.; Yu, J.; Gersh, B.J.; Mehran, R.; Stone, G.W. Incidence and angiographic characteristics of patients with apical ballooning syndrome (takotsubo/stress cardiomyopathy) in the HORIZONS-AMI trial: An analysis from a multicenter, international study of ST-elevation myocardial infarction. *Catheter. Cardiovasc. Interv.* **2014**, *83*, 343–348. [CrossRef] [PubMed]
6. Wittstein, I.S.; Thiemann, D.R.; Lima, J.A.; Baughman, K.L.; Schulman, S.P.; Gerstenblith, G.; Wu, K.C.; Rade, J.J.; Bivalacqua, T.J.; Champion, H.C. Neurohumoral features of myocardial stunning due to sudden emotional stress. *N. Engl. J. Med.* **2005**, *352*, 539–548. [CrossRef]
7. Gianni, M.; Dentali, F.; Grandi, A.M.; Sumner, G.; Hiralal, R.; Lonn, E. Apical ballooning syndrome or takotsubo cardiomyopathy: A systematic review. *Eur. Heart J.* **2006**, *27*, 1523–1529. [CrossRef]
8. Pelliccia, F.; Kaski, J.C.; Crea, F.; Camici, P.G. Pathophysiology of Takotsubo Syndrome. *Circulation* **2017**, *135*, 2426–2441. [CrossRef]
9. Paur, H.; Wright, P.T.; Sikkel, M.B.; Tranter, M.H.; Mansfield, C.; O'Gara, P.; Stuckey, D.J.; Nikolaev, V.O.; Diakonov, I.; Pannell, L.; et al. High levels of circulating epinephrine trigger apical cardiodepression in a β2-adrenergic receptor/Gi-dependent manner: A new model of Takotsubo cardiomyopathy. *Circulation* **2012**, *126*, 697–706. [CrossRef]
10. Cimarelli, S.; Sauer, F.; Morel, O.; Ohlmann, P.; Constantinesco, A.; Imperiale, A. Transient left ventricular dysfunction syndrome: Patho-physiological bases through nuclear medicine imaging. *Int. J. Cardiol.* **2010**, *144*, 212–218. [CrossRef]
11. Limongelli, G.; Masarone, D.; Maddaloni, V.; Rubino, M.; Fratta, F.; Cirillo, A.; Ludovica, S.B.; Pacileo, R.; Fusco, A.; Coppola, G.R.; et al. Genetics of Takotsubo Syndrome. *Heart Fail Clin.* **2016**, *12*, 499–506. [CrossRef] [PubMed]
12. Di Vece, D.; Citro, R.; Cammann, V.L.; Kato, K.; Gili, S.; Szawan, K.A.; Micek, J.; Jurisic, S.; Ding, K.J.; Bacchi, B.; et al. Outcomes Associated With Cardiogenic Shock in Takotsubo Syndrome. *Circulation* **2019**, *139*, 413–415. [CrossRef] [PubMed]
13. Jurisic, S.; Gili, S.; Cammann, V.L.; Kato, K.; Szawan, K.A.; D'Ascenzo, F.; Jaguszewski, M.; Bossone, E.; Citro, R.; Sarcon, A.; et al. Clinical Predictors and Prognostic Impact of Recovery of Wall Motion Abnormalities in Takotsubo Syndrome: Results From the International Takotsubo Registry. *J. Am. Heart Assoc.* **2019**, *8*, e011194. [CrossRef] [PubMed]
14. Wilson, H.M.; Cheyne, L.; Brown, P.A.; Kerr, K.; Hannah, A.; Srinivasan, J.; Duniak, N.; Horgan, G.; Dawson, D.K. Characterization of the Myocardial Inflammatory Response in Acute Stress-Induced (Takotsubo) Cardiomyopathy. *JACC Basic Transl. Sci.* **2018**, *3*, 766–778. [CrossRef] [PubMed]
15. Kastaun, S.; Gerriets, T.; Tschernatsch, M.; Yeniguen, M.; Juenemann, M. Psychosocial and psychoneuroendocrinal aspects of Takotsubo syndrome. *Nat. Rev. Cardiol.* **2016**, *13*, 688–694. [CrossRef]

16. Y-Hassan, S. Catecholamine Levels and Cardiac Sympathetic Hyperactivation-Disruption in Takotsubo Syndrome. *JACC Cardiovasc. Imaging* **2017**, *10*, 95–96. [CrossRef]
17. Y-Hassan, S.; Sörensson, P.; Ekenbäck, C.; Lundin, M.; Agewall, S.; Brolin, E.B.; Caidahl, K.; Cederlund, K.; Collste, O.; Daniel, M.; et al. Plasma catecholamine levels in the acute and subacute stages of takotsubo syndrome: Results from the Stockholm myocardial infarction with normal coronaries 2 study. *Clin. Cardiol.* **2021**, *44*, 1567–1574. [CrossRef]
18. Y-Hassan, S.; Falhammar, H. Clinical features, complications, and outcomes of exogenous and endogenous catecholamine-triggered Takotsubo syndrome: A systematic review and meta-analysis of 156 published cases. *Clin. Cardiol.* **2020**, *43*, 459–467. [CrossRef]
19. Imori, Y.; Yoshikawa, T.; Murakami, T.; Isogai, T.; Yamaguchi, T.; Maekawa, Y.; Sakata, K.; Mochizuki, H.; Arao, K.; Otsuka, T.; et al. Impact of Trigger on Outcome of Takotsubo Syndrome—Multi-Center Registry From Tokyo Cardiovascular Care Unit Network. *Circ. Rep.* **2019**, *1*, 493–501. [CrossRef]
20. Yerasi, C.; Koifman, E.; Weissman, G.; Wang, Z.; Torguson, R.; Gai, J.; Lindsay, J.; Satler, L.F.; Pichard, A.D.; Waksman, R.; et al. Impact of triggering event in outcomes of stress-induced (Takotsubo) cardiomyopathy. *Eur. Heart J. Acute Cardiovasc. Care* **2017**, *6*, 280–286. [CrossRef]
21. Ghadri, J.R.; Kato, K.; Cammann, V.L.; Gili, S.; Jurisic, S.; Di Vece, D.; Candreva, A.; Ding, K.J.; Micek, J.; Szawan, K.A.; et al. Long-Term Prognosis of Patients With Takotsubo Syndrome. *J. Am. Coll Cardiol.* **2018**, *72*, 874–882. [CrossRef] [PubMed]
22. Lau, C.; Chiu, S.; Nayak, R.; Lin, B.; Lee, M.S. Survival and risk of recurrence of takotsubo syndrome. *Heart* **2021**, *107*, 1160. [CrossRef] [PubMed]

Journal of
Clinical Medicine

MDPI

Article

Hypertrophic Cardiomyopathy in a Latin American Center: A Single Center Observational Study

Juan David López-Ponce de Leon [1,2,*], Mayra Estacio [3], Natalia Giraldo [1,2], Manuela Escalante [3], Yorlany Rodas [3], Jessica Largo [3], Juliana Lores [2], María Camila Victoria [3], Diana Argote [2], Noel Florez [1,2], Diana Carrillo [1,2], Pastor Olaya [1,2], Mauricio Mejia [4] and Juan Esteban Gomez [1,2]

1 Departamento de Cardiología, Fundación Valle del Lili, Cali 760032, Colombia; natalia.giraldo@fvl.org.co (N.G.); noel.florez@fvl.org.co (N.F.); diana.carrillo@fvl.org.co (D.C.); pastor.olaya@fvl.org.co (P.O.); juan.gomez@fvl.org.co (J.E.G.)
2 Facultad de Ciencias de la Salud, Universidad Icesi, Cali 760031, Colombia; juliana.lores@javerianacali.edu.co (J.L.); diana.argote.ri@fvl.org.co (D.A.)
3 Centro de Investigaciones Clínicas, Fundación Valle del Lili, Cali 760032, Colombia; mayraestacio1@gmail.com (M.E.); manuela.escalante@fvl.org.co (M.E.); jessica.largo.oc@fvl.org.co (J.L.); camilavictoriareyes@gmail.com (M.C.V.)
4 Departamento de Radiología, Fundación Valle del Lili, Cali 760032, Colombia; mauricio.mejia@fvl.org.co
* Correspondence: juan.lopez.po@fvl.org.co

Abstract: Background: Hypertrophic cardiomyopathy (HCM) is a complex disorder that includes various phenotypes, leading to different manifestations. It also shares different disadvantages typical of rare diseases, including limited recognition, lack of prospective studies assessing treatment, and little or delayed access to advanced treatment options. Reliable data about the prevalence and natural history of cardiomyopathies in South America are lacking. This study summarizes the features and management of patients with HCM in a university hospital in Colombia. Methods: This was an observational retrospective cohort study of patients with HCM between January 2010 and December 2021. Patient data were analyzed from an institutional cardiomyopathy registry. Demographic, paraclinical, and outcome data were collected. Results: A total of 82 patients during the study period were enrolled. Of these, 67.1% were male, and the mean age at diagnosis was 49 years. Approximately 83% were in NYHA functional class I and II, and the most reported symptoms were dyspnea (38%), angina (20%), syncope (15%), and palpitations (11%). In addition, 89% had preserved left ventricular ejection fraction (LVEF) with an asymmetric septal pattern in 65%. Five patients (6%) had alcohol septal ablation and four (5%) had septal myectomy. One patient required heart transplantation during follow-up. Sudden cardiovascular death was observed in 2.6%. The overall mortality during follow-up was 7.3%. Conclusions: HCM is a complex and heterogeneous disorder that presents with significant morbidity and mortality. Our registry provides comprehensive data on disease courses and management in a developing country.

Keywords: cardiomyopathies; hypertrophic cardiomyopathy

Citation: López-Ponce de Leon, J.D.; Estacio, M.; Giraldo, N.; Escalante, M.; Rodas, Y.; Largo, J.; Lores, J.; Victoria, M.C.; Argote, D.; Florez, N.; et al. Hypertrophic Cardiomyopathy in a Latin American Center: A Single Center Observational Study. *J. Clin. Med.* **2023**, *12*, 5682. https://doi.org/10.3390/jcm12175682

Academic Editor: Stefan Peters

Received: 8 June 2023
Revised: 17 July 2023
Accepted: 20 July 2023
Published: 31 August 2023

1. Introduction

Cardiomyopathies are a heterogeneous group of disorders in which the heart muscle is structurally and functionally abnormal in the absence of obstructive coronary artery disease, hypertension, valvular disease, and congenital heart disease sufficient to explain the observed myocardial abnormality [1,2]. The main phenotypes are dilated cardiomyopathy (DCM), hypertrophic cardiomyopathy (HCM), restrictive cardiomyopathy (RCM), left ventricular noncompaction (LVNC), and arrhythmogenic cardiomyopathy (ACM) [3]. In general, cardiomyopathy is an important problem, as it is associated with sudden death in young adults and is one of the main causes of heart transplantation.

The incidence and prevalence of inherited cardiomyopathies have been derived from screening studies and can vary by type and by geographic region. Reliable epidemiology of cardiomyopathies is primarily accessible from developed nations where accurate prevalence statistics based on the use of established diagnostic evaluations and criteria are collected [4,5].

HCM is a genetic disorder of cardiac myocytes characterized by unexplained cardiac hypertrophy without the presence of other pathologies that increase loading conditions. For a clinical diagnosis, a left ventricle (LV) wall thickness in diastole >15 mm must be present or >13 mm if there is a family member with HCM. A disease prevalence of 1:250 to 500 for HCM in adults seems to be similar in all races, and disease expression usually occurs in adolescents and young adults [4]. Unfortunately, South America lacks reliable data about the prevalence and incidence of cardiomyopathies [6,7].

In relation to the information on hypertrophic cardiomyopathy in Latin America, there are two studies, the first carried out in Argentina by Fernandez et al. in which they evaluated prevalence, clinical course, and pathological findings of left ventricular systolic impairment in patients with HCM [8] and the second in which Nilda Espínola-Zavaleta et al. in Mexico evaluated the survival and clinical behavior of hypertrophic cardiomyopathy in a cohort [9].

Cardiomyopathies are associated with high morbidity and mortality associated with premature death from arrhythmia, progressive heart failure, or stroke [10]. Most information about the presentation and natural history of cardiomyopathies has been derived from cohort studies in Europe and North America [11–13]. Information about the clinical profile and management of the disease at a national level is very limited.

This study summarizes the features and management of patients with HCM in a center that provides highly complex health services in Colombia.

2. Methods

This is an observational retrospective cohort study of patients with HCM that are included in the institutional cardiomyopathy registry (RIM) that have information on five cardiomyopathy subtypes, DCM, HCM, LVNC, ARVC, and RCM, diagnosticated between January 2010 and December 2021 in Fundación Valle del Lili in Cali, Colombia.

The patients with HCM had to meet the following criteria: evidence of left ventricular hypertrophy with a wall thickness of $\geq$15 mm (or >13 mm if there is a family member with HCM) in one or more myocardial segments in the absence of loading conditions, such as hypertension or valve disease, documented by echocardiography or cardiac magnetic resonance imaging (CMR) [14]. Eighty-two patients (27%) of the registry met the inclusion criteria for HCM.

Information obtained from the database included demographics, clinical and paraclinical comorbidities (NT-proBNP, Troponin, electrocardiogram), family history for HCM or SCD, and pharmacological and non-pharmacological treatments. The comorbidities evaluated were atrial fibrillation, stroke, diabetes mellitus, arterial hypertension, dyslipidemia, overweight, obesity, chronic kidney disease, hypothyroidism, and smoking. NYHA functional class and symptoms, such as angina, dyspnea, palpitations, and syncope, were recorded from the clinical history of admission.

Positive family history for HCM was defined as the documented presence of the disease in a first-degree relative, whereas positive family history for sudden cardiac death (SCD) was defined as the unexpected death of a first-degree relative younger than 40 years old. Cardiac dimensions and function were based on echocardiographic and CMR measurements.

All included patients had at least one follow-up visit, and those visits varied in timeframes for each patient. Atrial fibrillation and ventricular tachycardia (sustained or not sustained) were diagnosed based on an electrocardiogram (ECG) or 24 h ECG monitor recording or by an established history of the arrhythmias. Interpretations of the 12-lead electrocardiogram and 24 h ECG monitor were performed by a cardiologist or electrophysiologist. The outcomes of the study were mortality by any cause during the follow-up period, including SCD.

Institutional echocardiograms were performed following the ASE guidelines [15]. Extra institutional echocardiograms could not be evaluated in relation to the performance techniques used.

The baseline echocardiogram includes a screening assessment of ventricular function, chamber sizes, left ventricular wall thicknesses, aortic root diameter, pericardial effusions, and gross valvular structure and function, including an estimate of pulmonary arterial systolic pressure using the peak tricuspid regurgitation velocity.

The highest end-diastolic wall thickness was measured in the parasternal long-axis view and correlated with the same segment in the parasternal short-axis view, depending on the MHC phenotype, to avoid overestimations in quantification. They were classified depending on the location of the highest thickening and the number of segments involved in asymmetric septal, concentric, and predominantly apical. A description of the echocardiographic findings was made regarding the presence of primary mitral regurgitation, number, and location of papillary muscles, presence of anterior systolic movement of the SAM mitral valve, dynamic obstruction of the left ventricular outflow tract, or the presence of significant midventricular gradient. Echocardiographic phenotypes can be seen in Figure 1. Apical aneurysms and left ventricular thrombus were diagnosed by echocardiography or CMR.

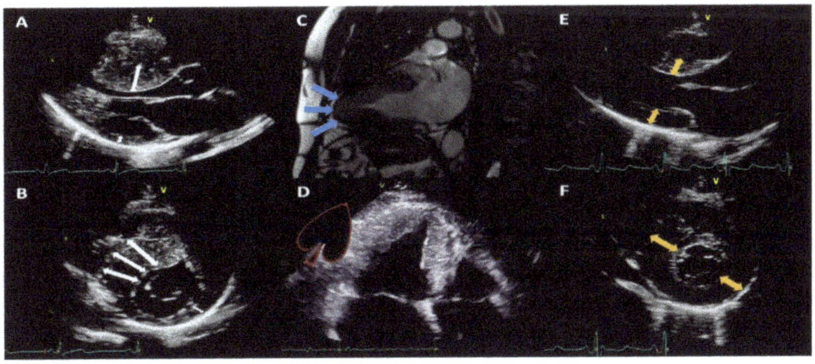

Figure 1. Echocardiographic and CMR images representing various phenotypic expressions of hypertrophic cardiomyopathy (**A**,**B**) from a patient with septal asymmetric hypertrophy (white double-headed arrows); (**C**) (CMR) and (**D**) in a patient with an apical HCM, which in systole produces a classic spade-shaped ventricular cavity (blue arrows); (**E**,**F**) in a concentric phenotype (yellow double-headed arrows). CMR: magnetic resonance imaging; HCM: hypertrophic cardiomyopathy.

Most of the CMRs were performed in the institution, using either 1.5 or 3.0 Tesla CMR scanners. LV measures of geometry and function were analyzed using standardized protocols. The asymmetric LV wall thickness was measured using the maximal end-diastolic wall thickness divided by the indexed LV end-diastolic volume (wall thickness/volume ratio), a useful discriminator between wall thickening due to exercise, pathological thickening-related HCM, or increased afterload conditions [14,15]. Myocardial T1 mapping was used to assess for diffuse myocardial fibrosis.

The patient data and laboratory findings were collected from the institutional medical records; each patient had an assigned ID number for confidentiality, and information was stored in REDCap (Research Electronic Data Capture). The study protocol was approved by the Institutional Review Board Ethics Committee of the Fundación Valle del Lili.

Statistical Analyses

A univariate descriptive analysis was performed. The normality of the continuous variables was analyzed using the Shapiro–Wilk test, with a statistical significance level of 5%. Variables that did not meet the normality assumption are presented as median and interquartile range (RIC) and the remaining variables as mean and standard deviation. Qualitative variables are presented as absolute frequencies and percentages. Data analysis was performed with the statistical software R V.4.2.1 (R Foundation for Statistical Computing) through RStudio 2022.07.0+548.

3. Results

Three hundred-five patients with cardiomyopathies were enrolled in the registry. Most patients had DCM (n = 199), followed by HCM (n = 82), LVNC (n = 11), ACM (n = 8), and RCM (n = 5) (Figure 2). In this study, 82 patients with HCM met the inclusion criteria. Baseline characteristics and outcomes are summarized in Table 1. The median age at diagnosis was 49 years (IQR 38–61), and most patients were male (67%) Figure 3.

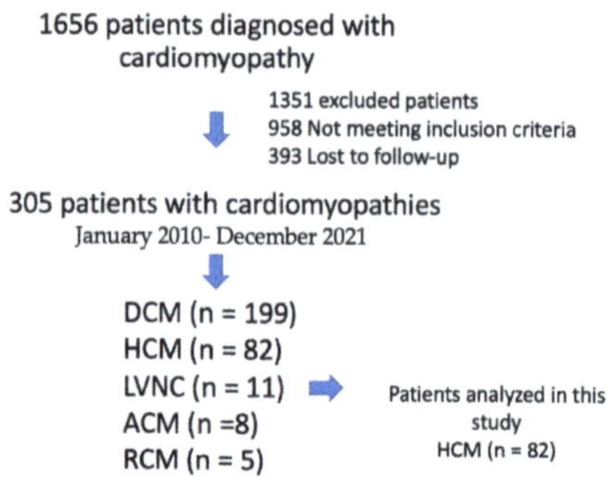

Figure 2. Flowchart describing patients in the study.

Table 1. Baseline characteristics and treatment.

Variable	HCM (n = 82)
Age at clinical diagnosis, n Median (IQR)	49.0 (37.5–61.0)
Gender, n Male, n (%)	55 (67.1%)
Family history of cardiomyopathy, n, (%)	12 (25.0%)
Family history of cardiomyopathy by level of consanguinity, n	
First degree, n (%)	8 (66.7%)
Second degree, n (%)	3 (25.0%)
NYHA functional class, n (%)	
Class I	43 (59.7%)
Class II	17 (23.6%)
Class III	10 (13.9%)
Class IV	2 (2.8%)
Angina, n (%)	16 (19.5%)
Dyspnea, n (%)	31 (37.8%)
Palpitations, n (%)	9 (11.0%)
Syncope, n (%)	12 (14.6%)
Personal history and comorbidities, n (%)	
Atrial fibrillation	11 (15.1%)
Stroke	7 (9.5%)
Diabetes mellitus type 2	9 (11.2%)

Table 1. *Cont.*

Variable	HCM (n = 82)
Arterial hypertension	24 (30.4%)
Dyslipidemia	17 (21.2%)
Overweight/Obesity	6 (7.6%)
Chronic kidney disease	3 (3.8%)
Hypothyroidism	7 (8.8%)
Smoking	9 (17.0%)
Pharmacologic treatment, *n* (%)	
Beta-blockers	58 (85.3%)
Diuretics, oral	13 (19.1%)
ACE-inhibitors	1 (1.5%)
Angiotensin II receptor blockers	17 (25.0%)
Mineralocorticoid receptor antagonists	7 (10.3%)
Calcium channel blockers	19 (27.9%)
Acetylsalicylic acid	8 (11.8%)
SGLT2 inhibitors	1 (1.5%)
ARNI	2 (2.9%)
Statins	13 (19.1%)
Oral anticoagulants Vitamin K antagonists Apixaban Rivaroxaban Non-specified	14 (20.5%) 4 (5.9%) 5 (7.4%) 4 (5.9%) 1 (1.5%)
Non-pharmacological treatment *n* (%)	
Angiography	7 (19.4%)
Alcohol septal ablation	5 (6.1%)
Septal myectomy	4 (4.9%)
Ventricular assist device	1 (1.3%)
Cardiac resynchronization therapy	2 (2.4%)
Implantable cardioverter-defibrillators	29 (35.4%)

NYHA: New York Heart Association; ACE: angiotensin-converting enzyme); SGLT-2: sodium-glucose cotransporter-2; ARNI: angiotensin receptor/neprilysin inhibitor.

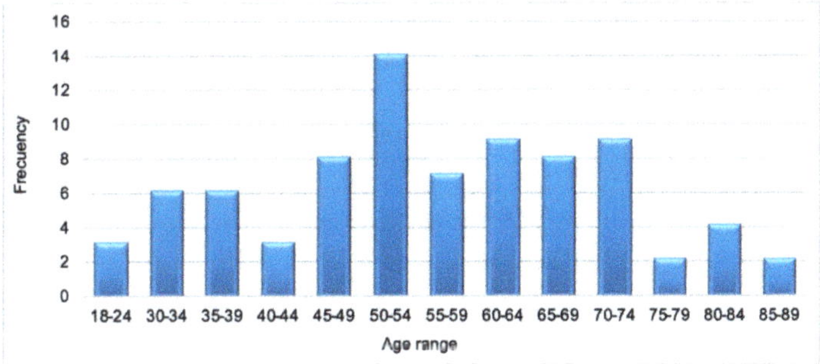

Figure 3. Age at the time of diagnosis.

The most frequent comorbidities were hypertension (30%), dyslipidemia (21%), atrial fibrillation (15%), type 2 diabetes mellitus (11%), stroke (9.5%), overweight or obesity (8%), hypothyroidism (8%), and chronic kidney disease (4%). Approximately 25% of the patients reported a family history of cardiomyopathy of which 67% were first-degree relatives, and 26% reported a history of sudden cardiac death (SCD) in any family member.

At enrollment, 60 patients (83%) were in the New York Heart Association (NYHA) I-II functional class. The most common symptoms were dyspnea (38%), angina (20%), syncope (15%), and palpitations (11%). Approximately 58% of the patients had an electrocardiogram record; the most frequent finding was atrial fibrillation (AF) in 12.5% and ventricular hypertrophy in only 8%. The NT-proBNP was measured in only 11 patients (13%), with a value > 1.200 pg/mL in 54.5% of the cases (negative if 125 pg/mL).

Table 1 describes pharmacologic and nonpharmacologic treatment before enrollment. Beta-blockers were the most frequently prescribed treatment (85%), followed by angiotensin-converting enzyme inhibitors (ACEi) and angiotensin II receptor blockers (ARBs) (26.5%). Sodium-glucose cotransporter-2 (SGLT-2) inhibitors were used in 1.5% of patients and angiotensin receptor-neprilysin inhibitors (ARNI) in 2.9%. For nonpharmacological therapy, the use of an implantable cardioverter-defibrillator was reported in 29 patients (35%); five patients (6%) underwent alcohol septal ablation; and four patients (5%) underwent septal myectomy.

The echocardiographic characteristics are described in Table 2. Most patients had a preserved ejection fraction (89%). Atrial dilatation > 34 mL/m^2 was documented in 45 patients (85%), and resting or provoked left ventricular outflow obstruction (LVOTO) with a gradient > 30 mmHg was present in 29 (52.7%) patients. Systolic anterior motion (SAM) of the mitral valve was present in 21 (47.7%) patients. The most common pattern was asymmetric septal hypertrophy in 37 (64.9%) patients, followed by concentric hypertrophy in 16 (28.1%) and only four (7%) patients with a predominantly apical pattern. One patient had a left ventricular thrombus, and none had an apical aneurysm formation.

Table 2. Echocardiographic Characteristics.

Variable, *n* (%)	**HCM (*n* = 82)**
Ejection fraction *n* = 73	
Reduced (<40%)	4 (5.8%)
Slightly reduced (40–49%)	4 (5.8%)
Preserved (>50%)	65 (89%)
Global longitudinal strain, median (IQR)	−13.4 (−18.1, −11.7)
Wall diameters	
Abnormal interventricular septum (>9 mm female; >10 mm male)	63 (100%)
Abnormal posterior wall (>9 mm female; >10 mm male)	36 (76.6%)
HCM subtype according to LV hypertrophy pattern	
Asymmetric septal	37 (64.9%)
Concentric	16 (28.1%)
Predominantly apical	4 (7.0%)
No data	25/82 (30.5%)
Left atrial volume indexed	53 (65.4%)
Normal: 16 to 34 mL/m^2	8 (15.1%)
Slightly abnormal: 35 to 41 mL/m^2	20 (37.7%)
Moderately abnormal: 42 to 48 mL/m^2	9 (17.0%)
Severely abnormal: >48 mL/m^2	16 (30.2%)
E/A ratio	
Normal (0.8–2)	20 (69%)
Abnormal (>2)	9 (31.0%)

Table 2. *Cont.*

Variable, *n* (%)	HCM (*n* = 82)
Right atrial area	
Normal $\leq$19 cm^2	23(57.5%)
Abnormal >19 cm^2	17(42.5%)
TAPSE	
Normal >17	32 (91.4%)
Decreased <17	3 (8.6%)
S′ wave	
Normal	18 (78.3%)
Abnormal	5 (21.7%)
Valvular heart disease	
Mitral regurgitation	43 (52.4%)
Aortic insufficiency	6 (7.3%)
Tricuspid insufficiency	34 (41.5%)
Aortic stenosis	4 (4.9%)
Mitral stenosis	0 (0.0%)
LV outflow tract gradient	
Normal	15 (27.3%)
<30 mmHg	11 (20.0%)
30–49 mmHg	8 (14.5%)
>50 mmHg	21 (38.2%)
Unreported	27/82 (32.9%)
SAM	21 (47.7%)
Pericardial effusion	2 (3.7%)

Asymmetric septal hypertrophy is considered when there is a pattern of septal thickness with the free LV wall >1.3/1.0. TAPSE: acronym for measurement of the tricuspid ring systolic excursion; LV: left ventricle; SAM: acronym for systolic anterior motion of the mitral valve.

CMR was performed on 34% of the patients. The predominant pattern was also asymmetric septal hypertrophy in 64%, concentric hypertrophy in 7.4%, and apical hypertrophy in 14.8%. SAM was present in five (22.7%) patients. Wall thickness/volume ratio > 0.15 mm $\times$ m^2 $\times$ mL (-1) was present in all patients.

Targeted sequencing of HCM genes and defining pathogenic variants was performed only in three patients who were sequenced using Illumina MiSeq (v2 kit) or NextSeq 500 (Mid Output v2 kit). The variants of genes encoded were TTN, TNNI3, and TTR.

During follow-up, heart transplantation was performed in one patient. SCD was observed in 2.6%. A history of AF was recorded in 22% of patients, and eight (10.7%) patients had an episode of sustained ventricular tachycardia. Eight patients were hospitalized during this period due to heart failure. The overall mortality during follow-up was 7.3% (six patients).

4. Discussion

This study provides a detailed contemporary assessment of the clinical profile, management strategies, and outcomes of HCM in a Latin American center. The clinical spectrum of HCM is complex and includes a variety of phenotypes, leading to different manifestations.

The most common type of LV hypertrophy was asymmetrical (64.9%), followed by concentric (28.1%) and apical (7.0%), with a similar trend to other studies [16]. Apical hypertrophic cardiomyopathy (AHCM) is a rare form of HCM that usually involves the left ventricle's apex and is also known as Yamaguchi syndrome. Asian countries exhibit the highest prevalence of AHCM. Historically, this condition was thought to be confined to this population, but it is also found in other populations [17]. The prevalence of AHCM in China is reported to be as high as 41% and more than 15% in Japan, whereas in the USA, the prevalence is 1–3% [18]. In our study, AHCM was relatively common (7%), in Latin America; there are few studies evaluating the frequency of the disease as well as the predominant phenotypic expression. In 2015, Nilda Espinola-Zavaleta et al. reported a cohort of 77 Mexican patients with HCM, finding that 11% had an apical phenotype and this was associated with poorer survival [9]. In this sense, more studies are needed to determine the outcomes in this subgroup since in series from other regions of the world, such as Asian populations, apical HCM is an atypical phenotype and usually has an apparently benign course.

LVOTO is described in the literature with a prevalence near 70%, addressing the importance of provocation maneuvers that augment the gradient to >30 mmHg in more than half of the patients with low gradients at rest [19,20]. Our LVOTO had a prevalence of only 52.7%, but considering the type of study, we cannot assure all gradients were evaluated in resting and provoked conditions with either Valsalva maneuvers or stress echocardiography, also taking into consideration that this variable is highly dynamic and influenced by factors that alter cardiac contractility and loading conditions.

Most patients received medical treatment. The proportion of patients on diuretics and ARBs was high although most of the patients had preserved LVEF; 30% had arterial hypertension. Current U.S. and European guidelines recommend ACEi and ARBs as a suitable first choice for hypertension treatment together with calcium channel blockers and thiazide diuretics [21]. Alcohol septal reduction (ASA) therapy was performed in 8% of our cohort, and 4.9% had a surgical septal myectomy. In adult patients with obstructive HCM who remain severely symptomatic despite medical treatment, septal reduction therapies are indicated. Even though recent studies keep showing better outcomes with septal myectomy in eligible patients in whom surgery is contraindicated or the risk is considered unacceptable because of comorbidities or advanced age, ASA is an option in experienced centers [22]. Despite these recommendations, 43% of United States patients undergo ASA instead of myectomy, and these numbers are known to be even higher in Europe [23,24]. In our center, the use of these techniques is still low.

Atrial fibrillation was the most common arrhythmia, recorded in 22% during the study follow-up, similar to what the evidence states where AF is present in 25–53%, with an annual incidence of 4%/year contributing to a decreased quality of life and risk of systemic thromboembolism [22,25,26]. These patients do not tolerate losing the atrial kick in addition to the frequent diastolic dysfunction; therefore, aggressive rate control or restoration of sinus rhythm is crucial. In this setting, oral anticoagulation is mandatory (unless contraindicated) for patients with HCM irrespective of risk-scoring systems due to the higher risk of thromboembolism [27].

Cardiovascular mortality in these patients is most frequently due to HF, followed by SCD and stroke-related death. During follow-up, six patients (7.3%) died. These data are comparable to previous studies [11,12]. Mortality varies according to the genotype; patients with sarcomeric HCM are diagnosed earlier in life and have the worst prognosis [28]; also in addition, women tend to be diagnosed later in life, with more symptomatic heart failure and a higher mortality rate. Ventricular arrhythmias and SCD were presented in 10.7% and 2.4% of patients, respectively, the latter with reported annual rates of approximately 0.5–1% [29].

In the study by Fernandez et al. in which they evaluated patients with hypertrophic cardiomyopathy and left ventricular systolic impairment (ILVSF), it was found that during follow-up, 14 patients (58%) with ILVSF reached the combined end point (one patient [4.2%] died from heart failure and thirteen [54%] underwent heart transplant) compared to three patients (0.8%) with normal systolic function (p = 0.001) [8]. In our cohort, the rate of these outcomes is not high, probably because most of the patients had a preserved ejection fraction.

HCM has predominantly been considered an autosomal dominant genetic disease, although de novo mutations explain some cases and, less frequently, autosomal recessive heredity. The genetic study may play a role in stratifying the prognosis of HCM patients. Genetic testing was only performed on three patients. The 2018 Heart Failure Society of America guideline on cardiomyopathies recommends genetic counseling for all patients with cardiomyopathy and their family members and that genetic testing should be offered to all patients diagnosed with all recognized forms of cardiomyopathy [30]. Our study has patients evaluated since 2010. The genetic tests in our country at that time were limited, and currently, access to these tests is still difficult due to the cost.

HCM is caused by a variety of mutations in genes encoding contractile proteins of the cardiac sarcomere, especially in cardiac myosin heavy chain beta (MYH7), myosin binding protein C (MYBPC3), and cardiac troponin T (TNNT2). To date, over 700 individual mutations have been identified [31]. With respect to specific genes in our study, pathogenic TTR variants are rare in carefully assessed HCM patients and may occur in double heterozygosity with pathogenic sarcomere variants [32]. About 2–7% of familial cardiomyopathy cases are caused by a mutation in the gene encoding cardiac troponin I (TNNI3). A. van den Wijngaard et al. described in their study the majority of Dutch TNNI3 mutations were associated with a HCM phenotype [33]. One patient had TTN mutation. While TTN truncation mutations are common in DCM, there is evidence that TTN truncations are rare in the HCM phenotype, with a frequency similar to control populations [34]. Using high-throughout sequencing in 142 HCM probands, Lopes et al. found 219 TTN rare variants with 209 being novel missense variants [35]. However, this cohort of individuals potentially had a sarcomeric gene mutation that likely caused HCM, and the actual pathogenic role of these TTN variants is unknown.

Several limitations should be considered when interpreting our data, including the retrospective cohort design, which is more susceptible to the effects of confounding and bias, and the fact that it is a single-institution study. We think that dilated cardiomyopathy is more common than HCM because our hospital is a center for patients with advanced heart failure; this could account for the low frequency of HCM and add extra selection bias to the population. Due to the observational nature of this study, we cannot exclude the presence of infiltrative cardiomyopathies, such as amyloidosis, sarcoidosis, Fabry disease, and Dannon disease.

Future studies, providing complete clinical information in combination with family history, echocardiographic and CMR parameters, and genetic testing would better clarify and characterize the HCM phenotype. A register of HCM patients should be established through multicenter efforts to identify the unique characteristics of this illness in Latin America and contribute to the reduction of morbidity and mortality in this population.

5. Conclusions

HCM is a complex and heterogeneous disorder, presenting significant morbidity and mortality. This registry provides comprehensive data on the disease course and management in a developing country.

Author Contributions: Conceptualization, J.D.L.-P.d.L., N.F., D.C., P.O., M.M., J.E.G. and N.G.; methodology, M.E. (Manuela Escalante), Y.R. and J.L. (Jessica Largo); writing—original draft preparation, J.L. (Juliana Lores), M.C.V. and D.A.; writing—review and editing, M.E. (Mayra Estacio). All authors have read and agreed to the published version of the manuscript.

Funding: This research received no external funding.

Institutional Review Board Statement: The study was conducted in accordance with the Declaration of Helsinki and approved by the Institutional Review Board.

Informed Consent Statement: Informed consent was obtained from all subjects involved in the study.

Data Availability Statement: Data supporting this study are included within the article and/or supporting materials.

Conflicts of Interest: The authors declare no conflict of interest.

References

1. Elliott, P.M.; Anastasakis, A.; Borger, M.A.; Borggrefe, M.; Cecchi, F.; Charron, P.; Hagege, A.A.; Lafont, A.; Limongelli, G.; Mahrholdt, H.; et al. 2014 ESC Guidelines on diagnosis and management of hypertrophic cardiomyopathy: The Task Force for the Diagnosis and Management of Hypertrophic Cardiomyopathy of the European Society of Cardiology (ESC). *Eur. Heart J.* **2014**, *35*, 2733–2779. [CrossRef]
2. Elliott, P.; Andersson, B.; Arbustini, E.; Bilinska, Z.; Cecchi, F.; Charron, P.; Dubourg, O.; Kühl, U.; Maisch, B.; McKenna, W.J.; et al. Classification of the cardiomyopathies: A position statement from the european society of cardiology working group on myocardial and pericardial diseases. *Eur. Heart J.* **2008**, *29*, 270–276. [CrossRef]
3. Zipes, D.P. Braunwald's Heart Disease: A Textbook of Cardiovascular Medicine. *BMH Med. J.* **2018**, *5*, 63.
4. McKenna, W.J.; Judge, D.P. Epidemiology of the inherited cardiomyopathies. *Nat. Rev. Cardiol.* **2021**, *18*, 22–36. [CrossRef]
5. Marian, A.J.; Braunwald, E. Hypertrophic Cardiomyopathy: Genetics, Pathogenesis, Clinical Manifestations, Diagnosis, and Therapy. *Circ. Res.* **2017**, *121*, 749–770. [CrossRef]
6. Bocchi, E.A.; Arias, A.; Verdejo, H.; Diez, M.; Gómez, E.; Castro, P. The Reality of Heart Failure in Latin America. *J. Am. Coll. Cardiol.* **2013**, *62*, 949–958. [CrossRef]
7. Bocchi, E.A. Heart Failure in South America. *Curr. Cardiol. Rev.* **2013**, *9*, 147–156. [CrossRef] [PubMed]
8. Fernández, A.; Vigliano, C.A.; Casabé, J.H.; Diez, M.; Favaloro, L.E.; Guevara, E.; Favaloro, R.R.; Laguens, R.P. Comparison of Prevalence, Clinical Course, and Pathological Findings of Left Ventricular Systolic Impairment Versus Normal Systolic Function in Patients with Hypertrophic Cardiomyopathy. *Am. J. Cardiol.* **2011**, *108*, 548–555. [CrossRef]
9. Espinola-Zavaleta, N.; Vega, A.; Basto, D.M.; Alcantar-Fernández, A.C.; Lans, V.G.; Soto, M.E. Survival and Clinical Behavior of Hypertrophic Cardiomyopathy in a Latin American Cohort in Contrast to Cohorts from the Developed World. *J. Cardiovasc. Ultrasound* **2015**, *23*, 20–26. [CrossRef]
10. Maron, B.J.; Towbin, J.A.; Thiene, G.; Antzelevitch, C.; Corrado, D.; Arnett, D.; Moss, A.J.; Seidman, C.E.; Young, J.B. Contemporary definitions and classification of the cardiomyopathies: An American Heart Association Scientific Statement from the Council on Clinical Cardiology, Heart Failure and Transplantation Committee; Quality of Care and Outcomes Research and Functional Genomics and Translational Biology Interdisciplinary Working Groups; and Council on Epidemiology and Prevention. *Circulation* **2006**, *113*, 1807–1816. [CrossRef]
11. Ho, C.Y.; Day, S.M.; Ashley, E.A.; Michels, M.; Pereira, A.C.; Jacoby, D.; Cirino, A.L.; Fox, J.C.; Lakdawala, N.K.; Ware, J.; et al. Genotype and Lifetime Burden of Disease in Hypertrophic Cardiomyopathy: Insights from the Sarcomeric Human Cardiomyopathy Registry (SHaRe). *Circulation* **2018**, *138*, 1387–1398. [CrossRef]
12. Cardim, N.; Brito, D.; Lopes, L.R.; Freitas, A.; Araújo, C.; Belo, A.; Gonçalves, L.; Mimoso, J.; Olivotto, I.; Elliott, P.; et al. The Portuguese Registry of Hypertrophic Cardiomyopathy: Overall results. *Rev. Port. Cardiol.* **2018**, *37*, 1–10. [CrossRef]
13. Neubauer, S.; Kolm, P.; Ho, C.Y.; Kwong, R.Y.; Desai, M.Y.; Dolman, S.F.; Appelbaum, E.; Desvigne-Nickens, P.; DiMarco, J.P.; Friedrich, M.G.; et al. Distinct Subgroups in Hypertrophic Cardiomyopathy in the NHLBI HCM Registry. *J. Am. Coll. Cardiol.* **2019**, *74*, 2333–2345. [CrossRef]
14. Maron, B.J.; Desai, M.Y.; Nishimura, R.A.; Spirito, P.; Rakowski, H.; Towbin, J.A.; Rowin, E.J.; Maron, M.S.; Sherrid, M.V. Diagnosis and Evaluation of Hypertrophic Cardiomyopathy: JACC State-of-the-Art Review. *J. Am. Coll. Cardiol.* **2022**, *79*, 372–389. [CrossRef]
15. Lang, R.M.; Badano, L.P.; Mor-Avi, V.; Afilalo, J.; Armstrong, A.; Ernande, L.; Flachskampf, F.A.; Foster, E.; Goldstein, S.A.; Kuznetsova, T.; et al. Recommendations for Cardiac Chamber Quantification by Echocardiography in Adults: An Update from the American Society of Echocardiography and the European Association of Cardiovascular Imaging. *Eur. Heart J. Cardiovasc. Imaging* **2015**, *16*, 233–271. [CrossRef]
16. Wigle, E.D.; Rakowski, H.; Kimball, B.P.; Williams, W.G. Hypertrophic Cardiomyopathy: Clinical spectrum and treatment. *Circulation* **1995**, *92*, 1680–1692. [CrossRef] [PubMed]
17. Jan, M.F.; Todaro, M.C.; Oreto, L.; Tajik, A.J. Apical hypertrophic cardiomyopathy: Present status. *Int. J. Cardiol.* **2016**, *222*, 745–759. [CrossRef]
18. Kitaoka, H.; Doi, Y.; A Casey, S.; Hitomi, N.; Furuno, T.; Maron, B.J. Comparison of prevalence of apical hypertrophic cardiomyopathy in Japan and the United States. *Am. J. Cardiol.* **2003**, *92*, 1183–1186. [CrossRef]
19. Huang, G.; Fadl, S.A.; Sukhotski, S.; Matesan, M. Apical variant hypertrophic cardiomyopathy "multimodality imaging evaluation". *Int. J. Cardiovasc. Imaging* **2020**, *36*, 553–561. [CrossRef]
20. Maron, M.S.; Olivotto, I.; Zenovich, A.G.; Link, M.S.; Pandian, N.G.; Kuvin, J.T.; Nistri, S.; Cecchi, F.; Udelson, J.E.; Maron, B.J.; et al. Hypertrophic Cardiomyopathy Is Predominantly a Disease of Left Ventricular Outflow Tract Obstruction. *Circulation* **2006**, *114*, 2232–2239. [CrossRef]
21. Unger, T.; Borghi, C.; Charchar, F.; Khan, N.A.; Poulter, N.R.; Prabhakaran, D.; Ramirez, A.; Schlaich, M.; Stergiou, G.S.; Tomaszewski, M.; et al. 2020 International Society of Hypertension Global Hypertension Practice Guidelines. *Hypertension* **2020**, *75*, 1334–1357. [CrossRef] [PubMed]
22. Lee, P.T.; Dweck, M.R.; Prasher, S.; Shah, A.; Humphries, S.E.; Pennell, D.J.; Montgomery, H.E.; Payne, J.R. Left Ventricular Wall Thickness and the Presence of Asymmetric Hypertrophy in Healthy Young Army Recruits: Data from the LARGE heart study. *Circ. Cardiovasc. Imaging* **2013**, *6*, 262–267. [CrossRef]

23. Ommen, S.R.; Mital, S.; Burke, M.A.; Day, S.M.; Deswal, A.; Elliott, P.; Evanovich, L.L.; Hung, J.; Joglar, J.A.; Kantor, P.; et al. 2020 AHA/ACC Guideline for the Diagnosis and Treatment of Patients with Hypertrophic Cardiomyopathy. *J. Am. Coll. Cardiol.* **2020**, *76*, e159–e240. [CrossRef]
24. Maron, B.J.; Yacoub, M.; Dearani, J.A. Benefits of surgery in obstructive hypertrophic cardiomyopathy: Bring septal myectomy back for European patients. *Eur. Heart J.* **2011**, *32*, 1055–1058. [CrossRef]
25. Kim, L.K.; Swaminathan, R.V.; Looser, P.; Minutello, R.M.; Wong, S.C.; Bergman, G.; Naidu, S.S.; Gade, C.L.F.; Charitakis, K.; Singh, H.S.; et al. Hospital Volume Outcomes After Septal Myectomy and Alcohol Septal Ablation for Treatment of Obstructive Hypertrophic Cardiomyopathy. *JAMA Cardiol.* **2016**, *1*, 324–332. [CrossRef]
26. van Velzen, H.G.; Theuns, D.A.; Yap, S.-C.; Michels, M.; Schinkel, A.F. Incidence of Device-Detected Atrial Fibrillation and Long-Term Outcomes in Patients With Hypertrophic Cardiomyopathy: US nationwide inpatient database, 2003–2011. *Am. J. Cardiol.* **2017**, *119*, 100–105. [CrossRef]
27. Wilke, I.; Witzel, K.; Münch, J.; Pecha, S.; Blankenberg, S.; Reichenspurner, H.; Willems, S.; Patten, M.; Aydin, A. High Incidence of De Novo and Subclinical Atrial Fibrillation in Patients with Hypertrophic Cardiomyopathy and Cardiac Rhythm Management Device. *J. Cardiovasc. Electrophysiol.* **2016**, *27*, 779–784. [CrossRef]
28. Guttmann, O.P.; Rahman, M.S.; O'Mahony, C.; Anastasakis, A.; Elliott, P.M. Atrial fibrillation and thromboembolism in patients with hypertrophic cardiomyopathy: Systematic review. *Heart* **2014**, *100*, 465–472. [CrossRef] [PubMed]
29. Moore, B.; Semsarian, C.; Chan, K.H.; Sy, R.W. Sudden Cardiac Death and Ventricular Arrhythmias in Hypertrophic Cardiomyopathy. *Heart Lung Circ.* **2019**, *28*, 146–154. [CrossRef]
30. Hershberger, R.E.; Givertz, M.M.; Ho, C.Y.; Judge, D.P.; Kantor, P.F.; McBride, K.L.; Morales, A.; Taylor, M.R.; Vatta, M.; Ware, S.M. Genetic Evaluation of Cardiomyopathy—A Heart Failure Society of America Practice Guideline. *J. Card. Fail.* **2018**, *24*, 281–302. [CrossRef]
31. Colombo, M.G.; Botto, N.; Vittorini, S.; Paradossi, U.; Andreassi, M.G. Clinical utility of genetic tests for inherited hypertrophic and dilated cardiomyopathies. *Cardiovasc. Ultrasound* **2008**, *6*, 62. [CrossRef]
32. Lopes, L.R.; Futema, M.; Akhtar, M.M.; Lorenzini, M.; Pittman, A.; Syrris, P.; Elliott, P.M. Prevalence of *TTR* variants detected by whole-exome sequencing in hypertrophic cardiomyopathy. *Amyloid* **2019**, *26*, 243–247. [CrossRef] [PubMed]
33. Wijngaard, A.v.D.; Volders, P.; Van Tintelen, J.P.; Jongbloed, J.D.H.; Berg, M.P.v.D.; Deprez, R.H.L.; Mannens, M.M.A.M.; Hofmann, N.; Slegtenhorst, M.; Dooijes, D.; et al. Recurrent and founder mutations in the Netherlands: Cardiac Troponin I (TNNI3) gene mutations as a cause of severe forms of hypertrophic and restrictive cardiomyopathy. *Neth. Heart J.* **2011**, *19*, 344–351. [CrossRef]
34. Gigli, M.; Begay, R.L.; Morea, G.; Graw, S.L.; Sinagra, G.; Taylor, M.R.G.; Granzier, H.; Mestroni, L. A Review of the Giant Protein Titin in Clinical Molecular Diagnostics of Cardiomyopathies. *Front. Cardiovasc. Med.* **2016**, *3*, 21. [CrossRef] [PubMed]
35. Lopes, L.R.; Zekavati, A.; Syrris, P.; Hubank, M.; Giambartolomei, C.; Dalageorgou, C.; Jenkins, S.; McKenna, W.; Plagnol, V.; Elliott, P.M.; et al. Genetic complexity in hypertrophic cardiomyopathy revealed by high-throughput sequencing. *J. Med. Genet.* **2013**, *50*, 228–239. [CrossRef]

MDPI
St. Alban-Anlage 66
4052 Basel
Switzerland
www.mdpi.com

Journal of Clinical Medicine Editorial Office
E-mail: jcm@mdpi.com
www.mdpi.com/journal/jcm

www.ingramcontent.com/pod-product-compliance
Lightning Source LLC
LaVergne TN
LVHW070359100526
838202LV00014B/1348